MASTERING DYSRHYTHMIAS:
A PROBLEM-SOLVING
GUIDE

MASTERING DYSRHYTHMIAS: A PROBLEM-SOLVING GUIDE

KEVIN R. BROWN, M.P.H., E.M.T.-P.

Paramedic Instructor, Institute of Emergency Medicine
Albert Einstein College of Medicine

Formerly, Supervisor of Paramedic Training
New York City Emergency Medical Services

Presently completing Doctor of Medicine Degree
Albert Einstein College of Medicine
Bronx, New York

SHELDON JACOBSON, M.D., F.A.C.E.P.

Medical Director, Emergency Services Department,
Hospital of the University of Pennsylvania

Associate Professor of Medicine
University of Pennsylvania School of Medicine

Associate Professor of Medicine in Surgery
University of Pennsylvania
Philadelphia, Pennsylvania

 F. A. DAVIS COMPANY • Philadelphia

Library of Congress Cataloging-in-Publication Data

Brown, Kevin R., 1953–
    Mastering dysrhythmias.

    Includes bibliographies and index.
    1. Arrhythmia—Diagnosis—Problems, exercises, etc.   2. Electrocardiography—Problems, exercises, etc.   I. Jacobson, Sheldon, 1938–   .   II. Title.
[DNLM: 1. Arrhythmia—diagnosis—programmed instruction.   2. Electrocardiography—programmed instruction.
WG 18 B878m]
RC685.A65B75   1987   616.1′28   87-15448
ISBN 0-8036-1251-6

To my brothers, Ed, Ron, Gene, and Tim

K.B.

FOREWORD

There is no question that we have seen a revolution in emergency and critical care in recent years, and perhaps nowhere is this more evident than in the area of advanced coronary care.

The proliferation of available services to the patient with a cardiac emergency has placed new demands on all levels of health care practitioners, and we have seen both individual and collective efforts to meet these challenges. The work of the American Heart Association in promoting ACLS training is but one example, and such courses for physicians and nurses are now commonplace. In addition, many communities have brought advanced life support to the streets through the development of paramedic training and soundly constructed Emergency Medical Service (EMS) systems.

Central to the treatment of cardiac emergencies is the ability of the clinician to immediately respond to changes in ECG rhythms, to correlate the rhythm with its hemodynamic effects, and to initiate the appropriate treatment modalities based on the analysis. It goes without saying that the necessary skill levels in interpreting ECGs accurately can only be achieved through constant practice, in both initial and continuing education programs, and in actual clinical conditions.

Mastering Dysrhythmias is thus a welcome addition for the student and educator alike, providing a diverse array of tracings for analysis and review, all the while keeping the focus that we are treating patients as a whole and not just the ECG. Beginning practitioners will appreciate the systematic approach to dysrhythmia recognition, and advanced clinicians will have found a valuable new reference and teaching tool.

Mr. Brown and Dr. Jacobson have given us a readable, accessible text that will surely challenge learners and enhance their ability to provide the best care for the patients they serve.

Gene Iannuzzi, RN, CEN, EMT-P

PREFACE

Our goal in writing this workbook is to improve the reader's ability to interpret dysrhythmia by providing ECG strips for practice along with answers that illustrate a standard process of analysis. Our first task was to justify adding another book to the already swollen shelves of dysrhythmia publications. Our belief is that *Mastering Dysrhythmias* incorporates a novel approach and fills a void in dysrhythmia instruction. The need for such a book became apparent when we realized that we were spending several hours photocopying ECG tracings for each class of students to provide practice in ECG interpretation. We soon learned that other instructors were doing the same, no matter which text was being used or how competent the classroom teaching was. *Mastering Dysrhythmias* remedies the problem by being primarily a workbook that contains over two hundred self-assessment tracings in addition to a multitude of illustrative examples that are likely to be encountered in practice. Its use is compatible with and will complement almost any text or lecture format.

The book is divided into two parts. A systematic analysis of ECGs is presented in the first chapter of Section 1. The next four chapters group the dysrhythmias into supraventricular dysrhythmias, atrioventricular heart blocks, ventricular dysrhythmias, and artificial pacemakers and artifacts. The first half of each of these chapters consists of a review of the characteristics and examples of specific dysrhythmias; in the second half, we provide self-assessment ECG tracings limited to the types discussed earlier. At the end of each chapter, we offer a thorough interpretation of these self-assessment tracings, which provides a step-by-step discussion of specific ECG features, including the logic leading to an answer's selection. Section 2 consists of five chapters containing a large variety of self-assessment tracings in a random sequence; again, interpretations of these tracings are provided at the end of each chapter.

In this text, an emphasis on the practical aspects of the recognition, the significance, and the acute therapy of dysrhythmia complements the ECG tracings. We deliberately limited the type and complexity of information in order to achieve a straightforward and rational presentation.

The appendix includes a glossary to clarify any terms that may be unfamiliar and a list of abbreviations. We have also provided blank forms that the reader can duplicate and use in the self-assessment exercises.

The rhythm strips are reproduced in their actual size, and except for the removal of artifacts or the emphasis of detail, they appear in original form. The ECGs were culled from the clinical services of the affiliated institutions of the Albert Einstein College of Medicine and the Emergency Medical Service of the City of New York.

In the final analysis, we are all striving to improve our clinical skills in a way that is meaningful to patient care. In the current technologic explosion in medicine, it is easy to become overly dependent on machines and the data bases that they produce. In this text, we have tried to maintain our focus directly on the patients and have attempted to use the ECG machine in a manner that will enhance the bedside management of patients.

In spite of the fact that ECGs have been used throughout the world for many years, a standard method of interpretation and standard terminology still do not exist. Students are bewildered by the fact that many terms are used to describe the same finding (for instance, premature atrial complexes, ectopic atrial beats, atrial extrasystoles, and atrial premature complexes to describe an ectopic atrial focus occurring early), or that authors use different criteria for classifying dysrhythmias. We even had to debate whether the term arrhythmia or dysrhythmia should be employed in this work, since both are widely used. We chose the term dysrhythmia because it means "disordered rhythm," whereas arrhythmia is defined as "without rhythm," which is true for only a few dysrhythmias, such as asystole or atrial fibrillation. For instance, ventricular trigeminy is not without rhythm; it has a definite disordered rhythm. Both terms are used interchangeably in common usage, however.

A large part of dysrhythmia analysis is subjective, which is why it is not uncommon to hear cardiologists disagreeing about an interpretation of the same tracing. For instance, ventricular tachycardia can be indistinguishable from supraventricular tachycardia (SVT) with aberrant conduction. When more than one possible explanation exists, we have includeed both in the answer section. Students, therefore, should regard the interpretations provided—especially those in the rationale section—as *suggested* answers and should realize that alternate choices do exist for certain strips. Teachers may provide an alternate list if desired.

We would gratefully appreciate any comments or suggestions to improve the effectiveness of *Mastering Dysrhythmias*.

Many hands went into shaping this project and making it a success. Our gratitude goes to our contributors: Dr. Martin Cohen, who wrote the section on pacemakers, Dr. Michael G. Kiengle, who wrote the treatment sections, Dr. Gary E. Lombordi, who wrote all the sections on concepts about dysrhythmias, and Dr. Richard L. Siegel, who contributed to Chapter 1. We also have received a great deal of professional assistance from our colleagues and would like to express our gratitude to Aracelia Augila, M.D.; Wallace Carter, Jr., M.D., EMT-P; Joseph Cirino, EMT-P; MacNeil Cross, EMT-P; Maggie Dubris, EMT-P; Edward Gabriel, EMT-P; Patricia Gabriel, R.N.; Paul Gennis, M.D.; Roosey Khawly, M.D.; Leo Leung, EMT-P; Ronald Maffei, EMT-P, Jean Menter, ECG Technician, Josephine Mirra, R.N.; Art Romano, EMT-P; Mark Starkman, EMT-P; Fritz Streuli, M.D.; William Toon, EMT-P; Mark Weiss, EMT-P; and Lucy Winton, EMT-P. We are grateful to Alan Metrick for having read the manuscript and making many suggestions on improving the presentation, and to Diane Carpenter, R.N., James Paturas, EMT-P, and Gene Ianuzzi, EMT-P, R.N., who reviewed the entire draft and the revisions of the manuscript: their comments were invaluable.

The staff at F.A. Davis deserve a large measure of credit for their help and expertise, especially Herb Powell, Bill Donnelly, Margaret King, and Philip Ashley. Our editor, Jean-François Vilain, deserves special acknowledgment for his diligence and advice. Mrs. Rita Rogers is to be commended for her excellent manuscript preparation throughout the many revisions. Also, Kevin Brown wants to thank Helen and Peggy Brown for their love and encouragement.

K.R.B.
S.J.

CONTRIBUTORS

MARTIN COHEN, M.D., F.A.C.C.

Professor of Medicine
Albert Einstein College of Medicine

Director of EKG Service
Bronx Municipal Hospital Center
Bronx, New York

MICHAEL G. KIENZLE, M.D.

Assistant Professor of Medicine
Department of Internal Medicine
Cardiovascular Division
University of Iowa
Iowa City, Iowa

GARY E. LOMBARDI, M.D.

Medical Director, Institute of Emergency Medicine
Albert Einstein College of Medicine

Associate Director, Emergency Department
Bronx Municipal Hospital Center
Bronx, New York

RICHARD L. SIEGEL, M.D.

Medical Director, Emergency Department
Newark Beth Israel Medical Center
Newark, New Jersey

CONTENTS

Section 1
DYSRHYTHMIA CHARACTERISTICS AND SELF-ASSESSMENT TRACINGS

Chapter One
DEVELOPING A SYSTEMATIC APPROACH TO DYSRHYTHMIA ANALYSIS

Faced with a complex dysrhythmia to interpret, students often become as pale, cool, and diaphoretic as the patient who is attached to the ECG machine. They flounder and are anxious because they have not yet learned to apply a standard, common-sense approach in evaluating disordered cardiac rhythms.

Some, in fact, approach dysrhythmia interpretation solely by rote memorization of individual patterns. Pattern recognition techniques not only are boring but also can lead to serious mistakes. A more effective method is to develop a logical and systematic analytic approach. In that way, the basic approach to identifying each dysrhythmia is the same, no matter how many dysrhythmia types may be present.

Essentially, dysrhythmias are analyzed just as we do with a physical examination: inspection followed by interpretation of findings. We make measurements and then we compare them to normal values—the ECG standard being the normal sinus rhythm (NSR). We identify the P waves and QRS complexes, sorting out their relationship to one another. We then deduce information about the pacemaker(s), the rate, the rhythm, and status of atrioventricular (AV) conduction.

It is assumed that you will be using this workbook in conjunction with a textbook or classroom instruction to learn the characteristics of each dysrhythmia, along with its electrophysiology and treatment. A summary of the ECG features and treatment for different dysrhythmias are contained in the chapters in Section 1. In this chapter we will look briefly at the cardiac conduction system and its activity in generating normal sinus rhythm, and then we will discuss the analysis of dysrhythmias.

CARDIAC CONDUCTION SYSTEM

The components of the cardiac conduction system are shown in Figure 1–1. One of the characteristics of some myocardial cells is **automaticity,** the ability to initiate spontaneous depolarization of the resting cell membrane. Normally, the process arises in the **sinoatrial (SA) node,** usually referred to as the pacemaker, which discharges 60 to 100 times each minute. The impulse then radiates in a fast traveling wave across the right atrium and left atrium, depolarizing the atria and followed shortly by mechanical systole. The impulse arrives at the **atrioventricular (AV) node,** through which it passes slowly, delaying activation of the ventricles until the atria have finished contraction. The impulse exits the AV node through a continuation of fibers called the **AV bundle** (His bundle), travels down the left and right **bundle branches,** and passes through the **Purkinje fibers** to terminate in the ventricular muscle. After depolarization of the muscle, the ventricles contract, ejecting blood. Impulses arising from sites other than the SA node are termed **ectopic** pacemakers.

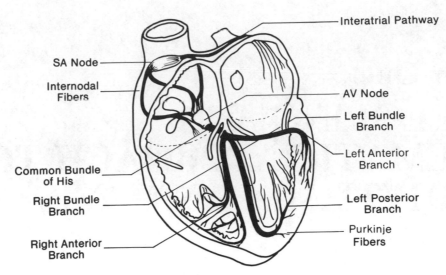

FIGURE 1–1. Myocardial conduction system.

CORRESPONDING ECG DEFLECTIONS

Normally, three major deflections are recorded, and these are labeled **P, QRS, and T** (Fig. 1–2). The **P wave** is due to atrial depolarization, and the tall, sharp **QRS deflection** is caused by ventricular depolarization. Repolarization of the ventricles is represented by the **T wave**. No wave is noticed for atrial repolarization because the QRS complex obscures it. The **P-R interval** is measured from the beginning of

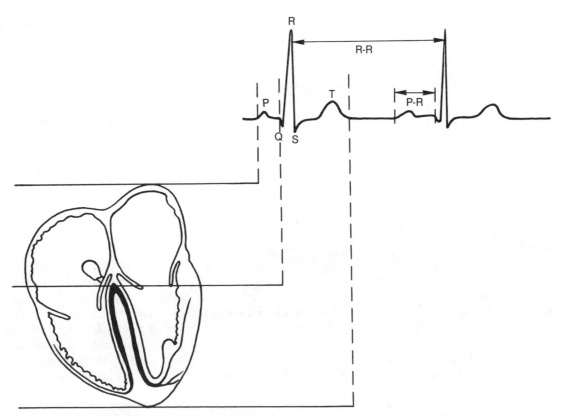

FIGURE 1–2. Relationship of ECG complex to conduction pathway.

the P wave to the start of the QRS complex and corresponds to the time it takes following atrial activation until the start of ventricular depolarization. This period is useful in gauging the speed of impulse transmission. A delay in the atria or AV node will be reflected by a longer than normal P-R interval. Likewise, a delay in depolarization of the ventricle will change the shape and duration of the QRS complex. A **U wave** is sometimes observed following the T wave and is thought to represent late repolarization of the ventricles.

NORMAL SINUS RHYTHM (NSR)
(Regular Sinus Rhythm)

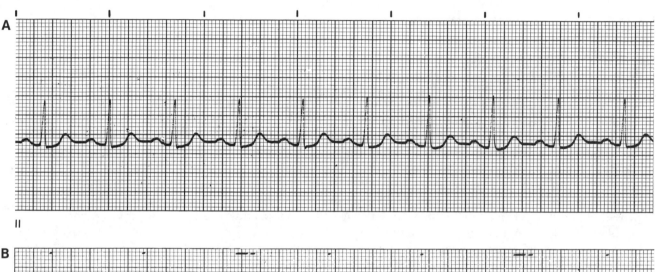

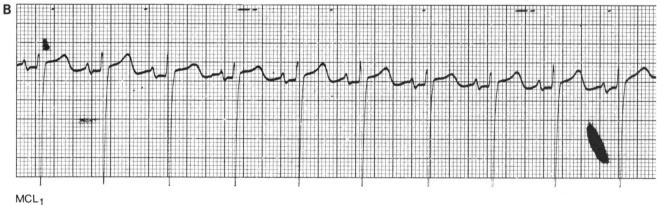

FIGURE 1–3. Normal sinus rhythm shown in the two leads commonly used for continuous monitoring.

Ventricular Rate:	60–100/minute.
Ventricular Rhythm:	Regular R-R intervals.
QRS Configuration:	Normal: all are the same size and shape with sharp, smooth waves.
QRS Duration:	Normal (0.10 sec or less).
Atrial Rate:	Same as ventricular rate.
Atrial Rhythm:	Regular P-P intervals.

P Wave Configuration:	Normal: all are the same size and shape, and are upright in lead II and biphasic or upright in MCL_1.
P-R Interval:	0.12–0.20 second.
Conduction Ratio:	One P wave to each QRS complex (1:1).
Significant Findings:	The R-R interval may be slightly irregular (0.04 to 0.08 second) due to changes in parasympathetic tone that accompanies breathing. Inspiration increases the heart rate slightly.
Interpretation:	Normal sinus rhythm is present because all findings are within normal limits.

CHOICE OF LEAD FOR CONTINUOUS MONITORING

There is no single lead that is ideal for detecting dysrhythmias. Lead I, for instance, provides notoriously poor representation of atrial activity in ectopic dysrhythmias. Therefore, it is important to utilize several leads when evaluating a cardiac rhythm. Particularly vexing rhythm disturbances sometimes require special electrode placement in addition to the standard 12 leads.

However, we are limited to relying on a single lead for continuous monitoring due to practical considerations. So we must choose a monitor lead that will provide the most useful data. Traditionally, **lead II** (utilizing a positive electrode at the left lower costal border and negative electrode placed inferior to the right midclavicular point) has been used as the classical "rhythm strip" since the advent of coronary care units. In general, it has been satisfactory since it provides tall, positive atrial and ventricular complexes which allows easy assessment of AV conduction. A significant disadvantage is the limited detail provided about abnormal ventricular conduction aside from making it easy to identify the wide, bizarre complex. It is of no help in recognizing bundle branch blocks, or in distinguishing supraventricular impulses that are aberrantly conducted from ectopic ventricular complexes.

The right precordial chest lead, popularized by Marriott, overcomes these problems and has gained favor as the lead for continuous monitoring. Termed MCL_1, or modified chest lead$_1$, this lead is a variation of V_1 and utilizes the positive electrode in the fourth intercostal space at the right sternal border and a negative electrode placed inferior to the left midclavicular point. Leads II and MCL_1 offer different views that complement each other. Although PVCs show well in both leads, only MCL_1 aids in determining which ventricle it is likely to have come from. The P wave shape in lead MCL_1 is highly variable as shown in Figure 1–4.

The shape and polarity of the P-QRS-T complex components are found in Table 1–1. It is important to know how normal sinus rhythm (see Fig. 1–3) will appear in both leads.

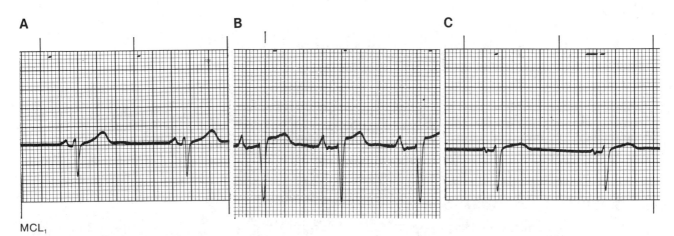

MCL$_1$

FIGURE 1–4. In lead MCL_1 the P wave shape is variable.

TABLE 1–1. Comparison of Lead II and MCL$_1$

Wave	Lead II	Lead MCL$_1$
P	POSITIVE	VARIABLE: BIPHASIC (+/−COMPONENT) OR POSITIVE
QRS	POSITIVE	MAINLY NEGATIVE
T	POSITIVE	VARIABLE

SEQUENCE OF STEPS IN ANALYSIS

Where to begin? ECG interpretation is approached in different ways: some prefer to begin by looking at the P waves and then moving on to the QRS complexes—this follows the physiologic sequence of cardiac conduction. Others follow the reverse order. Which is correct? They both are; it makes no difference where you start as long as you apply a consistent approach.

In this book we will always follow the same sequence of steps. We chose to start by inspecting the QRS complexes, then move on to the P waves, look at the atrioventricular relationship, and then form an interpretation. Our rationale is that the QRS complexes are the tallest and most easily detectable feature and that ventricular activity is the most important consideration in determining heart rate and cardiac output. The atria may be fibrillating wildly, but as long as the ventricular rate and output are adequate, the patient can usually tolerate the dysrhythmia. In contrast, if the ventricles should fibrillate, the pumping action of the heart will suddenly cease. Generally, atrial dysrhythmias are less serious than ventricular ones, which is why we prefer to look at the QRS complexes first, especially if we suspect our patient is seriously ill. The tall QRS complex also serves as a reference, and we know where the P and T waves should be in relation to it.

The steps in the analysis are listed in the following outline, after which each is described in more detail.

1. General inspection
2. Identification of specific waves
3. Analysis of ventricular activity
   a. Rate
   b. Rhythm
   c. Shape
4. Analysis of atrial activity
   a. Rate
   b. Rhythm
   c. Shape
5. Assessment of atrioventricular relationship
   a. Conduction ratio
   b. Discharge sequence (P:QRS or QRS:P)
   c. P-R interval
6. Formulation of interpretation
7. Evaluation of dysrhythmia in terms of patient's clinical status

STEP ONE: GENERAL INSPECTION

To start, briefly make a general inspection of the tracing and note any gross abnormalities, such as extra beats, pauses, or obvious disturbances in rhythm. Quickly check to see if the beats are all identical or if some come early and are abnormally shaped. This will help to pinpoint areas for closer inspection later.

STEP TWO: IDENTIFICATION OF SPECIFIC WAVES

Next, scan several typical complexes and identify each of the wave components. Determine if the parts of the complexes are constant from one beat to the next. Normally, this will be easy to do because the QRS complexes are usually tallest and are easy to distinguish from the P waves. But sometimes more care is needed because nonconducted P waves may be hidden in the ST segments or in the T waves if an AV block is present. Also, as the heart rate increases and the cardiac cycles get closer together, the P waves may merge with and be hidden by the T waves that precede them.

After mentally labeling the QRS complexes, sort out the P waves. In normal sinus rhythms they occur just ahead of the R waves at a fixed P-R interval of three to five small boxes on the grid. Then look at the T waves, which immediately follow the R waves. ST segment deviations and U waves may distort their appearance.

So far, our goal has been simply to identify each individual ECG component so we can make a closer inspection later.

STEP THREE: ANALYSIS OF VENTRICULAR ACTIVITY

Now inspect the rate, rhythm, and configuration of the ventricular depolarizations.

Rate

Calculate the rate of QRS complexes. This will determine if the rate falls within normal limits for NSR (60 to 100/minute), is below 60/minute (bradycardia), or faster than 100/minute (tachycardia). The QRS, or R wave, rate usually corresponds to the ventricular contractions and should equal the pulse rate.

Calculating rates. There are several reliable techniques available for calculating rates. The first one can be used for irregular and regular rhythms. The last two methods can be used *only* for regular rhythms. Although we speak about R waves (QRS complexes) in the examples below, the techniques are the same for counting P waves.

Method one: Counting the cycle lengths in a 6-second period. A cycle length is the distance between a wave in one complex and the corresponding wave in the following cardiac cycle, for example, the R-R interval. After counting the number of R-R intervals in a 6-second strip, simply multiply the number by 10 to get the rate per minute. Standard ECG paper has marks every 1 to 3 seconds to facilitate rate determination (Fig. 1–5). In Figure 1–6 the rate is 80/minute because the 6-second period contains exactly eight cycle lengths.

Also include in your calculations any fractions of cycle lengths (a half a cycle, a third of a cycle, a quarter of a cycle) for the 6-second period. For example, if a 6-second interval included seven and one-half R-R cycles, the rate would be determined by multiplying 7.5 by 10 = 75/min (see Fig. 1–7). What would the rate be if we counted four and one-third cycles in 6 seconds as in Figure 1–8? It would be about 43/minute (4.3 multiplied by 10 = 43).

Although these values are only approximate, the quick determination is useful to see if the rate is within a normal range (60 to 100/minute), is bradycardiac (less than six cycles in 6 seconds), or is tachycardiac (more than 10 cycles in 6 seconds).

Method two: Count the number of whole (and parts of) large boxes that separate any two consecutive R waves and divide that number into 300 (which is the paper speed per minute). This method is accurate only for regular rhythms, that is, those with constant R-R intervals.

Number of Large Boxes in R-R Interval	Division into 300		Rate/Minute
1	300 ÷ 1	=	300
2	300 ÷ 2	=	150
3	300 ÷ 3	=	100
4	300 ÷ 4	=	75
5	300 ÷ 5	=	60
6	300 ÷ 6	=	50
7	300 ÷ 7	=	43

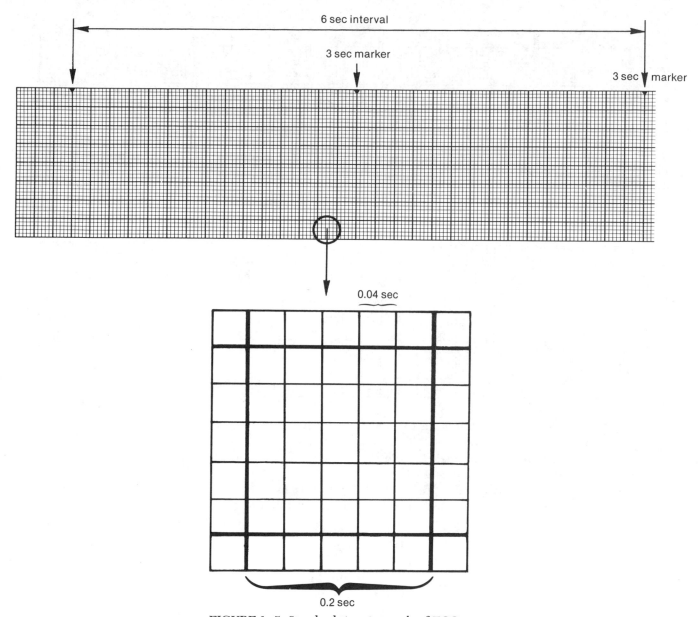

FIGURE 1–5. Standard time intervals of ECG paper.

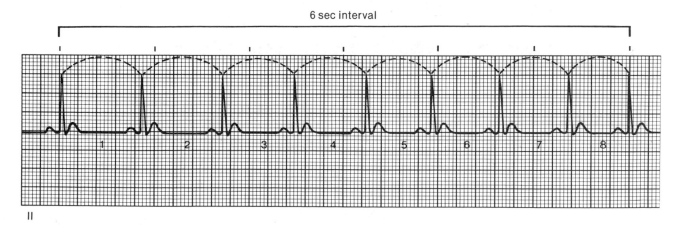

FIGURE 1–6. Cardiac cycle rate of 80/minute (8 R-R intervals multiplied by 10).

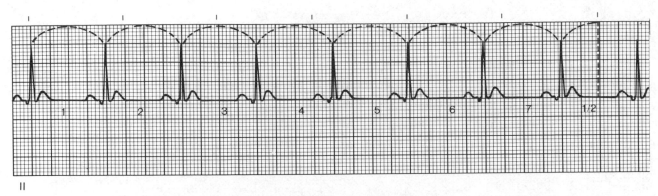

FIGURE 1–7. Cardiac cycle rate of 75/minute ($7\frac{1}{2}$ R-R intervals multiplied by 10).

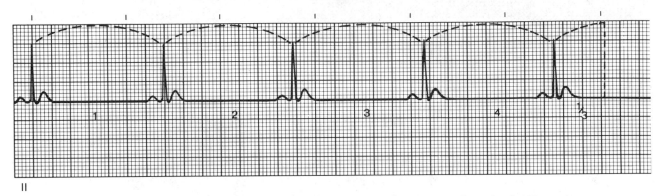

FIGURE 1–8. Cardiac cycle rate of 43/minute ($4\frac{1}{3}$ R-R intervals multiplied by 10).

Figure 1–9 has two and one-half large boxes in one R-R interval. Therefore, the rate is about 120 complexes per minute ($300 \div 2.5 = 120$).

Method three: The corresponding rate multiples for every large box in an R-R interval are memorized. Again, the R-R intervals must be constant. The values are as follows:

300 (for one box)
150 (for two boxes)
100 (for three boxes)
75 (for four boxes)
60 (for five boxes)
50 (for six boxes)
43 (for seven boxes)

The values can be counted off as the ECG strip is examined (see Fig. 1–10).

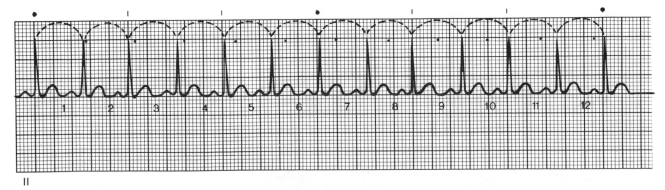

FIGURE 1–9. Cardiac cycle rate of 120/minute (12 R-R intervals multiplied by 10).

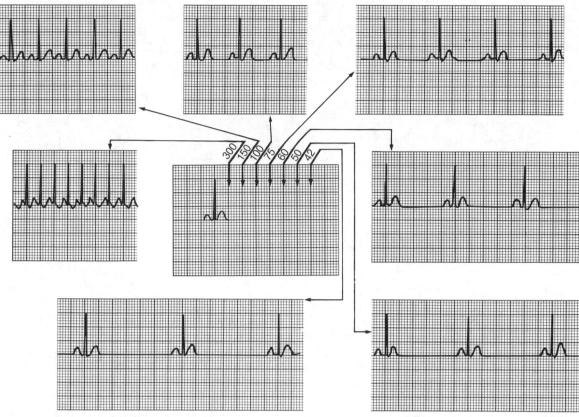

FIGURE 1–10. Cardiac cycle rates determined by the number of large ECG boxes between consecutive QRS complexes.

Rhythmicity

Next, assess the regularity of the R-R intervals. Is the ventricular rhythm regular, as expected for a normal sinus rhythm, or irregular, as occurs in a dysrhythmia (Fig. 1–11)? If irregular, we must see if it occurs in one of the following patterns:

Intermittently irregular. The generally regular rhythm is occasionally disrupted. Premature complexes are the most common causes.

Regularly irregular. The rhythmicity of the R-R interval waxes and waves in a cycle. A regular pattern between the QRS complexes emerges even though the general rhythmicity is disrupted.

Irregularly irregular. No recurring pattern exists. The spacing of the R-R intervals occurs as if by chance, giving a grossly disrupted ventricular rhythm.

QRS Configuration

See if the shapes of the QRS complexes are identical to one another and whether the contours of the strokes are sharp and even. The shape as well as the duration of the complex will help tell the origin of the ventricular depolarization. The normal QRS range is 0.06 to 0.10 sec. If they are narrow and within 0.10 second or less it **indicates a supraventricular origin** with normal intraventricular conduction (Fig. 1–12). If the QRS complexes are wide, 0.12 sec or more in duration, and their contour distorted (bizarre, notched, slurred), it represents one of two conditions (Fig. 1–13):

1. The origin is **within the ventricle,** or
2. The beat arose from a supraventricular focus (SA node, atria, or AV junction) **but follows an aberrant intraventricular conduction path.**

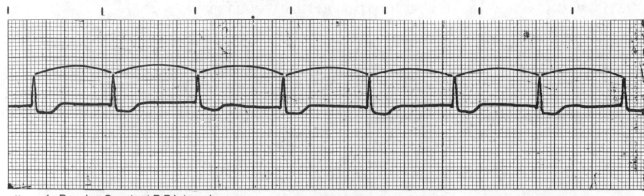

II 1. Regular: Constant R-R intervals

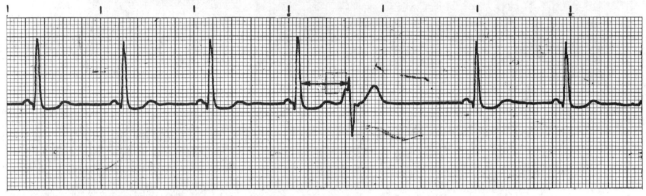

II 2. Intermittently irregular: Occasional variations in R-R interval

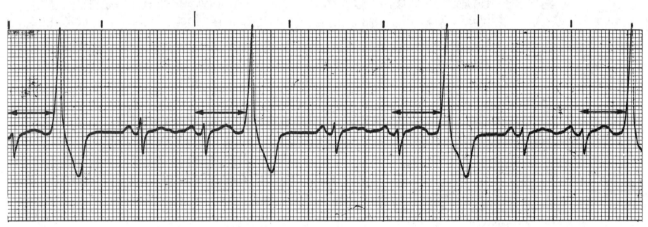

II 3. Regularly irregular: Every third R-R interval varies

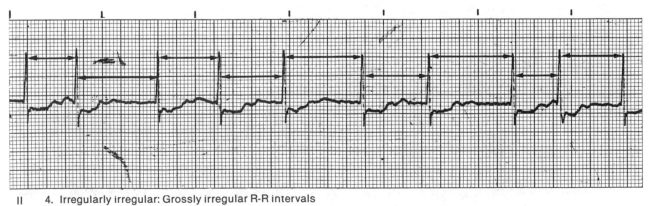

II 4. Irregularly irregular: Grossly irregular R-R intervals

FIGURE 1–11. Ventricular rhythm patterns.

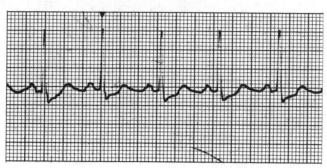

1. Sinus

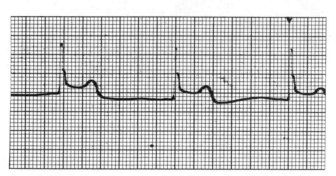

2. Sinus

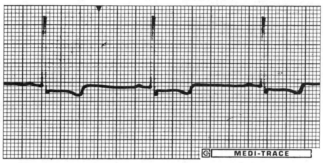

3. AV junctional

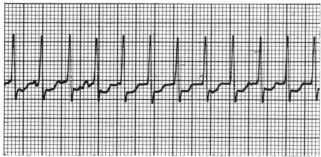

4. Supraventricular: Atrial or AV junctional

FIGURE 1–12. Rhythms with normal QRS durations.

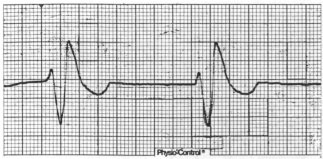

1. Idioventricular complexes

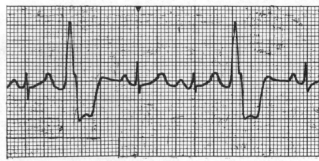

2. Premature ventricular complexes

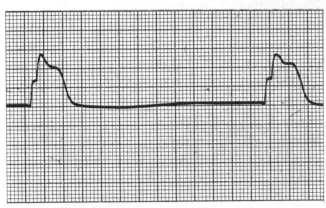

3. Idioventricular complexes

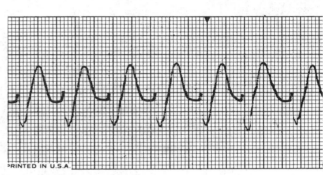

4. Ventricular tachycardia

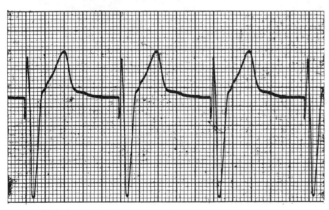

5. Artificial ventricular pacemaker

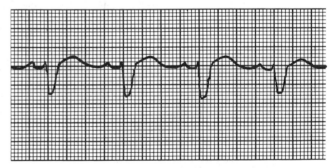

6. Normal sinus rhythm with abnormal intraventricular conduction

FIGURE 1–13. Rhythms with wide, distorted QRS complexes.

STEP FOUR: ANALYSIS OF ATRIAL ACTIVITY

Perform the same inspection of atrial depolarization as for the ventricular activity. First, are there P waves? If not, the rhythm did not originate in the sinus node, and therefore, an ectopic pacemaker is controlling the heart activity. See if there are abnormally shaped atrial waves present, such as fibrillatory (f) waves, flutter (F) waves, or P prime (P′) waves, which indicate ectopic pacemakers. **P′ waves** are atrial depolarizations of ectopic origin that differ in shape or size from normal P waves and are seen in PACs. If atrial activity is entirely missing, as evidenced by an isoelectric (flat) baseline between QRS complexes, it means the pacemaker is originating in the AV junction or within the ventricles.

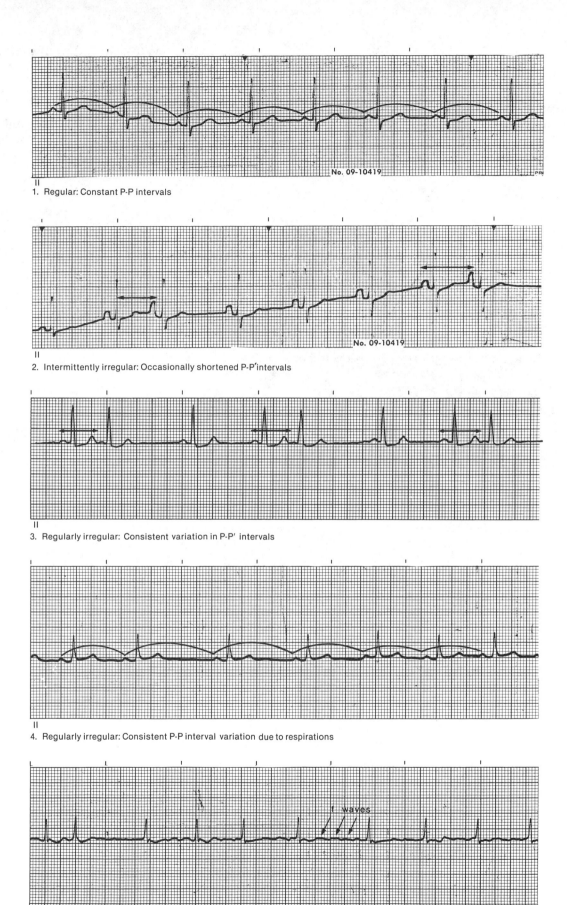

1. Regular: Constant P-P intervals

2. Intermittently irregular: Occasionally shortened P-P′intervals

3. Regularly irregular: Consistent variation in P-P′ intervals

4. Regularly irregular: Consistent P-P interval variation due to respirations

5. Irregularly irregular: Grossly irregular atrial activity

FIGURE 1–14. Atrial rhythm patterns.

15

Rate

Calculate the rate of atrial waves, using the same methods described for QRS complexes. The P wave rate should be exactly the same as the QRS complexes if sinus activity is present and 1:1 AV conduction exists. If there are more atrial waves than QRS complexes, then not all the atrial waves are conducted. This frequently happens when the atrial rate is rapid, as in atrial flutter, where it is around 300/minute and the AV node does not conduct all the impulses.

Rhythm

Check the P-P intervals to determine if the pacemaker is discharging regularly or if a dysrhythmia exists. If the P-P interval is irregular, check to see if one of the following patterns exists (Fig. 1–14):

Intermittently irregular. The generally regular rhythm is occasionally disrupted. Premature complexes are the most frequent cause of occasionally disrupted P-P intervals.

Regularly irregular. The changing P-P intervals form a repetitive pattern. This often is seen with sinus dysrhythmias in which the P-P intervals gradually increase and decrease in association with breathing.

Irregularly irregular. No consistent atrial rhythm exists. Instead, the P-P pattern is replaced by randomly occurring atrial complexes, as most commonly seen in atrial fibrillation.

Configuration

For a rhythm to be labeled NSR, regularly occurring P waves with identical shapes must be observed. In lead II, P waves are small, positive deflections that have rounded, slightly asymmetric contours. In lead MCL_1, the P waves may be biphasic, meaning that they have both a positive and negative component, as well as being positive in lead II. Shifts in pacemaker sites are reflected in changes in P wave shapes (Fig.

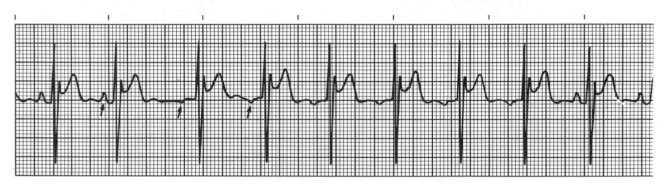

FIGURE 1–15. Alterations in P wave shapes.

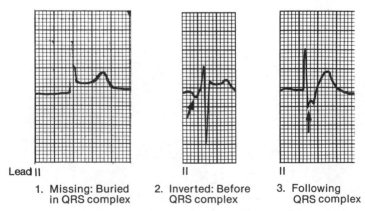

Lead II   II   II

1. Missing: Buried   2. Inverted: Before   3. Following
   in QRS complex   QRS complex   QRS complex

FIGURE 1–16. Position of P' wave in AV junctional complexes.

1–15). Supraventricular dysrhythmias have altered or absent P waves. The P waves seen in AV junctional dysrhythmias show three general appearances illustrated in Figure 1–16. The term P′ is applied to atrial waves that differ in shape from sinus P waves.

STEP FIVE: ASSESSMENT OF THE AV RELATIONSHIP

Establish the relationship of the atrial waves to the QRS complexes. Is the AV conduction ratio **1:1**, that is, one P wave for each QRS complex, as in sinus rhythm? If it is greater than 1:1, such as 3:2, or 2:1, not all atrial impulses are being conducted to the ventricles. (The ratios 3:2 and 2:1 indicate that every third or second P wave is blocked, respectively.) Conduction may be totally disrupted, in which case the Ps and QRSs would be unrelated.

The best way to determine AV conduction ratio is to ask two questions:

1. Is every P wave followed by a QRS complex?
2. Is every QRS complex preceded by a single P wave?

If the answer to these questions is "no," look at the rhythm to determine if a pattern exists (Fig. 1–17). For instance, in repetitive cycles, the sequence of nonconducted P waves will be constant, for example, every other P wave is blocked. A convenient way to determine this is to measure the P-R intervals to see if that value is fixed or changing.

P-R Interval

This interval is measured from the beginning of the P wave to the start of the QRS complex. It reflects the time that the impulse takes from the start of atrial depolarization until the ventricles begin to be stimulated. In regular sinus rhythm, the P-R interval is **constant** from beat to beat and is **no greater than 0.20 sec (200 msec)**. The most common disturbance is a P-R interval greater than 0.20 sec (Fig. 1–18) due to delayed AV conduction. The P-R interval may be shorter than normal, as in accelerated AV conduction. The P-R interval may show a cyclic progressive increase in duration, as in one type of heart block (see Fig. 1–17).

STEP SIX: FORMULATION OF AN INTERPRETATION

Now, we are ready to make a judgment—a rhythm interpretation which is based on the review of the data. First look at all the parts—the P waves, QRS complexes, AV conduction ratio, and so on—and then assemble the facts into a plausible account for what has been observed. If there are no variations from the standards of NSR, the yardstick by which all tracings are compared, then the ECG tracing is normal. If deviations exist, our interpretation must convey *all* the needed information about the mechanism of the cardiac cycle, including site(s) of impulse formation and conduction activity.

Here are examples of interpretations that could be phrased better or that **lack** information:

Example 1
Interpretation: Rapid atrial fibrillation.
Atrial fibrillation is always rapid; after all, it is an atrial tachydysrhythmia. The reference made is to the ventricular rate, but the term "rapid" is too general. It could be interpreted to mean 180/minute as well as 110/min. It is better to note the average ventricular rate in the interpretation.
Rephrased interpretation: Atrial fibrillation with an average ventricular response of 130/minute.

Example 2
Interpretation: First degree AV block.
This interpretation omits a location of the pacemaker site.
Rephrased interpretation: Sinus rhythm with a first degree AV block.

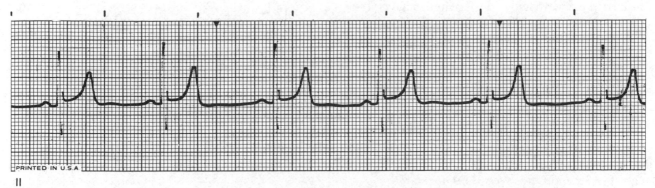

1. Normal 1:1 AV conduction: All P waves are conducted

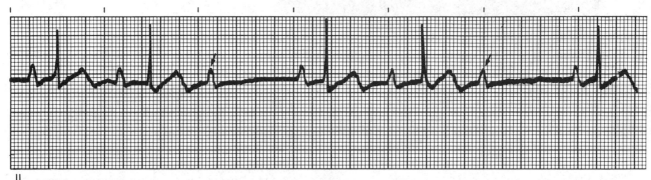

2. Heart block with 3:2 AV conduction: Arrows indicate blocked P wave

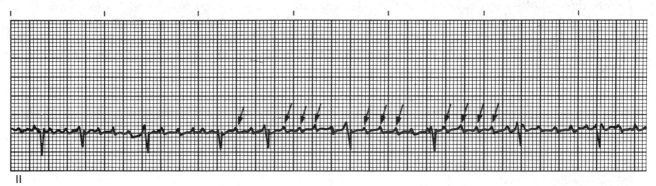

3. Variable (4:1, 5:1, 3:1) AV conduction: Atrial tachydysrhythmia

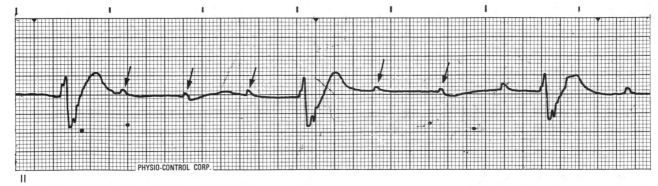

4. No AV conduction: Complete heart block

FIGURE 1–17. Examples of different atrioventricular conduction patterns.

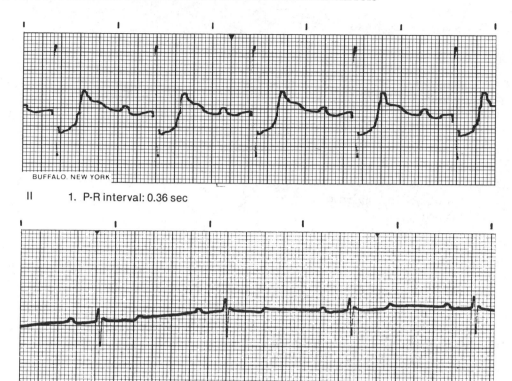

II   1. P-R interval: 0.36 sec

II   2. P-R interval: 0.32 sec

FIGURE 1–18. Examples of prolonged P-R intervals (>0.20 sec).

Example 3
Interpretation: AV junctional rhythm.

An AV junctional rhythm is similar to a symptom, and the underlying defect (a failure in sinus node activity) must be included.

Rephrased interpretation: Sinus arrest with an AV junctional escape rhythm at 50/min.

Example 4
Interpretation: Premature Ventricular Complexes.

This interpretation omits the underlying rhythm (from which the ventricular beats are premature) as well as the frequency of ectopic beats. A complete interpretation also should describe the shapes of the ectopic beats.

Rephrased interpretation: Sinus rhythm with an average of six unifocal PVCs per minute

Example 5
Interpretation: Second degree AV heart block, Mobitz type 2.

In all cases of heart block in which one or more beats are not conducted, it is important to list the conduction ratio and the average ventricular response because these factors convey the severity of the disorder. Suppose the patient has a sinus rate of 90/minute. In 3:2 conduction the ventricular rate would be 60, but in 3:1 it would be only 30! The conduction ratio makes quite a difference.

Rephrased interpretation: Second degree AV heart block, Mobitz type 2; 3:2 AV conduction, with a ventricular rate of 60/minute.

Example 6
Interpretation: Artificial pacemaker rhythm.

When artificial pacemakers are involved, the interpretation should tell whether or not the patient's natural pacemaker is functioning, and whether the artificial device is capturing the heart and also whether it is discharging appropriately (that is, not competing with the sinus node).

Rephrased interpretation: Artificially paced rhythm with 1:1 capture; no evidence of sinus activity.

Hypothetical Interpretation Examples

The data below were obtained from a review of *hypothetical* ECG tracings showing common dysrhythmias. Without viewing the tracings, we will formulate the information provided into an interpretation. After we finish making interpretations for these six cases, we will begin to analyze actual tracings using the same approach. The reasoning will be much clearer after you study the specific types of dysrhythmias in the following chapters.

Case 1 Data:

Ventricular activity
Rhythm: Regular
Duration: 0.08 second, narrow
Shape: Normal
Rate: 80/minute

Atrial activity
Rhythm: Regular
Shape: Normal
Rate: 80/min

AV relationship
Conduction ratio: 1:1, that is, one P wave for each QRS complex
P-R interval   0.12 second

Case 1 Interpretation:

The ventricular activity is normal: the QRS shape is as expected and the rhythm is regular. Atrial activity is also without variation from NSR. Each cycle has a single P wave that is followed by a QRS; conduction is 1:1. The P-R interval indicates that the time between the start of atrial and ventricular depolarization is normal.

Therefore, we can conclude from the duration of activation and the narrow shape that the QRS complex has a **supraventricular origin.** The P waves identify the pacemaker as the **sinus node,** and it is discharging within a normal limit (60 to 100/minute). The AV conduction is **1:1,** meaning that no form of AV block is present. This, then, is regular sinus rhythm; no abnormalities in impulse formation or conduction exist. Our reasoning started with the general (it is supraventricular) and went to the specific (it is sinus).

Case 2 Data:

Ventricular activity
Rhythm: Regular
Rate: 150/minute
Shape: Wide and bizarre

Atrial activity
Rhythm: Infrequently seen
Rate: Infrequent
Shape: Distorted by QRSs

AV relationship
Conduction ratio: Unrelated Ps and QRSs

Case 2 Interpretation:

We have found that the QRS complexes have an abnormal shape and occur at a rate **faster** than normal. The wide QRS complexes with prolonged activation times tell us that the complex is either of ventricular origin, or that a supraventricular impulse follows an abnormal intraventricular path. Because P waves are unrelated to the QRSs, the dominant pacemaker cannot be the sinus node, **nor can 1:1 AV conduction exist.** The wide QRSs must be due to a rapid ectopic pacemaker **located within the ventricle,** since the P waves are not conducted. Therefore, this dysrhythmia is ventricular tachycardia.

Case 3 Data:

> **Ventricular activity**
> Shape: Absent
> Rate: Absent
> Rhythm: Absent
>
> **Atrial activity**
> Shape: Absent
> Rhythm: Absent
> Rate: Absent
>
> **AV relationship**
> Conduction ratio: Absent
>
> **Significant findings**
> The ECG resembles a flat line.

Case 3 Interpretation:

Ventricular activity is totally **lacking.** The atria, likewise, show **no activity.** Complete cardiac stand-still exists. The isoelectric baseline indicates nonfunctioning sinus and latent pacemakers. As a result, asystole develops in this dying heart.

Case 4 Data:

> **Ventricular activity**
> Rhythm: Grossly irregular
> Rate: About 130/minute
> Shape: 0.08 second, narrow, consistent
>
> **Atrial activity**
> Rhythm: Absent
> Rate: Absent
> Shape: Wavy baseline, P′ waves are too numerous to count and have varying shapes.
>
> **AV relationship**
> No fixed AV conduction ratio exists.

Case 4 Interpretation:

The ventricular shapes are narrow yet the rhythm is irregular. The beats must be **supraventricular** because of the short QRS duration. Missing P waves **rule out the sinus node** as pacemaker. The wavy baseline with atrial waves of varying sizes and shapes is typical of a rapid ectopic atrial focus. The lack of a fixed AV conduction ratio indicates that we are dealing with atrial fibrillation.

Case 5 Data:

> **Ventricular activity**
> Rhythm: Regular
> Rate: 50/minute
> Shape: Narrow
>
> **Atrial activity**
> Rhythm: Regular
> Shape: Inverted P waves
> Rate: 50/minute
>
> **AV relationship**
> 1:1 but the P waves are found to have a P-R interval of only 0.06 second.

Case 5 Interpretation:

Ventricular activity consists of narrow QRS complexes pointing toward a **supraventricular focus.** The rate is bradycardiac. Regular atrial activity is present, but the P wave is **inverted** and has a **shortened** P-R interval. The rate is the same as the QRS complexes. No AV block exists. We can conclude that the sinus node is **not** the pacemaker; the rhythm originates in the AV junction at a bradycardiac rate. This is an **escape** pacemaker that developed when the sinus node either failed to discharge, or did discharge, but more slowly than the AV junction. The inherent rate of automaticity for the AV junctional tissue is between 40 and 60/min. An escape pacemaker is a subsidiary focus that discharges when the normal pacemaker does not discharge.

Case 6 Data:

Ventricular activity

Rhythm:	Occasionally irregular, some beats occur early in the R-R intervals.
Rate:	130/minute
Shapes:	Two shapes: The dominant rhythm shows narrow QRS complexes of normal duration. Every third complex is wide and distorted with a duration of 0.14 sec.

Atrial activity

Shape:	Constant and upright before narrow QRS complexes, but the distorted QRS complexes have no P waves prior to them.
Rhythm:	Occasionally irregular when early beats occur.
Rate:	130/minute.

AV relationship

1:1 except for the wide QRS complexes.
P-R interval for narrow QRS complexes is 0.14 second.

Other findings

The early beats are followed by compensatory pauses and have T waves that slope in a direction opposite to that of the early QRS complexes.

Case 6 Interpretation:

The two shapes of the QRS complex point to **different sites** of ventricular activation. The narrow QRS complexes occur at a tachycardiac rate. Each is preceded by a P wave in a 1:1 AV relationship. The early beats occur prematurely but in a **pattern:** Two normal beats are followed by a distorted QRS complex. This is a **trigeminal** pattern. The abnormal QRS complexes lack P waves and have compensatory pauses. These are features of premature ventricular complexes (PVCs). The pattern creates the dysrhythmia of sinus tachycardia with ventricular trigeminy.

Interpretations of Actual ECG Tracings

Now we will apply the same format in analyzing actual ECG tracings. You are not expected to be able to correctly interpret these dysrhythmias yet. The purpose is to acquaint you with the thinking process involved in deducing the answers. The specific dysrhythmias will become more familiar after you read the following chapters. You **are** expected to be able to calculate the rates, measure the intervals, and determine the AV conduction ratios.

ECG 1

Interpretation:	Complete AV heart block (idioventricular escape rhythm at 30/minute).
Rationale:	**Ventricular activity** The QRS complexes are wide (0.12 second) and have a regular rhythm. The rate is very slow.

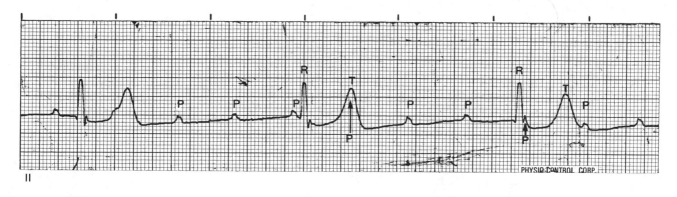

I. VENTRICULAR ACTIVITY
A. QRS
1. Rate: *below 30*/min
2. Shape: *WIDE* ☐ NL
3. Duration: *0.12* sec
B. R-R Interval ☒ regular

II. ATRIAL ACTIVITY
A. P wave
1. Rate: *100* /min
2. Shape: ☒ NL
B. P-P Interval ☒ regular

II. AV RELATIONSHIP
A. P-R Interval *NONE* sec
B. Conduction Ratio
(P:R wave) *NONE* :
C. Pacemaker Site
1. Dominant: ☒ SA, ☐ Atrial, ☐ AV, ☐ Idioventricular
2. Other sites: ☐ SA, ☐ Atrial, ☐ AV, ☒ Idioventricular

Other Significant Findings:_____

Dysrhythmia Interpretation: *Complete AV heart block*

Clinical Significance/Comments:_____

FIGURE 1–19.

Atrial activity
The P waves are upright with a constant shape and rhythm (regular P-P intervals).

AV relationship
The P-R interval is not constant. It shows no pattern in its variability. The AV conduction ratio is nonexistent. No relationship between the P waves and the QRS complexes exists.

Reasoning
The slow ventricular rate and wide QRS complexes indicate a possible **idioventricular focus**. P waves are present but are unrelated to the ventricular activity. Therefore, AV dissociation exists. This rhythm is third degree AV block.

ECG 2

Interpretation:

Atrial fibrillation (ventricular response averages about 105/minute).

Rationale:

Ventricular activity
The QRS complexes are narrow (0.08 second) and the rhythm is grossly irregular.

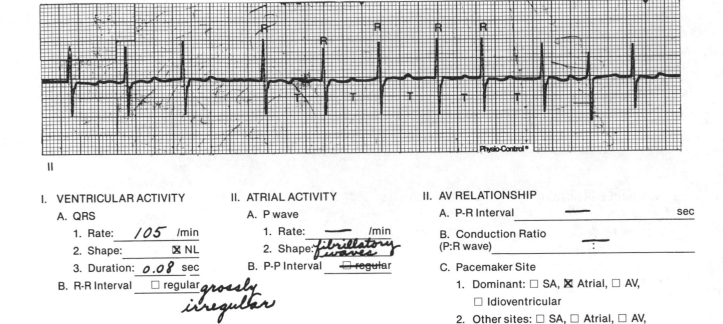

II

I. VENTRICULAR ACTIVITY

   A. QRS

      1. Rate: *105* /min

      2. Shape: ⊠ NL

      3. Duration: *0.08* sec

   B. R-R Interval   ☐ regular *grossly irregular*

II. ATRIAL ACTIVITY

   A. P wave

      1. Rate: —— /min

      2. Shape: *fibrillatory waves*

   B. P-P Interval   ☐ regular

II. AV RELATIONSHIP

   A. P-R Interval _____ —— _____ sec

   B. Conduction Ratio
   (P:R wave) _____ : _____

   C. Pacemaker Site

      1. Dominant: ☐ SA, ⊠ Atrial, ☐ AV,
         ☐ Idioventricular

      2. Other sites: ☐ SA, ☐ Atrial, ☐ AV,
         ☐ Idioventricular

Other Significant Findings:_____

Dysrhythmia Interpretation:___*atrial fibrillation*_____

Clinical Significance/Comments:_____

FIGURE 1–20.

Atrial activity

Consistent P waves are absent. Instead, we see a fine wavy, almost isoelectric baseline (fibrillatory or f waves).

AV relationship

We cannot calculate a P-R interval or a conduction ratio.

Reasoning

The grossly irregular ventricular rhythm is typical of the random conduction of the numerous f waves through the AV node. The narrow QRS duration indicates normal intraventricular conduction, and this means that the impulse must have originated from a **supraventricular focus**. The absence of P waves **eliminates the sinus node** as the site of impulse formation. The findings of a rapid atrial ectopic focus with a randomly occurring ventricular rhythm are typical of atrial fibrillation.

ECG 3

Interpretation:

Ventricular fibrillation.

Rationale:

Ventricular activity

No organized activity exists. Instead, only a chaotic baseline with complexes of changing sizes and shapes is found.

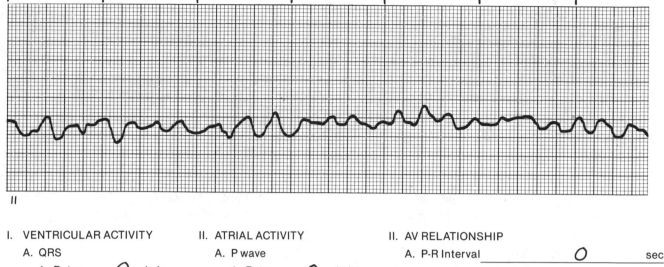

II

I. VENTRICULAR ACTIVITY
  A. QRS
    1. Rate: _O_ /min
    2. Shape: ☐ NL
    3. Duration: _____ sec
  B. R-R Interval ☐ regular

II. ATRIAL ACTIVITY
  A. P wave
    1. Rate: _O_ /min
    2. Shape: ☐ NL
  B. P-P Interval ☐ regular

II. AV RELATIONSHIP
  A. P-R Interval _____ _O_ ____ sec
  B. Conduction Ratio
  (P:R wave) _____:_____
  C. Pacemaker Site
    1. Dominant: ☐ SA, ☐ Atrial, ☐ AV,
      ☐ Idioventricular
    2. Other sites: ☐ SA, ☐ Atrial, ☐ AV,
      ☐ Idioventricular

Other Significant Findings: _No complexes – Just a wavy baseline_

Dysrhythmia Interpretation: _Ventricular fibrillation_

Clinical Significance/Comments: _____

FIGURE 1–21.

Atrial activity
None.

AV relationship
None.

Reasoning
The complete absence of organized P waves and QRS complexes **eliminates** normal atrial or ventricular activity. The bizarre and wavy baseline is characteristic of ventricular fibrillation.

ECG 4

Interpretation: Agonal idioventricular rhythm

Rationale:

Ventricular activity
The QRS complexes are wide and distorted—no T waves are seen. The rhythm is regular, but the rate is very slow.

Atrial activity
Missing.

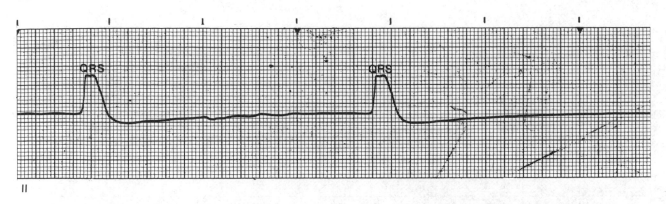

II

I. VENTRICULAR ACTIVITY
  A. QRS
    1. Rate: __20__ /min
    2. Shape: _Distorted_ ☐ NL
    3. Duration: _0.28_ sec
  B. R-R Interval ☒ regular

II. ATRIAL ACTIVITY
  A. P wave
    1. Rate: ___0___ /min
    2. Shape: _____ ☐ NL
  B. P-P Interval ☐ regular

II. AV RELATIONSHIP
  A. P-R Interval _____——_____ sec
  B. Conduction Ratio _____
     (P:R wave) _____:_____
  C. Pacemaker Site
    1. Dominant: ☐ SA, ☐ Atrial, ☐ AV,
       ☒ Idioventricular
    2. Other sites: ☐ SA, ☐ Atrial, ☐ AV,
       ☐ Idioventricular

Other Significant Findings:_____

Dysrhythmia Interpretation:___Idioventricular rhythm_____

Clinical Significance/Comments:_____

FIGURE 1–22.

AV Relationship
None.

Reasoning
The wide QRS complexes mean either that beats arise in the ventricles or that they are supraventricular but abnormally conducted. The missing P waves **rule out** a sinus pacemaker and enable us to **eliminate** the latter possibility. It is termed agonal because it is seen in dying hearts and represents highly unstable activity that is preterminal.

ECG 5

Interpretation: Normal sinus rhythm. No dysrhythmias are present.

Rationale: Let's see how this interpretation would be arrived at using the suggested analysis format.

Ventricular activity
The R-R intervals are regular and the shape and duration of the QRS complexes are normal. This indicates that ventricular activation occurs **along normal pathways.**

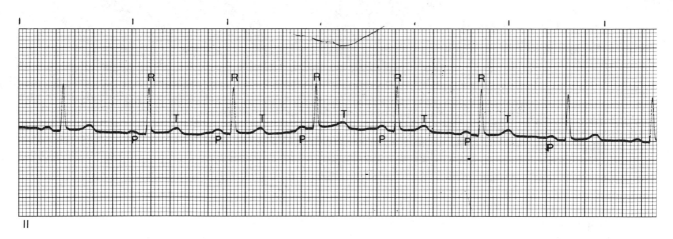

I. **VENTRICULAR ACTIVITY**
A. QRS
1. Rate: _68_ /min
2. Shape: ☒ NL
3. Duration: _0.08_ sec
B. R-R Interval ☒ regular

II. **ATRIAL ACTIVITY**
A. P wave
1. Rate: _68_ /min
2. Shape: ☒ NL
B. P-P Interval ☒ regular

II. **AV RELATIONSHIP**
A. P-R Interval _0.16_ sec
B. Conduction Ratio
(P:R wave) _1 : 1_
C. Pacemaker Site
1. Dominant: ☒ SA, ☐ Atrial, ☐ AV, ☐ Idioventricular
2. Other sites: ☐ SA, ☐ Atrial, ☐ AV, ☐ Idioventricular

Other Significant Findings: _None_

Dysrhythmia Interpretation: _(RSR) Regular or normal sinus rhythm_

Clinical Significance/Comments: _____

FIGURE 1–23.

Atrial activity
The P-P intervals are regular, indicating **normal atrial activation** by the sinus node. The shapes of the P waves are consistent and are upright in lead II, as expected.

AV relationship
Each QRS is preceded by a single P wave, and each P wave is followed by a QRS complex, indicating a uniform cycle. AV block is therefore **absent.**

Conclusion:
The pacemaker is sinus and the heart is activated in a normal manner. No defects in either impulse formation or conduction are present.

ECG 6

Interpretation: Ventricular tachycardia (170/minute).

Rationale: **Ventricular activity**
The QRS complexes are wide and distorted. The rhythm is

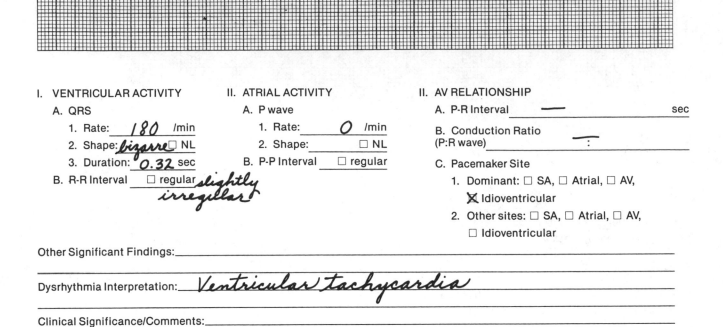

I. VENTRICULAR ACTIVITY
   A. QRS
      1. Rate: _180_ /min
      2. Shape: _bizarre_ ☐ NL
      3. Duration: _0.32_ sec
   B. R-R Interval   ☐ regular _slightly irregular_

II. ATRIAL ACTIVITY
   A. P wave
      1. Rate: _0_ /min
      2. Shape: ☐ NL
   B. P-P Interval   ☐ regular

II. AV RELATIONSHIP
   A. P-R Interval   ———   sec
   B. Conduction Ratio ———
   (P:R wave)   :
   C. Pacemaker Site
      1. Dominant: ☐ SA, ☐ Atrial, ☐ AV,
         ☒ Idioventricular
      2. Other sites: ☐ SA, ☐ Atrial, ☐ AV,
         ☐ Idioventricular

Other Significant Findings:_____

Dysrhythmia Interpretation: _Ventricular tachycardia_____

Clinical Significance/Comments:_____

FIGURE 1–24.

slightly irregular. The QRS complexes do not resemble normal activity, and the rate is extremely fast.

Atrial activity
No P waves or other atrial activity is visible.

AV relationship
We cannot calculate a P-R interval or a conduction ratio.

Reasoning
The wide and distorted QRS complexes indicate two possibilities: a ventricular focus or an aberrantly conducted supraventricular impulse. We eliminate the latter choice because atrial waves are absent. The rapid wide-QRS rhythm is a ventricular tachycardia.

ECG 7

Interpretation:

Sinus bradycardia (50/minute).

Rationale:

The ventricular complexes are within the time limits for normal intraventricular conduction. QRS complexes occur regularly and have a normal shape, each of which has a single P wave ahead of it. The atrial activity shows normal P waves, each fol-

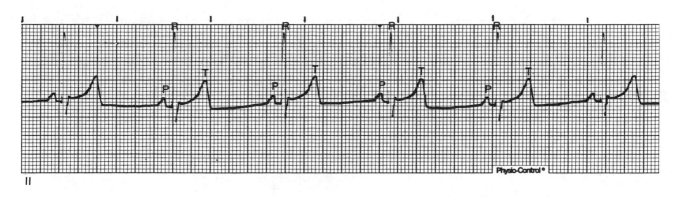

I. VENTRICULAR ACTIVITY
  A. QRS
    1. Rate: _52_ /min
    2. Shape: ☒ NL
    3. Duration: _0.08_ sec
  B. R-R Interval ☒ regular

II. ATRIAL ACTIVITY
  A. P wave
    1. Rate: _52_ /min
    2. Shape: ☒ NL
  B. P-P Interval ☒ regular

II. AV RELATIONSHIP
  A. P-R Interval _0.16_ sec
  B. Conduction Ratio
  (P:R wave) _1 : 1_
  C. Pacemaker Site
    1. Dominant: ☒ SA, ☐ Atrial, ☐ AV,
       ☐ Idioventricular
    2. Other sites: ☐ SA, ☐ Atrial, ☐ AV,
       ☐ Idioventricular

Other Significant Findings:_____

Dysrhythmia Interpretation:_*Sinus bradycardia*_____

Clinical Significance/Comments:_____

FIGURE 1–25.

lowed by a QRS complex. Therefore, the AV conduction ratio is 1:1. Because the SA node is discharging at a rate below 60/min, sinus bradycardia exists. The only deviation from NSR is the slowed rate of impulse formation.

ECG 8

Interpretation: Supraventricular tachycardia (170/minute).

Rationale:

Ventricular activity
The ventricular complexes are narrow (0.08 second) and have a regular rhythm (constant R-R intervals). The rate is tachycardiac because it exceeds 100/minute.

Atrial activity
No P waves or other ectopic atrial waves (P′, F, or f waves) are visible.

AV relationship
We cannot calculate a P-R interval or a conduction ratio.

Reasoning
A QRS duration of 0.10 second or less means that the depolarization of the ventricles must have followed normal pathways. That is to say, for the thick ventricles to have activated so

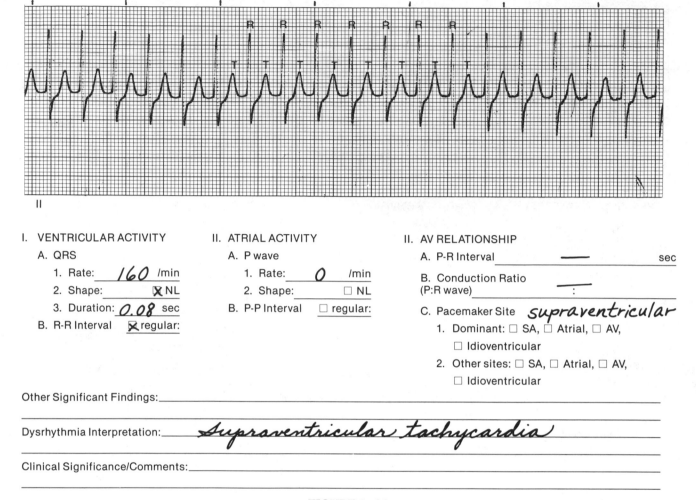

II

I. VENTRICULAR ACTIVITY
  A. QRS
    1. Rate: _160_ /min
    2. Shape: ☒ NL
    3. Duration: _0.08_ sec
  B. R-R Interval ☒ regular:

II. ATRIAL ACTIVITY
  A. P wave
    1. Rate: _0_ /min
    2. Shape: ☐ NL
  B. P-P Interval ☐ regular:

II. AV RELATIONSHIP
  A. P-R Interval _____——_____ sec
  B. Conduction Ratio
  (P:R wave) _____—_____ :
  C. Pacemaker Site _supraventricular_
    1. Dominant: ☐ SA, ☐ Atrial, ☐ AV,
       ☐ Idioventricular
    2. Other sites: ☐ SA, ☐ Atrial, ☐ AV,
       ☐ Idioventricular

Other Significant Findings: _____

Dysrhythmia Interpretation: _Supraventricular tachycardia_____

Clinical Significance/Comments: _____

FIGURE 1–26.

quickly, the impulse must have started from a **supraventricular site** (above the His bundle bifurcation) and proceeded along the normal His-Purkinje pathway. Otherwise, a wide and distorted QRS complex would have been inscribed. Absence of P waves rules out the sinus node as the dominant pacemaker, although ectopic P waves may be hidden in the QRS-T complexes. We **cannot** identify the precise site of origin for this rapid dysrhythmia, and thus, it is considered an SVT or supraventricular tachydysrhythmia.

STEP SEVEN: ASSESSMENT OF HEMODYNAMIC CONSEQUENCES AND NEED FOR TREATMENT

The last step and ultimate goal in analyzing a dysrhythmia includes evaluation of how the altered cardiac rhythm affects a patient's condition. Once we diagnose a dysrhythmia, what can we do about it? Does everyone with a dysrhythmia require treatment? If so, how quickly? Within minutes? Hours? Days? These are two basic principles to keep in mind when trying to answer these questions:

1. Is the dysrhythmia causing hemodynamic compromise or severe symptoms?
2. Are the circumstances such that the dysrhythmia is likely to become more serious in the immediate future?

Let's consider these principles one at a time: One good rule that, unfortunately, is often violated is TREAT THE PATIENT, NOT THE ECG. When someone asks, "How should PVCs be treated?" he really intends, "How should **patients** experiencing PVCs be treated?" Whether a particular dysrhythmia constitutes an emergency, whether it should be treated, and if so, how it should be treated can only be determined within the clinical setting. We can only assess the hemodynamic consequences of a particular dysrhythmia by evaluating the patient: testing the level of consciousness, obtaining vital signs, and examining skin color and temperature.

Remember, an identical dysrhythmia in two patients can have completely different effects on their cardiovascular systems. The classic example of this is the patient with a moderately rapid ventricular tachycardia, say, at 150/minute. A relatively young, otherwise healthy patient with this dysrhythmia may be sitting on the stretcher, talking coherently, complaining of nothing more than "palpitations." Yet, the same dysrhythmia in an elderly patient with underlying coronary artery disease and a past history of several myocardial infarctions could result in signs or symptoms of shock, severe ischemic chest pain, pulmonary edema, or—at its worst—cardiac arrest. Obviously, each of these patients will require a different approach to the treatment of their condition.

How Dysrhythmias Alter Hemodynamics

How do dysrhythmias affect a person's hemodynamic status? A few basic facts are worth quickly reviewing in order to answer this question:

1. We generally divide dysrhythmias into those resulting in a slow ventricular rate (bradydysrhythmias) and those resulting in a rapid ventricular rate (tachydysrhythmias), as shown in Figures 1–27 and 1–28.
2. Blood pressure (BP) is determined by cardiac output and peripheral vascular resistance (PVR).
3. Cardiac output is determined by stroke volume (SV), that is, the amount of blood pumped with each systolic contraction of the ventricles, and heart rate (HR).

These are related in the following formula: $BP = HR \times SV \times PVR$. When the heart rate speeds up, the systolic phase of the cycle changes very little; what primarily changes is a decreased time spent in diastole. Because this is the phase during which the ventricles fill with blood, **the shorter diastole, the less the volume is in the ventricle during the next systolic contraction and the smaller the stroke volume.** Because stroke volume is a major component of cardiac output, each person will have a unique combination of heart rate and stroke volume that will produce a maximal cardiac output. If the rate goes faster than this, the stroke volume will continue to decrease, cardiac output will fall, and—eventually—peripheral vascular resistance will be unable to compensate and blood pressure will fall. This is thus the effect of a tachydysrhythmia on the patient's hemodynamic status.

On the other hand, when a person's heart rate slows, the stroke volume can increase up to a point in order to compensate. Again, there will be a point for everyone where the stroke volume has increased to the maximum, such that **if the heart rate slows any more, the cardiac output begins to fall** and, again, eventually the blood pressure.

In this way **both** tachydysrhythmias and bradydysrhythmias are capable of causing hemodynamic compromise. The term "hemodynamic compromise" means those signs and symptoms resulting from the following:

1. Inability of the heart to pump blood in a forward direction; associated with symptoms of shock such as cool, clammy, pale skin, altered mental status, hypotension, and decreased urine output
2. A backup of pressure behind the ventricles, resulting in venous congestion in the pulmonary circulation, seen as congestive failure and pulmonary edema
3. An elevated central venous pressure, with distended neck veins, hepatic enlargement, and dependent edema

Rather than describing particular dysrhythmias as minor or serious, it is more useful to list their likely effects upon cardiac output. The classifications shown in Table 1–2 are useful for this purpose, although how a patient tolerates them can vary, and this is why a particular dysrhythmia is listed in more than one category.

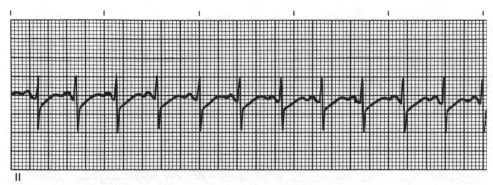

1. Sinus: Normal QRS complexes, P waves, SA nodal pacemaker

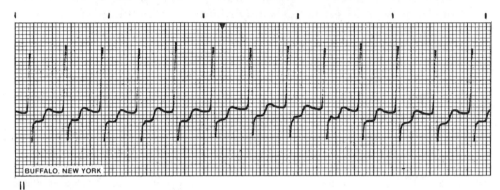

2. Supraventricular: Normal QRS complexes, missing P waves, atrial or junctional pacemaker

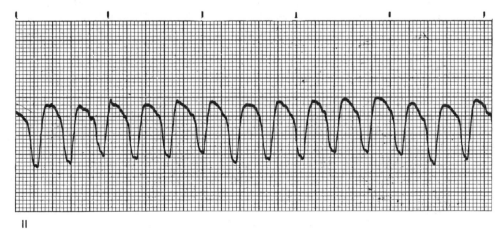

3. Ventricular: Wide, bizarre QRS complexes, missing P waves, His-Purkinje pacemaker

FIGURE 1–27. Tachydysrhythmias (rate >100/min).

Evaluating the Need to Treat a Patient with a Dysrhythmia

The degree to which the patient is hemodynamically unstable determines the urgency with which he or she needs to be treated. Obviously, if the person is in cardiac arrest, then no time may be wasted. The protocols used for treating this situation should be based on the currently accepted national "standard of care," namely, those prescribed by the American Heart Association in its Advanced Cardiac Life Support Course.

If the patient is *not* in cardiac arrest, then there are several questions that must be answered immediately:

1. Is the patient **conscious** or **unconscious?**
2. Are we able to detect a **blood pressure?** The BP may be detected by auscultation in some patients and **only** by palpation in others; most often, it is detectable by both methods. In some patients, special devices such as Doppler flowmeters or arterial lines are needed to accurately assess blood pressure.
3. What does the **pulse** feel like? Is it weak or strong? Does every QRS complex on the ECG monitor result in a palpable pulse beat, or is there a **pulse deficit**, meaning a difference between the heart rate counted by ECG monitor or auscultation and the peripheral pulse?

If the patient is unconscious, the pulse is weak, and the blood pressure is extremely low or undetectable, we know that such a patient has only seconds to minutes to be treated before a cardiac arrest is

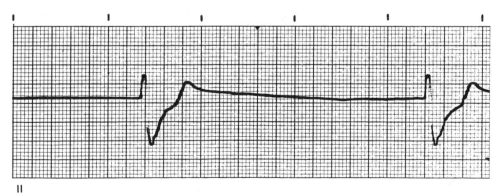

1. Sinus: P waves, normal QRS complexes

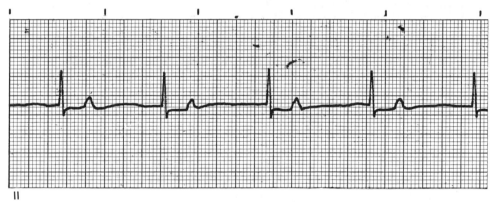

2. AV junctional: Absent P waves, normal QRS complexes

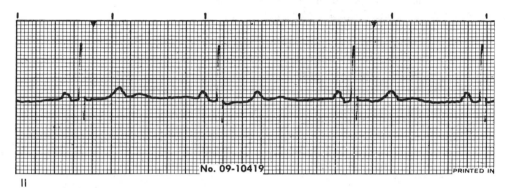

3. Idioventricular: Absent P waves, wide, bizarre QRS complexes

FIGURE 1–28. Bradydysrhythmias (rates <60/min).

TABLE 1–2. Dysrhythmias Classified by Their Effect on Cardiac Output°

Dysrhythmias associated with **normal or near normal** hemodynamics (generally benign):
1. Sinus rhythm with PACS
2. Sinus rhythm with PJCs
3. Artificial pacemaker rhythm with 1:1 capture
4. Atrial fibrillation with an average ventricular response between 60 and 100/min
5. Atrial flutter with an average ventricular response between 60 and 100/min
6. Sinus rhythm with first degree AV block
7. Sinus rhythm with occasional PVCs
8. Sinus bradycardia averaging 50 to 60/min
9. AV junctional rhythm averaging 50 to 60/min
10. Sinus rhythm with second degree AV block Mobitz type 1
11. Isorhythmic AV dissociation

Dysrhythmias with **normal or near normal** hemodynamics but potentially dangerous:
1. Sinus rhythm with short episodes of ventricular tachycardia
2. Sinus rhythm with short episodes of PSVT
3. Accelerated junctional rhythms
4. Artificial pacemaker rhythm with PVCs that are new, multifocal, or couplets
5. Sinus rhythm with second degree AV block Mobitz type 2
6. Atrial flutter or fibrillation with tachycardiac ventricular rates
7. Sinus rhythm with sinus arrest
8. Sinus bradycardia with rates below 50/min

Dysrhythmias with **significantly altered hemodynamics:**
1. Ventricular tachycardia (with pulses)
2. Sinus rhythm or atrial fibrillation with complete heart block
3. Very slow (40/min or below) sinus, junctional, or idioventricular rhythms
4. Malfunctioning artificial pacemakers with idioventricular rhythms

Dysrhythmias associated with **absent hemodynamics**—lethal conditions:
1. Ventricular fibrillation
2. Asystole
3. Pulseless ventricular tachycardia or flutter
4. Agonal idioventricular complexes
5. Electromechanical dissociation
6. Third degree AV heart block with ventricular standstill

°Classification devised by Fritz Streuli, M.D.

likely. If the patient is conscious, but is having significant signs and symptoms of hemodynamic compromise, such as chest pain, altered mental status, diaphoresis, and pulmonary rales, with a moderately low blood pressure, we know we must act quickly, but we have a bit more of a grace period than in the previous situation.

For instance, if the two patients noted above were both found to be in ventricular tachycardia, the first person would probably have to be electrically cardioverted immediately, while the second would be a candidate for a trial of drug therapy before having to resort to electrical conversion. In the one situation, we want to use the modality first that has the best chance of working, even though it may have more potential risks (for example, cardioversion precipitating ventricular fibrillation), while in the second, we can hold it in reserve until some of our more conservative methods have proved unsuccessful.

Thus, dysrhythmias can have a wide variety of effects on individual patients. There are more or less standard approaches for treating each of the more commonly encountered dysrhythmias. However, whether to utilize them at all, or—once deciding to—determining how quickly to progress from one step to the next must be a purely **clinical** decision, based on the appearance of the patient and all available historical information. Up to now, we have been talking about **sustained** dysrhythmias. At this point, we want to return to the question posed earlier concerning the need to treat patients with premature beats. The purpose is not to describe specific therapy—since this will be dealt with in a subsequent chapter—instead, we want to discuss the reasoning that is involved in deciding whether to institute treatment.

Another form of dysrhythmia that is even more common is seen in the patient having **periodic extrasystoles.** These extra beats may generate from virtually anywhere in the heart, such as the atrium, AV junction, or ventricle. They may come in a totally random pattern, or they may have a sustained regularity. It is most common to see them appear **early** in a given cardiac cycle, in which case we refer to them as **premature.** When they occur **late,** it is usually because the next expected normal beat did not appear on time, in which case we think of the extra beat as being **compensatory.** In this latter situation, the treatment of the extra beats is to correct the underlying deficit in the rhythm. In the former, treatment will consist of suppressing the extra beats, usually with specific antidysrhythmic drug therapy.

The question often arises, "Which patients should have these extra beats suppressed and which should not?" Who are we going to subject to these drugs—all of which have potential side effects—because the "risk" of the therapy is worth the "benefit" to the patient? It is uncommon for **supraventricular** premature beats (PACs and PJCs) to require treatment. They generally are considered to be benign and are best left alone—unless they are occurring so frequently that they either are affecting the person hemodynamically, or periodically triggering a more sustained dysrhythmia, or are causing such unpleasant palpitations that they are interfering with the person's life.

We are usually more concerned with premature ventricular complexes (PVCs), and there is still a great deal of controversy surrounding the best approach to these. Through studies of large numbers of volunteers in the military, it has been determined that most normal people have occasional PVCs. These are sometimes explainable on the basis of an increase in sympathetic nervous system tone or as a result of certain types of stimulants, such as nicotine, caffeine, and alcohol. Frequently, however, there is no such explanation and the PVCs are of "unknown" etiology. Does this mean that a large segment of the population should be on antidysrhythmia drug therapy? We hope not.

It is clear that, in the patient in whom we suspect active myocardial ischemia, the risk of PVCs triggering a sustained malignant dysrhythmia such as ventricular tachycardia or ventricular fibrillation is so well documented that an attempt should be made to suppress them. It has been found that certain patterns of PVCs have a more malignant potential than others (such as frequent PVCs, multiformed PVCs, runs of ventricular tachycardia, PVCs on a T wave), but even the ones not fitting these descriptions can have this effect. In recent years, the concept of "prophylactic" antidysrhythmic therapy in such patients has become popular, meaning treating the person with an appropriate history of a myocardial infarction with such medication **prior** to actually seeing PVCs. The rationale for this approach is that if someone is not constantly watching the patient's monitor, "warning" PVCs may be missed. Also, it is always possible that there will be no such "warning" PVCs but rather that the **first** ectopic beat to occur is the one that sets off the serious dysrhythmia. Whether one ascribes to this theory or not, the need to suppress PVCs in the face of acute myocardial ischemia is a concept that is well accepted.

The more difficult situation is the patient who is **not** having any signs or symptoms of active ischemia and who is discovered, while being monitored, to have PVCs. If the patient has had a recent syncopal episode, we like to assume a cause and effect relationship (although frequently this is not borne out after such patients have been thoroughly evaluated), and these patients will generally be admitted for further observation and workup. Likewise, in a patient with possible digitalis toxicity having PVCs, the patient may be otherwise asymptomatic. Again, because of the possible consequences of such an abnormality becoming progressively worse, this patient may also be admitted for further monitoring and possibly for treatment.

Aside from such specific situations, one we are often faced with is the asymptomatic patient with no obvious precipitating factors for PVCs, who may be having a routine ECG done or who may have been placed on a cardiac monitor for some other, noncardiac reason, in whom we see PVCs. As a general rule, the first question that needs to be asked in such patients is whether they have a **past history** that may be consistent with ischemic heart disease. Have they had a previous myocardial infarction? If so, when? Patients in the early post myocardial infarction period having PVCs are at high risk for sudden death. Have they had episodes that suggest angina? Do they have any significant risk factors for coronary artery disease?

In most such patients, **acute** antidysrhythmic therapy is not necessary, unless the patient has a strongly suggestive history and is having frequent or malignant runs of PVCs. In the majority of such patients, a more extensive workup will be necessary to determine the presence and extent of the person's coronary artery disease or the ease with which their PVCs may trigger a more sustained dysrhythmia in order to know whether and how to treat them.

Interpreting rhythm strips is an art that can be developed to almost any degree, from the most basic to the most sophisticated. Hopefully, the rest of this text will assist you in your development of this very useful and potentially lifesaving skill.

Chapter Two
SUPRAVENTRICULAR DYSRHYTHMIAS
DISORDERS OF SINUS, ATRIAL, AND AV JUNCTIONAL FUNCTION

SINUS DYSRHYTHMIA (ARRHYTHMIA)

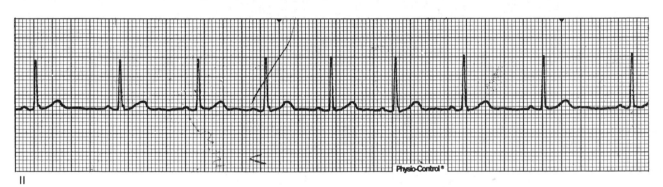

II

FIGURE 2–1. Sinus dysrhythmia.

Ventricular Rate:	Normal.
Ventricular Rhythm:	Regularly irregular R-R intervals.
QRS Shape:	Normal.
QRS Duration:	Normal.
Atrial Rate:	Same as ventricular.
Atrial Rhythm:	Regularly irregular P-P intervals (same as ventricular rhythm).
P Wave Shape:	Normal.
P-R Interval:	Normal and constant from beat to beat.
Conduction Ratio:	1:1 AV ratio; that is, one P wave to each QRS complex.
Significance:	None; this benign dysrhythmia is commonly seen in healthy people—there is no treatment necessary.
Etiology:	The variation in sinus rhythm is due to the effects of breathing upon the autonomic nervous system. Vagal tone is increased during expiration, thereby slowing the rate. It is common in children and patients with lung disease.

37

Acute Drug Therapy: No treatment required.

Concepts about This Dysrhythmia:
- Is simply a variation of NSR.
- The most common type is due to respiration and changes in vagal tone (normal cardiovascular reflexes).
- The heart rate increases during inspiration. As the rate increases, the R-R intervals shorten.
- The cycle rate slows during exhalation. As the rate decreases, the R-R intervals lengthen.
- Asking the patient to hold his or her breath will transiently abolish the arrhythmia.

SINUS TACHYCARDIA

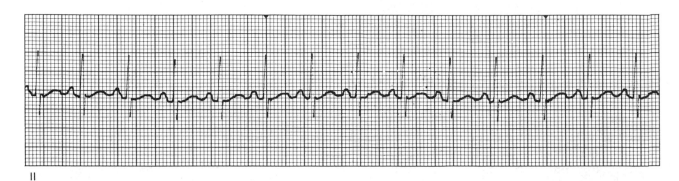

FIGURE 2–2. Sinus tachycardia (120/min).

Ventricular Rate: Greater than 100/min.°

Ventricular Rhythm: Regular R-R intervals.

QRS Shape: Normal.

QRS Duration: Normal.

Atrial Rate: Same as ventricular.

Atrial Rhythm: Regular P-P intervals.

P Wave Shape: Normal.

P-R Interval: Normal (at rapid rates, the P wave may appear to merge with the preceding T wave because the T-P interval shortens).

Conduction Ratio: 1:1 AV ratio.

Significance: Sinus tachycardia is caused by the increased secretion of epinephrine by the sympathetic nervous system or by decreased vagal tone. It is not dangerous in itself, and in certain stressful conditions such as exercise, fever, and anxiety, is a perfectly normal response. But in patients experiencing myocardial ischemia, sinus tachycardia causes an increase in myocardial oxygen demand.

°The upper limit varies, but at rates greater than 150/minute one is much more likely to be dealing with a supraventricular tachydysrhythmia other than sinus tachycardia.

In patients with coronary atherosclerosis and fixed obstruction to blood flow the increased oxygen delivery that is required to sustain rapid heart rates may not be possible. This may predispose to more serious rhythm disturbances.

Acute Therapy: Treatment is directed at the underlying cause. In myocardial ischemia, oxygen administration, analgesics, and beta-blocking agents are effective in slowing the heart rate and may limit the size of infarction.

SINUS BRADYCARDIA

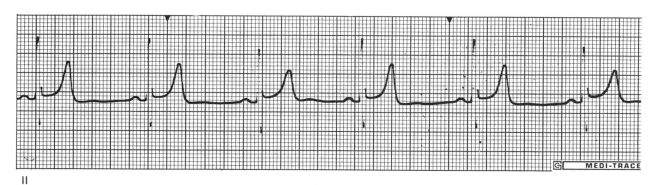

FIGURE 2–3. Sinus bradycardia (50/min).

Ventricular Rate: Below 60/min.

Ventricular Rhythm: Regular R-R intervals.

QRS Configuration: Normal.

QRS Duration: Normal.

Atrial Rate: Same as ventricular rate.

Atrial Rhythm: Regular P-P intervals.

P Wave Shape: Normal.

P-R Interval: Normal.

Conduction Ratio: 1:1 AV ratio.

Significance: The clinical importance depends on the cause of this dysrhythmia, how slow it is, and particularly on how the patient is tolerating it.

Etiology: The rate of impulse formation is slowed. Sinus bradycardia is due to increased vagal (parasympathetic) tone; it may be caused by drugs, particularly digitalis or morphine, which decrease the automaticity of the SA node. Sinus node dysfunction is common in acute inferior wall MIs, and may be due to direct ischemia or injury of the SA node or caused by a reflex mechanism rather than direct effect on the nodal tissue. In well conditioned athletes, a slow resting heart rate is common and normal, while in the elderly, it may be due to atherosclerotic degeneration of the nodal tissue.

Acute Drug Therapy: Usually does **not** require treatment. Treatment is indicated in ischemic heart disease when a slow rate allows ventricular escape beats or the patient becomes hemodynamically unstable.

1. Atropine, 0.5 to 1.0 mg IV
2. Isoproterenol, IV infusion at 2 to 20 µg/min (1 to 2 mg diluted in 500 ml of 5 percent dextrose in water and flow titrated to effect)
3. Artificial pacing

See treatment protocol shown in Figure 2–4.

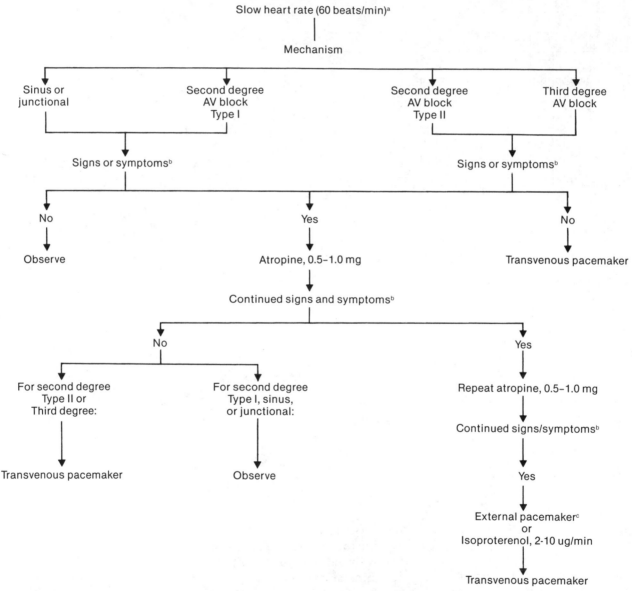

FIGURE 2–4. Bradycardia. This sequence was developed to assist in teaching how to treat a broad range of patients with bradycardia. Some patients may require care not specified here. This algorithm should not be construed to prohibit such flexibility. *Key:* [a]A solitary chest thump or cough may stimulate cardiac electrical activity and result in improved cardiac output and may be used at this point. [b]Hypotension (blood pressure <90 mm Hg), premature ventricular contractions, altered mental status or symptoms (e.g., chest pain or dyspnea), ischemia, or infarction. [c]Temporizing therapy.

Concepts about Sinus Bradycardia:

- Due to high vagal tone, the P-R interval may increase correspondingly.
- Slowing of SA nodal discharge may result in periods of AV junctional rhythms, or isorhythmic AV dissociation, wherein the atria and ventricles beat independently. This occurs when the slowed SA pacemaker allows an AV junctional focus to discharge and determine the ventricular rate. Retrograde conduction to the atria does not occur, so the SA node continues to control the atria. Since anterograde conduction through the AV node is unimpeded, a sinus impulse arriving to find the node nonrefractory will be normally conducted. The condition occurs because of the similar rates of discharge of the SA node and AV junction. It is important to remember that no intrinsic AV nodal conduction defect is present and that the AV dissociated state will end when the sinus node speeds up.

SINUS BLOCK/ARREST

A

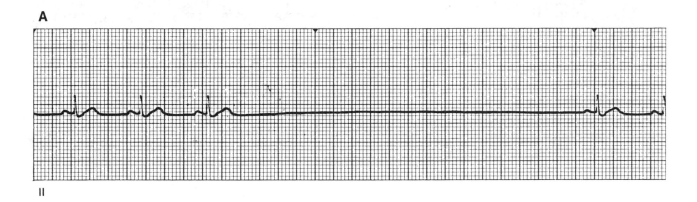

II

B

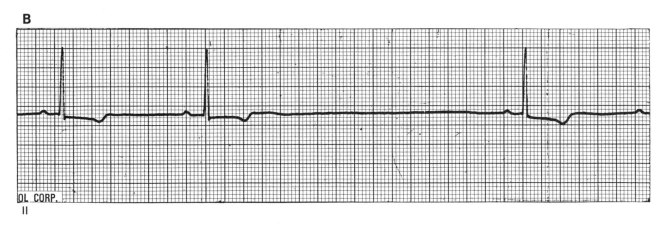

II

FIGURE 2–5. Sinus arrest.

Sinus block and arrest share the finding of intermittent failure of the atria to depolarize, resulting in missing cardiac cycles. The ECG shows transient asystolic pauses, which are often terminated by escape complexes. The disorders result from impairment of SA nodal function or the inability of the atrial tissue surrounding the node to respond to the stimulus.

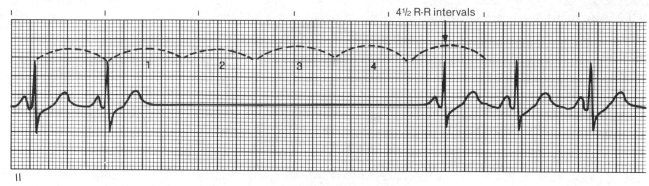

4½ R-R intervals

Arrest: The sinus beat following the pause is *not* a multiple of the normal R-R interval

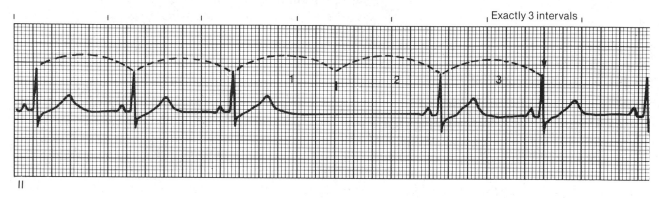

Exactly 3 intervals

Block: The sinus complex following the pause is an exact multiple of the normal R-R interval

FIGURE 2–6. ECG difference between sinus arrest versus block.

Ventricular Rate:	Depends on sinus rate and the frequency and length of the pauses.
Ventricular Rhythm:	Irregular R-R intervals.
QRS Configuration:	Normal.
QRS Duration:	Normal.
Atrial Rate:	Same as the ventricular rate.
Atrial Rhythm:	Irregular P-P intervals.
P Wave Configuration:	Normal.
P-R Interval:	Normal.
Conduction Ratio:	1:1 AV ratio.
Hallmark Finding:	The ECG shows asystolic pauses in which entire cardiac cycles (P-QRS-T waves) are missing. These pauses are usually terminated by escape complexes or rhythms.
Description and Terminology:	One or more sinus impulses fail to initiate a cardiac cycle. Consequently, no P-QRS-T complexes are inscribed for each of the missing cycles. The ECG records this as a sudden prolongation

of the P-P interval. If this pause is sufficiently long, it may permit latent pacemakers to discharge. **Therefore, the complex terminating sudden pauses should be examined to see if it is an escape beat.** There are several possible mechanisms by which the heart may remain unstimulated:

1. Sinus node fails to generate an impulse.
2. Sinus impulse is generated but is blocked and fails to exit the node (called SA exit block).
3. Sinus impulse fails to stimulate the atria because either the impulse is weaker than normal or the atrial tissue fails to respond to the stimulus.

Since the surface ECG records the same finding (prolonged P-P interval) for all three mechanisms, it is not possible to detect the cause. As a result, the terminology pertaining to sinus dysfunction is imprecise. Sinus **block** has come to mean an occasional SA dysfunction in which usually one or two cycles is missing, whereas sinus **arrest** implies that the SA node fails for a prolonged period. The prolonged P-P pause in block is usually a multiple of the underlying P-P cycle, whereas in arrest the pause is not a multiple.

It is a better practice to use the term sinus block to apply to all the possible dysfunctions, separating them into incomplete and complete forms, as is done for AV blocks.

In **incomplete SA block** there is an occasional loss of atrial stimulation, most commonly for one cycle. As a result, the P-P interval that includes the pause will equal exactly two normal P-P intervals.

In **complete SA block,** SA nodal activity fails for a sustained period and the prolonged P-P interval is considerable (can last for several seconds if not terminated by escape beats) but is not a multiple of the underlying P-P interval.

Although there is a less common form of incomplete block, all forms of this dysrhythmia are relatively rare and will not be discussed.

Etiology:

There is a variety of causes, including drug excess of digitalis and quinidine, increased vagal tone, carotid body hypersensitivity, carotid sinus massage, hyperkalemia, rheumatic heart (inflammatory) disease, coronary artery diseases including ischemia, injury, infarction, fibrosis, and other degenerative changes of the SA node.

Acute Drug Therapy:

Depends on underlying cause. If due to drug toxicity, withdraw offending agent. Additionally, atropine, isoproterenol, or an artificial pacemaker may be needed.

Concepts about This Dysrhythmia:

- **Warning:** Sinus nodal depression may be iatrogenically caused by vigorous carotid sinus massage (CSM) when treating cases of PSVT.
- To be complete the interpretation should include the duration of the arrest. For example: "Sinus arrest with a 4 sec period of asystole."
- Intrinsic disease of the sinus node can cause failure of sinus node impulse formation for variable periods of time, often of a duration long enough to cause syncope.

PREMATURE SUPRAVENTRICULAR COMPLEXES

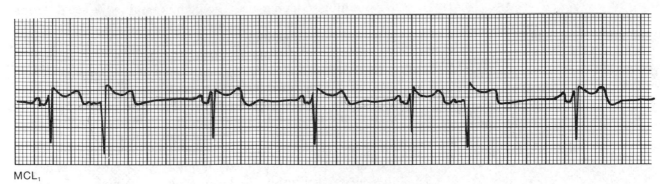

MCL₁

FIGURE 2–7. PACs (beats 2 and 6).

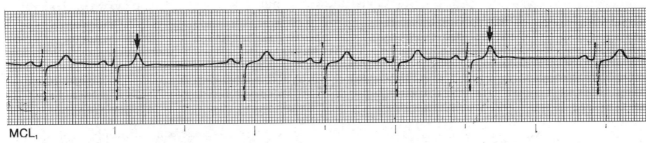

MCL₁

FIGURE 2–8. Nonconducted PACs. The ECG pauses are caused by the blocked P' waves (arrows) hidden in the T waves of the preceding sinus beats.

For convenience, and based on their similarities, we have included premature beats that arise from an ectopic atrial or AV junctional focus under the same heading.

PREMATURE ATRIAL COMPLEXES (PACs, ATRIAL EXTRASYSTOLES, ATRIAL PREMATURE BEATS)

Ventricular Rate:	Normal.
Ventricular Rhythm:	Irregular R-R intervals when PACs occur.
QRS Shape/Duration:	Normal. (However, if aberrantly conducted, the QRS complex may be wide and distorted, resembling a PVC.)
Atrial Rate:	Depends on sinus plus PACs.
Atrial Rhythm:	Intermittent irregularity when PAC occurs.
P Wave Shapes:	Vary. The P' waves of the PACs are of different shape and size than normal P waves. The P' wave can be buried in the preceding T wave, giving a peaked appearance to the T wave.
P-R Interval:	May be shorter or longer than sinus P-R interval.
Conduction Ratio:	1:1 ratio.
Significance:	These premature complexes are of minor clinical significance. Proper identification is important in order to distinguish them from the malignant PVCs. PACs cause little effect on cardiac output. Patients often are aware of them as palpitations or "skipped beats."

Etiology: This is a benign dysrhythmia. The ectopic supraventricular (atrial or junctional) pacemaker discharges and may be due to increased sympathetic stimulation or atrial irritability. This dysrhythmia may be associated with diseases that indirectly affect the atria, such as cor pulmonale (chronic pulmonary disease causing heart failure), pulmonary embolism, pneumonia, or atrial infarction.

Increased atrial automaticity may be due to increased sympathetic stimulation caused by excessive coffee intake (caffeine) or anxiety.

Acute Drug Therapy: Usually none.

Concepts about This Dysrhythmia:
- If the PAC occurs very early in the R-R interval, especially if it occurs during the previous ventricular repolarization (T wave), the P' wave may not be conducted (called blocked PACs).
- Nonconducted PACs cause pauses on the ECG and cause the preceding T wave to be peaked and taller than sinus beats.
- PACs may initiate episodes of paroxysmal supraventricular tachycardia.
- Can occur in grouped beatings such as atrial bigeminy, atrial trigeminy, etc.

Differentiation between PACs and PVCs

PACs usually
- Have normal shaped QRS complexes.
- Have associated P waves.
- Have T waves that are in the same direction (concordant) as the QRS complex of the PAC.
- Do **not** have a fully compensatory pause following the premature beats.
- Have QRS complex deflections that are in the same direction as normal beats.

PVCs, in contrast, usually
- Have wide and distorted QRS complexes.
- Lack P waves.
- Have T waves shaped opposite in direction (discordant) to the QRS complex of the PVC.
- Commonly have compensatory pauses following the premature beats.

PREMATURE JUNCTIONAL (NODAL) COMPLEXES (PJCs, PNCs)

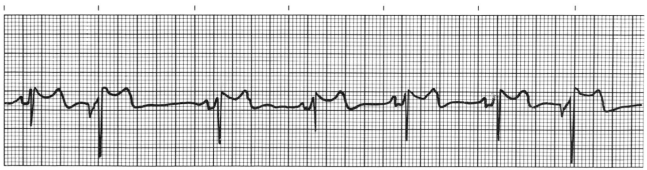

MCL₁

FIGURE 2–9. PJCs (beats 2 and 7).

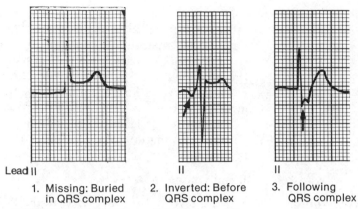

Lead II

1. Missing: Buried   2. Inverted: Before   3. Following
   in QRS complex   QRS complex   QRS complex

FIGURE 2–10. Position of P′ wave in AV junctional complexes.

The junctional area surrounding the AV node prematurely depolarizes before the next sinus impulse occurs. This junctional ectopic beat occurs **early** in the R-R interval and may or may not be followed by a compensatory pause. This is generally a benign dysrhythmia, similar to PACs. PJCs must be viewed within the patient's clinical appearance to determine the significance.

Ventricular Rate:	Normal.
Ventricular Rhythm:	Irregular R-R intervals when PJCs occur.
QRS Shape:	Normal.
QRS Duration:	Normal (unless aberrantly conducted).
Atrial Rate:	Normal.
Atrial Rhythm:	Irregular P-P intervals when PJCs occur.
P Wave Shape:	P′ wave can be upright, inverted, or biphasic, depending on lead being used. In lead II and MCL$_1$, the P′ waves are inverted. The position of the P′ wave in relation to the QRS complexes is quite variable. It can occur before or after the QRS complex or be absent. Most commonly it is absent, as in Figure 2–10.
P-R Interval:	Shortened or unable to detect.
Conduction Ratio:	If P′ waves can be identified, it is 1:1; otherwise more QRS complexes will be seen than P waves.
Etiology and Significance:	Same as for PACs.
Acute Drug Therapy:	Usually none.

PAROXYSMAL SUPRAVENTRICULAR TACHYCARDIA (PSVT, PAROXYSMAL ATRIAL TACHYCARDIA, PAT)

Ventricular Rate:	150 to 250/minute (commonly averages about 200/minute)
Ventricular Rhythm:	Regular R-R intervals.
QRS Shape:	Usually normal (unless aberrant conduction).
QRS Duration:	Normal.
Atrial Rate:	150 to 250/minute (same as ventricular).

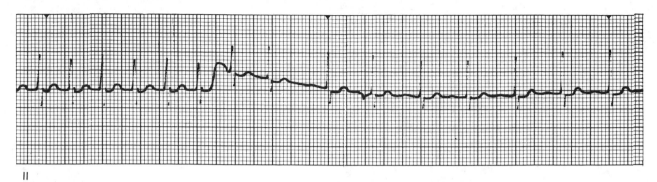

II

FIGURE 2–11. Abrupt conversion from PSVT to a sinus rhythm.

Atrial Rhythm:	The P wave is usually **not** visible; if seen, it has a different configuration than normal P waves. Position of P' wave in relation to the QRS complex is variable: sometimes it is before, but just as often, it follows QRS.
P-R Interval:	Shortened if P' waves visible.
Conduction Ratio:	Usually 1:1; if greater, then probably due to digitalis induced block or hypokalemia.
Significance:	Commonly observed in relatively healthy individuals without demonstrable heart disease aside from mitral valve prolapse. In younger individuals it is well tolerated except for palpitations and lightheadedness as long as the rate doesn't exceed 180/minute or persist for an extended length of time. Older individuals, on the other hand, may develop angina or a myocardial infarction, and in the face of preexisting heart disease this can lead to congestive heart failure and acute pulmonary edema.
Etiology:	This tachydysrhythmia is often precipitated by a PAC or PJC which reenters the AV node (or SA node, atria, or His bundle) and initiates a cycle of repetitive stimulation. The reentry loop is most often within the AV node but can involve the atria and the SA node. About 5 percent of the SVTs are actually due to a rapidly firing autonomous pacemaker within the atria.
Acute Drug Therapy:	Figure 2–12 shows the treatment flow chart.
Terminology:	SVT refers to a **group** of regular tachydysrhythmias originating above the ventricles. The term is applied because of the difficulty in separating sinus, atrial, and AV junctional tachycardias from one another based on the ECG findings of narrow QRS complexes and short R-R cycles in which P waves are not clearly seen. Paroxysmal SVT is only one dysrhythmia of the group. Chronic SVT is usually due to digitalis toxicity.
Concepts about PSVT:	• Has abrupt onset and cessation, unlike sinus tachycardia which has a gradual increase and decrease.
	• It may last for seconds to hours, or even days.
	• PSVT resembles a string of consecutive PACs at a rate greater than 100/minute.
	• Vagal maneuvers (CSM, etc.) are diagnostic as well as therapeutic (see Table 2–3). PSVTs are suddenly terminated by

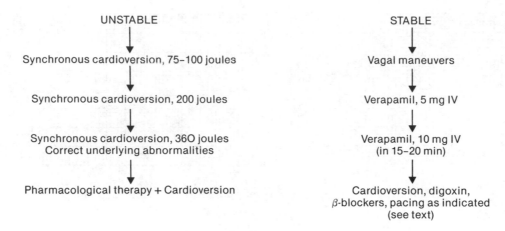

UNSTABLE	STABLE
Synchronous cardioversion, 75–100 joules	Vagal maneuvers
Synchronous cardioversion, 200 joules	Verapamil, 5 mg IV
Synchronous cardioversion, 36O joules Correct underlying abnormalities	Verapamil, 10 mg IV (in 15–20 min)
Pharmacological therapy + Cardioversion	Cardioversion, digoxin, β-blockers, pacing as indicated (see text)

If conversion occurs but PSVT recurs, repeated electrical cardioversion
is not indicated. Sedation should be used as time permits.

FIGURE 2–12. Paroxysmal supraventricular tachycardia (PSVT). This sequence was developed to assist in teaching how to treat a broad range of patients with sustained PSVT. Some patients may require care not specified here. This algorithm should not be construed as prohibiting such flexibility. Flow of algorithm presumes PSVT is continuing. (Courtesy of the American Heart Association ACLS.)

vagal maneuvers which slow the conduction velocity and thereby disrupt the reentry pathway. (In sinus tachycardia CSM produces only a gradual slowing and a return to rapid rate with release of pressure.)
- Unlike atrial flutter, AV conduction is usually 1:1.
- It may be impossible to distinguish PSVT with aberrant intraventricular conduction from ventricular tachycardia since the QRS complexes are distorted in both.

ATRIAL FIBRILLATION

Ventricular Rate: Usually 100 to 160/min; if medicated, usually less than 100/min.

Ventricular Rhythm: Irregularly irregular R-R intervals.

QRS Shape: Normal.

QRS Duration: Normal unless preexisting conduction disease exists.

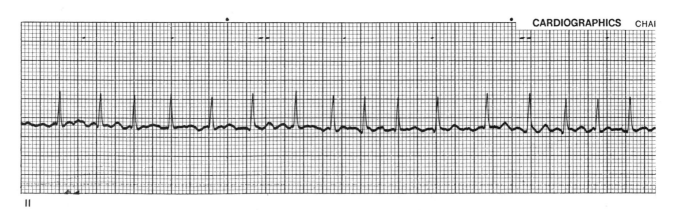

FIGURE 2–13. Atrial fibrillation with a tachycardiac (120/min) ventricular response.

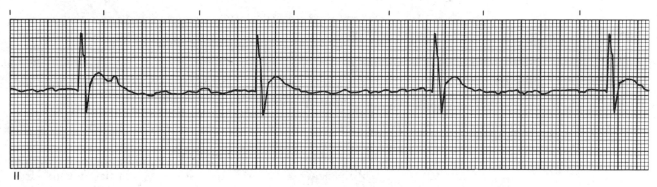

FIGURE 2–14. Atrial fibrillation with complete AV block. An idioventricular escape focus paces the heart at 32/min.

Atrial Rate:	350 to 600/min (not measurable on the ECG tracing).
Atrial Rhythm:	Irregular.
P Wave Shape:	No true P waves; instead small fibrillatory waves of different shapes, sizes and configurations. The f waves often appear as a wavy baseline.
P-R Interval:	Absent.
P-P Interval:	Absent.
Conduction Ratio:	No fixed AV ratio. Random conduction.
Significance:	The atria fail to contract in a coordinated manner. Although atrial fibrillation can be paroxysmal and does occur in the setting of a myocardial infarction, this dysrhythmia is usually a chronic condition and can be reasonably well tolerated. It may be due to chronic degenerative disease of the atria and is not infrequent in elderly patients, as well as those with valvular disease. In a damaged heart, the development of atrial fibrillation, while not life-threatening, may aggravate the ischemic state further. Patients with longstanding fibrillation often develop emboli which lead to strokes. This is caused by mural thrombi being dislodged from the walls of the atria which were formed from the stasis of blood in atrial fibrillation.
Etiology:	Rapid and irregular atrial depolarizations caused by multiple areas of reentry causing numerous wavelets.

Acute Drug Therapy:

1. Cardioversion for patients not tolerating the dysrhythmia.
2. Digitalization.
3. Slowing of ventricular response can be achieved with use of beta or calcium channel blockers.

NOTE: When atrial fibrillation is due to Wolff-Parkinson-White syndrome, Digitalis, Verapamil, and beta blockers can **increase** the ventricular response. Therapy for this situation is cardioversion; slowing can be achieved with intravenous 1) Lidocaine and 2) Procainamide.

Concepts about This Dysrhythmia:

- Lead MCL₁ is the best for detecting f waves. Lead I is **not** desirable because the f waves appear flat and this makes the baseline isoelectric.

- A complete interpretation should include the average ventricular rate per minute because this determines the seriousness of dysrhythmia, for example, "atrial fibrillation with a ventricular rate of about 120/min."
- Ventricular rates are termed "controlled" if under 100/minute, and "uncontrolled" if tachycardic.
- The loss of coordinated atrial systole ("atrial kick") corresponds to a 10 to 25 percent reduction in ventricular filling and cardiac output.
- The pulse is diagnostic: the rhythm is irregularly irregular with varying pulse pressures (since the cardiac output varies from beat to beat). Pulse deficits are common as a result of shortened cardiac cycle lengths.
- This dysrhythmia may exist for short periods and convert back to NSR spontaneously or be a chronic condition.
- May exist in a hybrid state as "fibrillation-flutter."
- Frequently reoccurs in spite of treatment.

ATRIAL FLUTTER

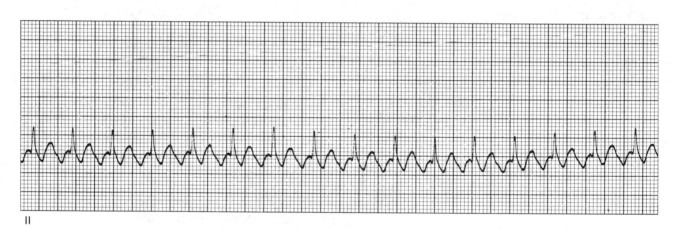

FIGURE 2–15. Atrial flutter with 2:1 AV conduction.

Ventricular Rate:	Depends on the atrial rate and conduction ratio. When 2:1 AV conduction exists, the range is 140 to 160/minute.
Ventricular Rhythm:	Regular (unless variable AV conduction exists).
QRS Shape:	Normal.
QRS Duration:	Normal.
Atrial Rate:	250 to 350/min (usually around 300/min).
Atrial Rhythm:	Regular.
P Wave Shape:	Absent, replaced by regular "sawtooth" shaped (F) waves.
P-R Interval:	F-R interval is constant for conducted F waves.
Conduction Ratio:	Usually a fixed ratio such as 2:1, 3:1, or 4:1 but may be variable. Unless accessory AV conduction pathways exist, a 1:1 ratio does **not** occur because the AV node is refractory.

Etiology: This regular tachydysrhythmia is caused by a reentry of a stimulus within the atria.

Acute Drug Therapy:

1. Patients not tolerating rhythm can be cardioverted at low energy.
2. Ventricular response can be slowed with a beta blocker, such as propranolol, or a calcium channel blocker, such as verapamil.
3. Conversion to NSR can be seen occasionally following digitalization.
4. Spontaneous reversion also common.

Concepts about This Dysrhythmia:

- A complete interpretation should also include the AV conduction ratio as well as the average ventricular rate, such as "atrial flutter with 3:1 conduction and an average ventricular rate of 100/min."
- The degree of AV conduction determines the pulse rate and the hemodynamic consequences. An atrial rate of 300/minute with a 4:1 AV conduction will produce a ventricular rate of 75 which is within a tolerable range; on the other hand, a 2:1 ratio produces a rate of 150/minute which may cause a fall in blood pressure and ischemic chest pain in a patient with diminished cardiac reserve.
- Avoid using the term "block" when referring to the AV conduction ratio because it is a normal functional consequence of the refractoriness of the AV node rather than a pathological condition.
- A 2:1 AV conduction produces a regular tachycardia (rate of 140 to 160/min), which is often misinterpreted as sinus tachycardia because the second F wave is often overlooked. Therefore, scrutinize the ST-T wave complexes for nonconducted atrial beats whenever encountering rhythm with this ventricular range.
- MCL$_1$ usually provides the best view of this dysrhythmia since the flutter waves are emphasized, while lead I provides the worst.
- The jagged baseline is usually the best due to this dysrhythmia. It has been described as a "picket-fence" (see Fig. 2–16) or "sawtooth" form.
- Carotid sinus massage or other vagal maneuvers in tachydysrhythmias may unmask hidden F waves by increasing AV nodal refractoriness.
- May be difficult to distinguish from ventricular tachycardia if aberrant ventricular conduction exists.
- Flutter may degenerate into atrial fibrillation and may be seen as the hybrid form "atrial flutter-fibrillation."
- Flutter may be an extremely unstable dysrhythmia if the AV conduction is unreliable. The conduction ratio in such cases

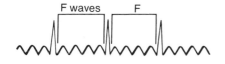
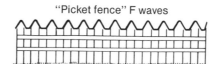

FIGURE 2–16. Flutter (F) waves are uniform in shape, unlike fibrillatory waves.

may change to 5:1, 8:1, 10:1, etc. These cases produce minimal cardiac output and the patients should be quickly converted to a more stable rhythm. Conduction ratios in excess of 4:1 usually result from medication toxicity.

AV JUNCTIONAL (NODAL) RHYTHMS

AV junctional rhythms are not a primary ECG interpretation; they are secondary to another defect, such as depression of the sinus node or increased automaticity of the AV junction.

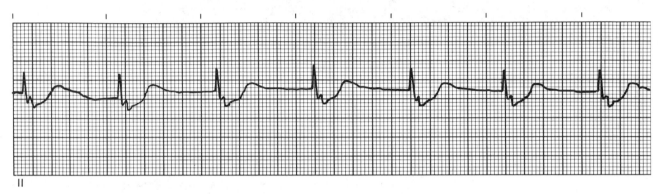

FIGURE 2–17. Sustained AV junctional rhythm.

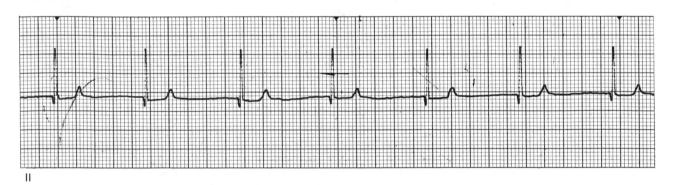

FIGURE 2–18. Sustained AV junctional rhythm.

Ventricular Rate:	Three common ranges depending on mechanism: Basic (escape) rhythm (40 to 60/minute); Accelerated junctional rhythm (60 to 100/minute); Junctional tachycardias (above 100/minute).
Ventricular Rhythm:	Regular R-R intervals.
Ventricular Shape:	Normal QRS configuration.
QRS Duration:	Normal.
Atrial Rate:	P′ waves are usually not seen. If they are, the rates conform to those listed above.
Atrial Rhythm:	Regular if visible.
P Wave Configuration:	P waves are replaced by P′ waves. Possible shapes in lead include:

1. P′ waves **precede** QRS but are inverted with a short P-R interval;
2. *no* evidence of P waves (hidden by QRS); and
3. P waves **follow** QRS complex.

In lead MCL$_1$, the biphasic shape changes, usually from a $+/-$ to a $-/+$.

P-R Interval: If present, less than normal.

Conduction Ratio: 1:1 but the order of occurrence may reverse if the atria are activated after the ventricles.

Hallmark Characteristics:
- Normal QRS.
- Abnormal, inverted or missing P waves.

Etiology: Junctional escape rhythms occur when the sinus node fails to discharge. The AV junctional pacemaker passively discharges at 40 to 60/min.

Junctional rhythms which **compete** with the SA node for pacemaker control occur at rates above 60/minute. The increased degree of AV junctional discharge is due to a reentry rhythm or a rapid ectopic focus.

Concepts about AV Junctional Rhythms:
- Although these are also known as nodal rhythms, the AV node does not have the inherent ability to form an impulse. The area of the AV junction that does have the property of automaticity is the tissue surrounding the AV node. Therefore, the use of the term "nodal rhythm" is a misnomer; such rhythms are really junctional ones that originate in the upper His bundle.
- AV junctional tachycardia is difficult to separate from other PSVTs by ECG characteristics, so it is included in that group.
- Slow junctional rhythms emerge when the sinus node is depressed. They are really secondary to another disorder so the ECG interpretation should include the primary defect, such as "sinus arrest with an AV junctional escape rhythm at 50/minute."

TABLE 2–1. Dysrhythmia Synopsis: Sinus Dysrhythmias

	P Waves	QRS Complexes	AV Relationship	Other Features
1. Sinus bradycardia	Normal	Normal	Normal	Rate below 60/min
2. Sinus tachycardia	Normal	Normal	Normal	Rate above 100/min
3. Sinus arrest/SA exit block	Missing in dropped cycles / Normal in conducted cycles	Missing in dropped cycles / Normal for conducted cycles	Missing in dropped cycles / Normal for conducted cycles	Long asystolic R-R intervals during periods of arrest
4. Sinus dysrhythmia	Normal shape	Normal shape	Normal	Benign variation of RSR / Varies with phases of respiration

TABLE 2–2. Dysrhythmia Synopsis: Supraventricular Tachycardias

	P Waves	QRS Complexes	AV Relationship	Key Features	Response to Vagal Maneuvers
Atrial flutter	Absent, replaced by regular F waves Atrial rate of 250–350/min	Normal Usually regular	Usually a fixed AV conduction greater than 1:1, e.g., 2:1, 3:1, 4:1	Sawtooth pattern	Stepwise decrease in rate with return to previous rate with offset of pressure
Atrial fibrillation	Absent; replaced by irregular f waves. Atrial rate of 350–600/min (not countable).	Normal Irregularly irregular; rate is under 100/min (treated) or above 100/min (untreated)	Random AV conduction	Fibrillatory/chaotic baseline Irregularly irregular R-R intervals	No response or transient slowing of ventricular response
Multifocal atrial tachycardia	Sinus P waves plus P′ waves of at least three shapes	Irregular rhythm	1:1	Changing shapes of ectopic P waves	None
Paroxysmal supraventricular tachycardia (PSVT)	Absent P′ waves are missing If present, found preceding, following, or in the QRS complex	Normal Regular R-R interval	1:1 if P′ wave visible S2:1, 3:1 conduction, suspect digitalis toxicity	Abrupt onset and termination Occur in bursts	No response or conversion to RSR
Sinus tachycardia	Normal	Normal	1:1	Gradual return to slower rates	None, or transient slowing
AV junctional tachycardia	See PSVT; unable to differentiate from PSVT				See Table 3–3

TABLE 2–3. Vagal Maneuvers

1. Valsalva maneuver.
2. Valsalva maneuver plus right carotid massage (before carotid massage ascertain that patient has strong bilateral carotid pulses and that there are no carotid bruits). Massage vigorous under angle of jaw with head hyperextended for no longer than 15 sec. Do not massage carotids in patients over the age of 60.
3. Gag reflex.
4. Diving reflex—the head is plunged into ice water for 10 to 15 sec. This works infrequently and should be reserved for young, healthy patients who will be cooperative and will not aspirate the water.
5. Tensilon (edrophonium) plus Valsalva maneuver, 8 to 10 mg IV. Used for differential diagnosis more than for conversion. Side effects are abdominal cramps, brochospasm, vomiting, and retching.
6. Neo-Synephrine plus Valsalva maneuver—1 mg in 50 ml administered over 2 min; reserved for patients who are hypotensive with their tachydysrhythmias. Should not be used in the elderly or in patients with cerebrovascular disease.

TABLE 2–4. Common Supraventricular Rates

Rhythm	Rate
Sinus tachycardia	100–150/min
Paroxysmal supraventricular tachycardia (PSVT)	140–250/min
Atrial flutter	250–350/min
Atrial fibrillation	350–600/min

EXERCISE A: SELF-ASSESSMENT ECG TRACINGS 1 TO 37

The following ECGs show a variety of supraventricular dysrhythmias. Analyze each tracing according to the systematic approach outlined in Chapter One and formulate an interpretation. Check your answers with the suggested interpretations beginning on page 72.

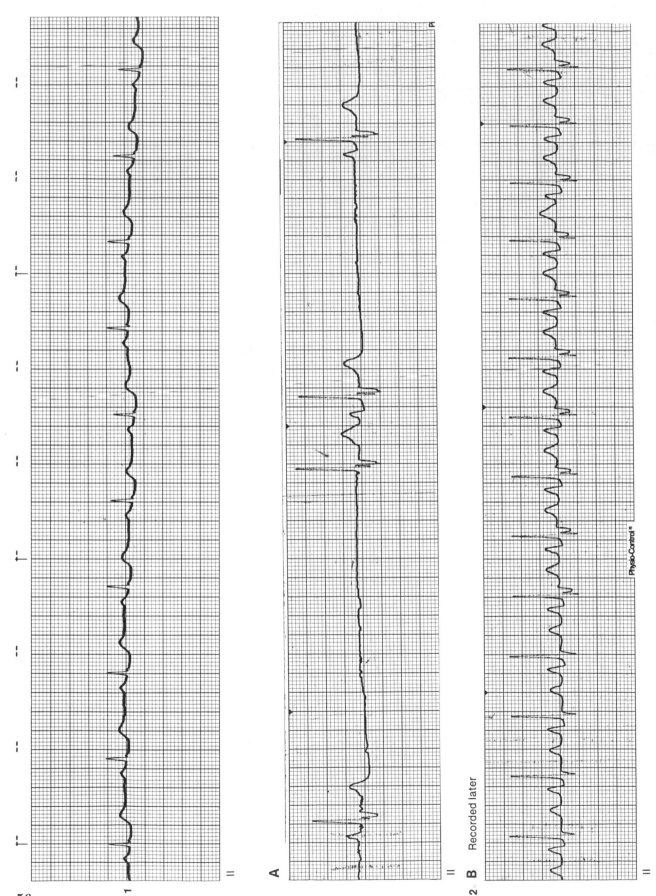

56

1

II

A

II

B   Recorded later

2

II

PhysioControl ®

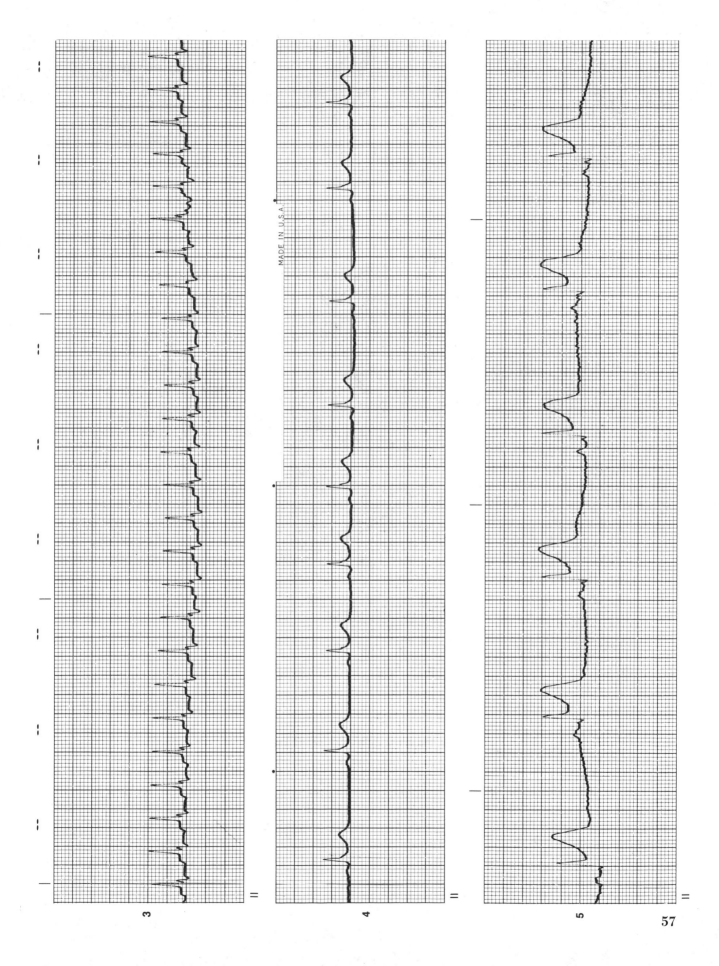

3

4

5

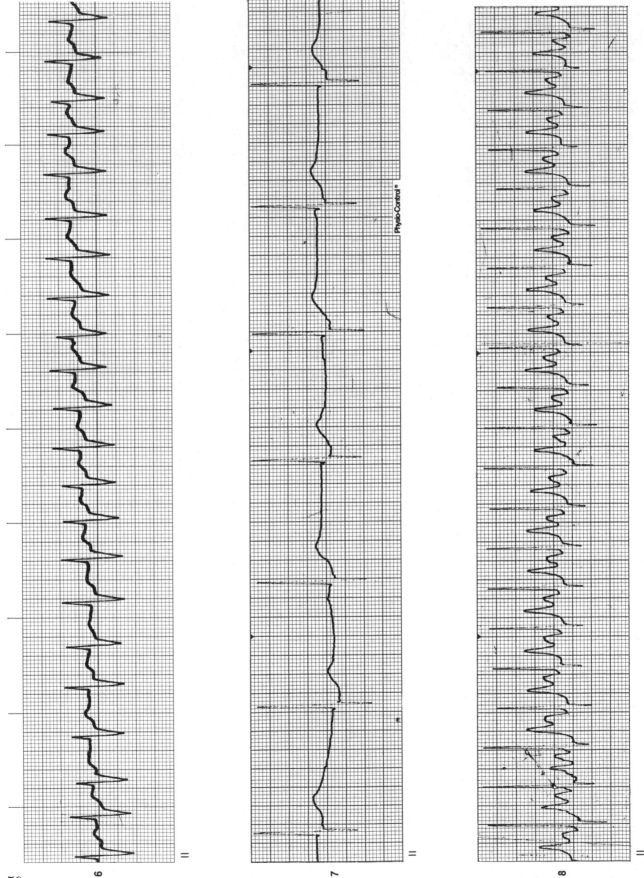

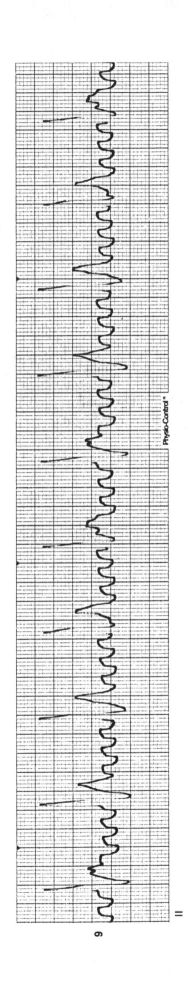

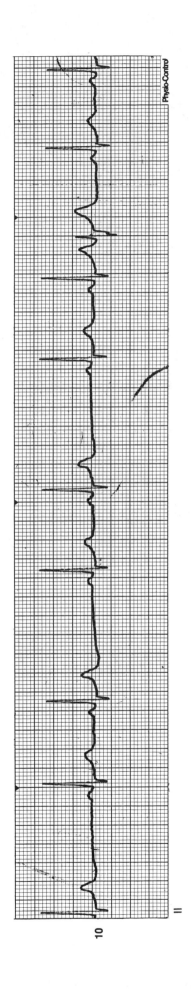

9

10

59

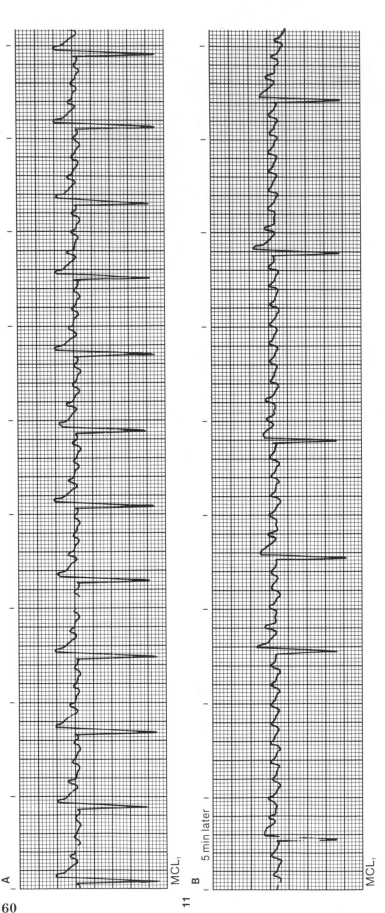

A

MCL₁

B

5 min later

MCL₁

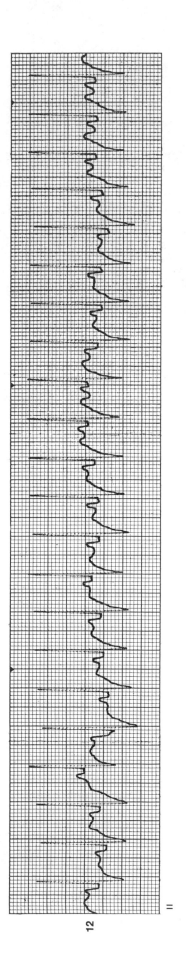

II

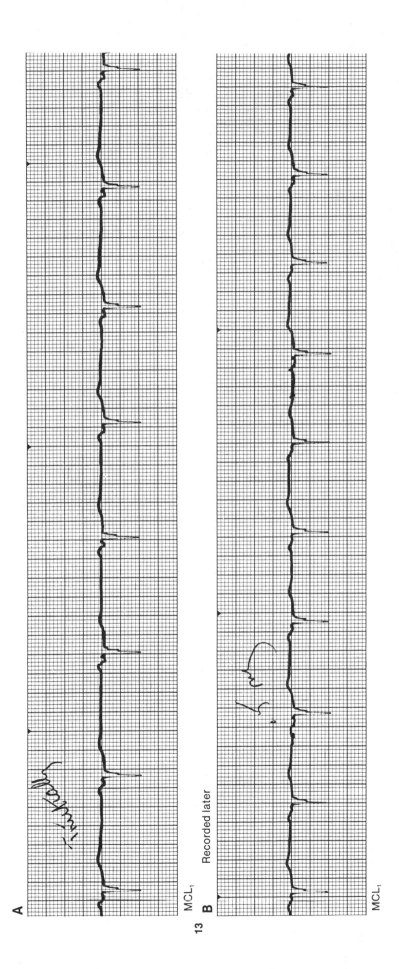

A

MCL₁

B   Recorded later

MCL₁

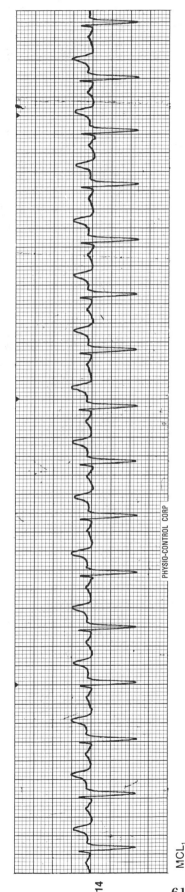

MCL₁

PHYSIO-CONTROL CORP

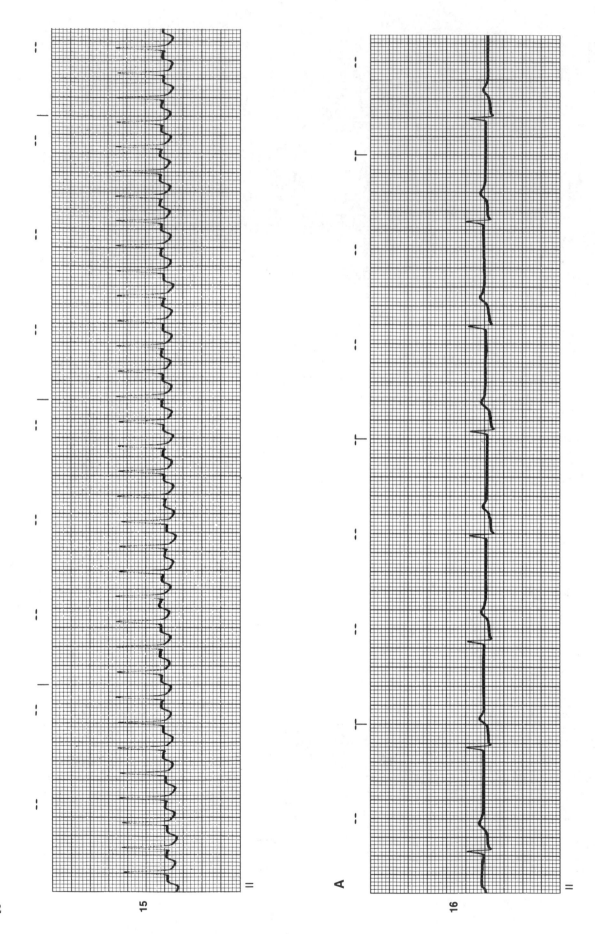

62

15

16

A

B   Recorded later

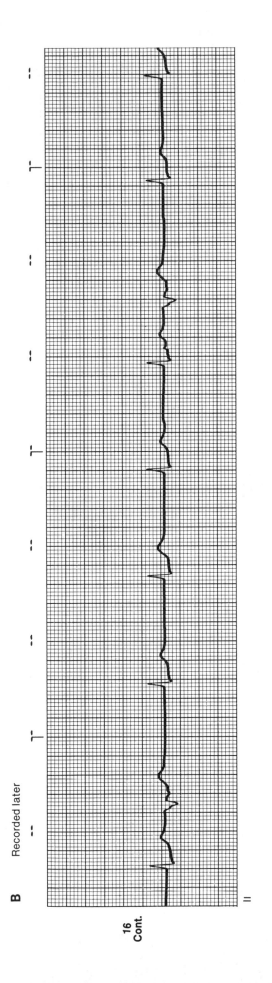

16
Cont.

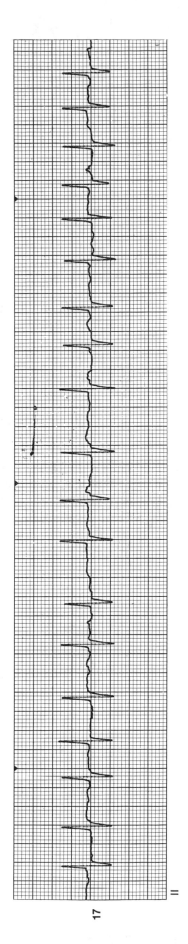

17

63

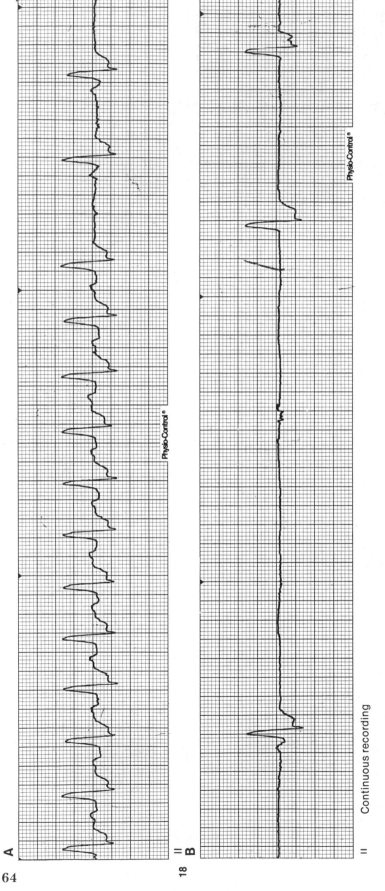

A

II

Physio-Control®

18 B

II

Physio-Control®

Continuous recording

II

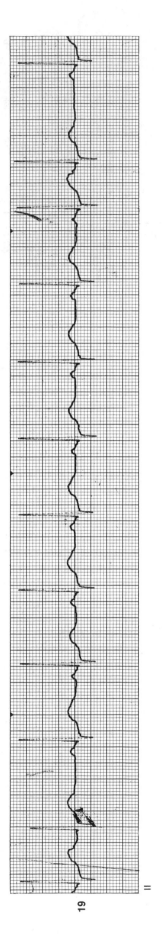

19

II

64

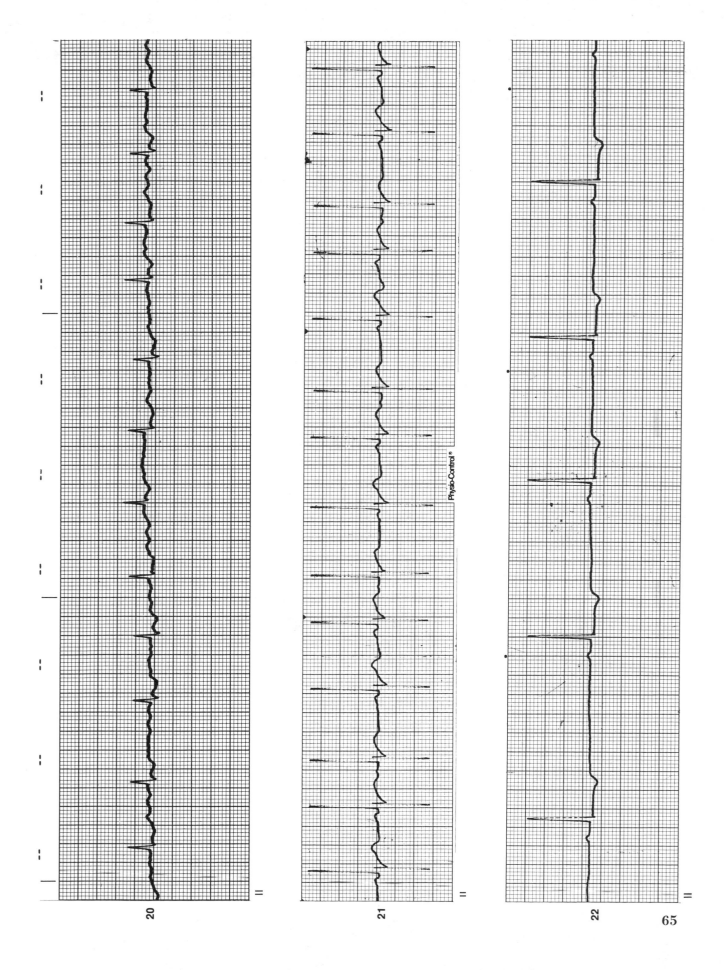

20

21

Physio-Control®

22

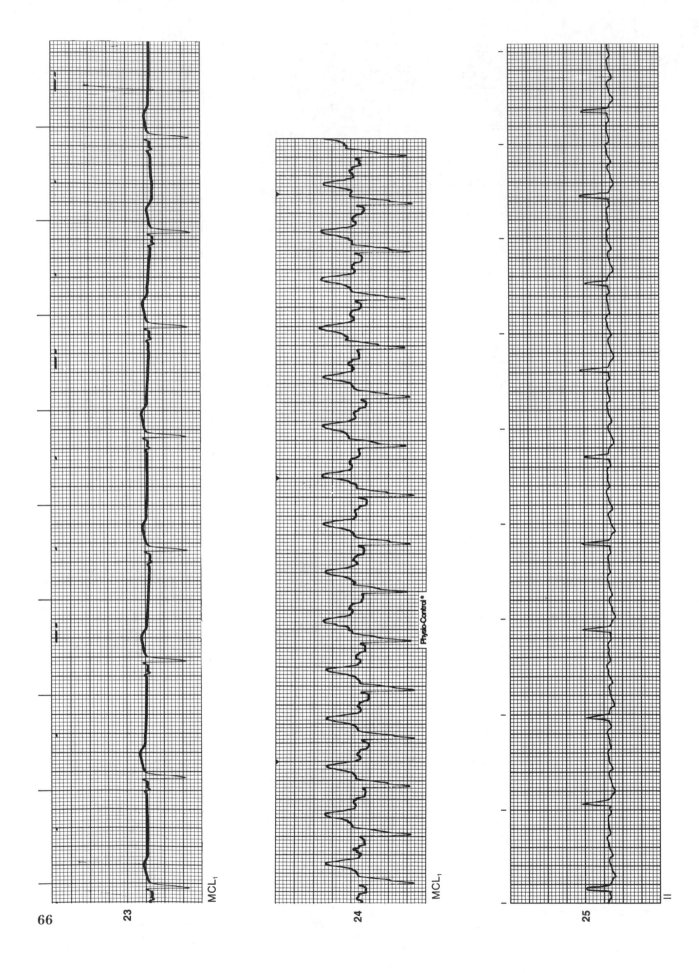

66

23

MCL₁

24

MCL₁

Physio-Control®

25

II

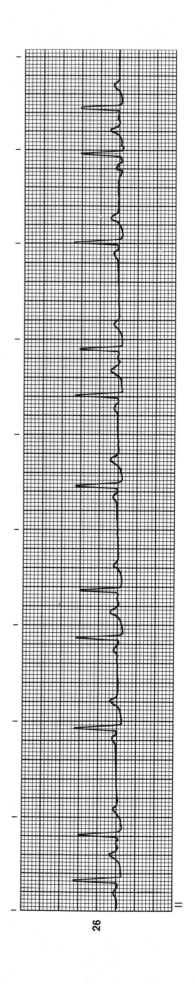

26

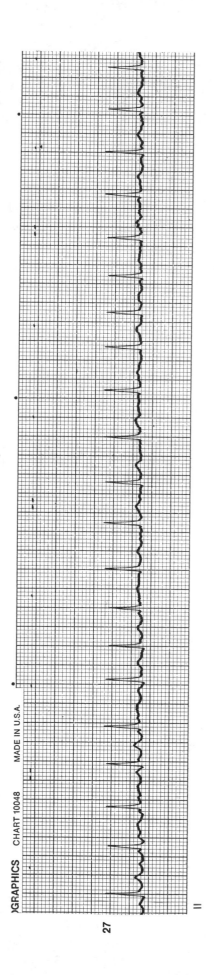

27

67

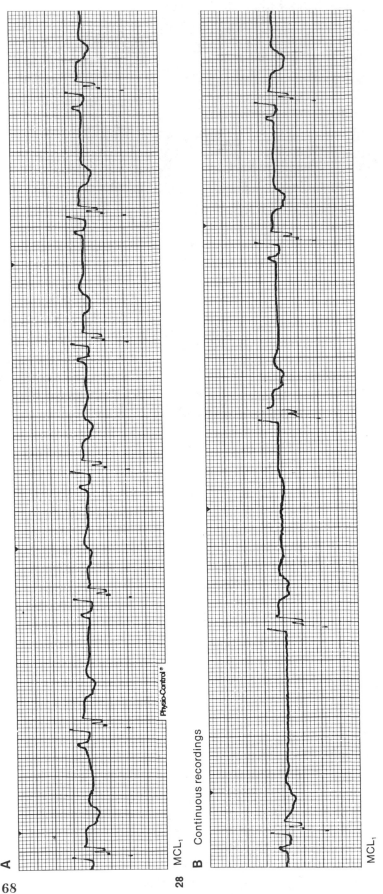

A

68

MCL₁

B Continuous recordings

MCL₁

28

Physio-Control®

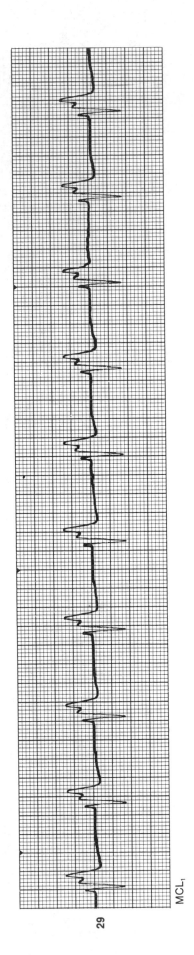

29

MCL₁

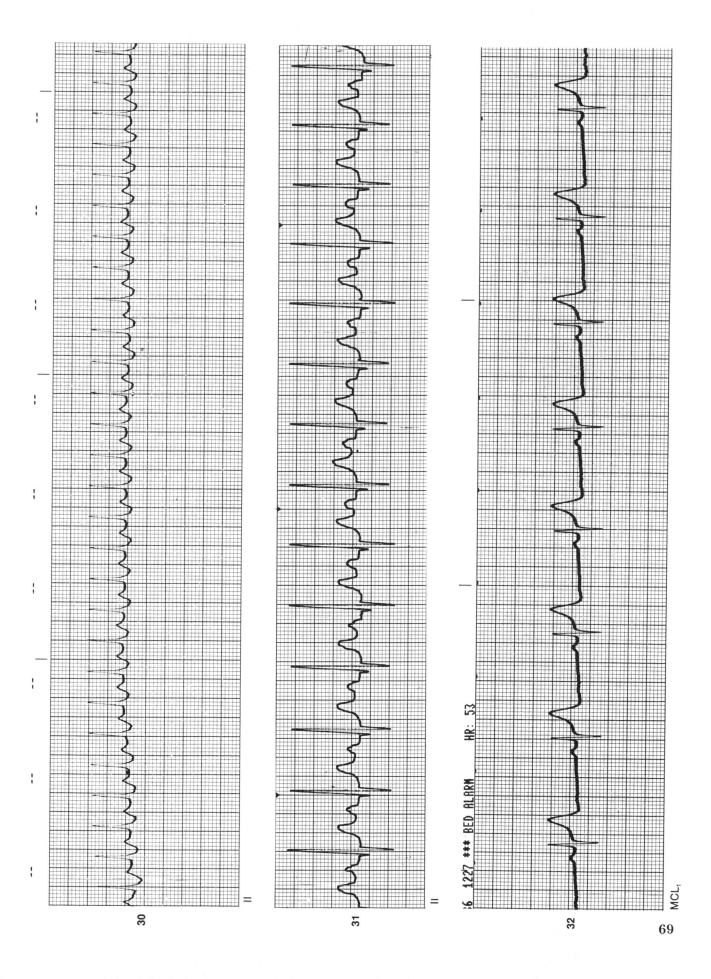

30

II

31

II

:6 1227 *** BED ALARM   HR: 53

32

MCL₁

69

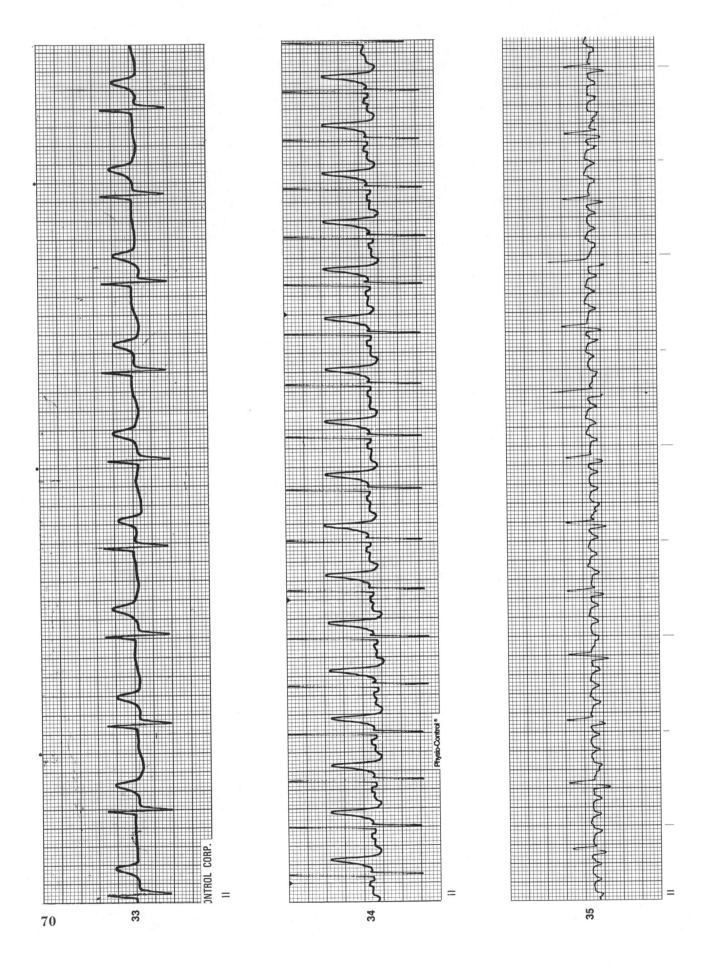

33

34

35

ONTROL CORP.

II

II

II

Physio-Control®

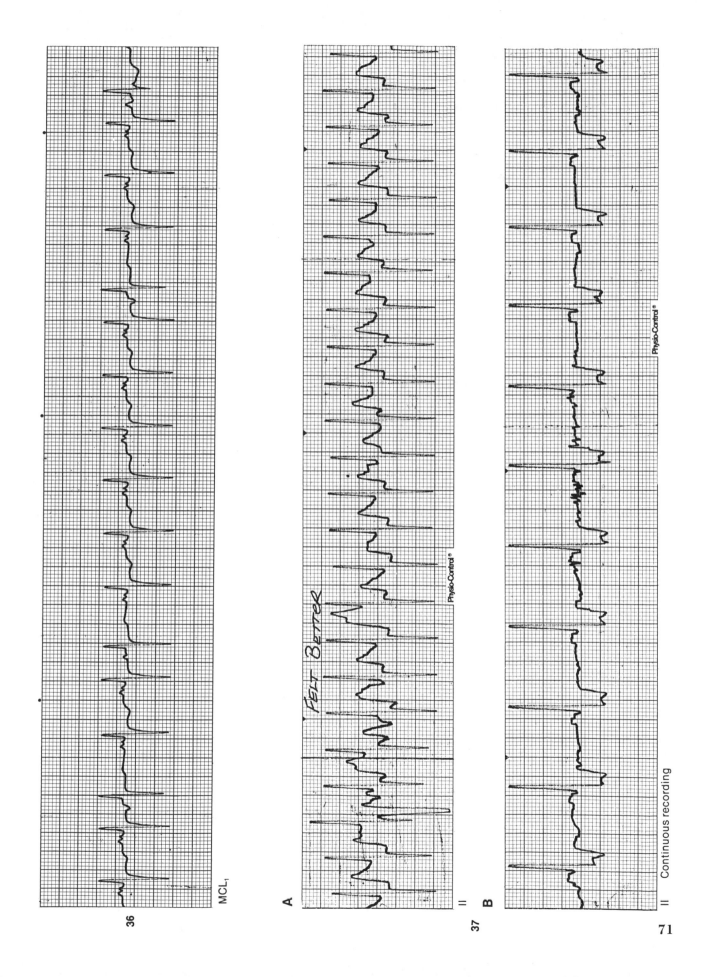

36

MCL₁

A

FELT BETTER

Physio-Control®

II

37

B

Physio-Control®

II

Continuous recording

71

ANSWERS TO PRACTICE ECG TRACINGS 1 TO 37

1

Rate __65__ /min. Rhythm __regular__

QRS Duration __0.08__ s. P-R Interval __0.16__ s.

AV Conduction Ratio __1:1__

Interpretation: **NORMAL SINUS RHYTHM (NSR).**

Rationale: Ventricular activity is normal and regular. The same is true for atrial activity; the P waves have a consistent shape and are upright in lead II. The P-R interval is normal. Each P wave is followed by a QRS complex, and every QRS is preceded by a single wave. This eliminates any AV conduction disturbances and tells us that the pacemaker is the sinus node. No delays in conduction or disturbances in rhythm are noted.

2

Rate __A) 20–30__ /min. Rhythm __A) irregular__
__B) 94__ __B) regular__

QRS Duration __A) 0.12–0.14__ s. P-R Interval __A) 0.20__ s.
__B) 0.12–0.14__ s. __B) 0.16__ s.

AV Conduction Ratio __A) 1:1__
__B)1:1__

Interpretation: **SINUS ARREST WITH A BRADYCARDIAC VENTRICULAR RATE.**

Rationale: The second complex in *A* is an AV junctional escape pacemaker that emerges after a delay of 3.8 seconds following the last sinus beat. The discharge of this latent pacemaker terminates a period of electrical and cardiac silence. Since the electrical stimulus for mechanical contraction is lacking, cardiac output ceases and loss of consciousness is common. In sinus arrest the sinus impulse fails to develop, and consequently, the atrial muscle and remainder of the heart remain unstimulated.

Strip *B* shows the resumption of normal sinus rhythm after treatment. In *B* ventricular and atrial activity is normal. The AV conduction ratio is 1:1. The sinus rate is just slightly under 100/minute.

The **hallmark finding** of sinus arrest is the sporadic absence of complete cardiac cycles (P waves, QRS complexes, T waves). As a result, we see prolonged periods of asystole, which show up as longer than normal P-P intervals.

3

Rate __170__ /min. Rhythm __regular__

QRS Duration __0.10__ s. P-R Interval __absent__

AV Conduction Ratio __1:1__

Interpretation: **SUPRAVENTRICULAR TACHYCARDIA (SVT).**

Rationale: The ventricular rhythm is regular and the QRS complexes are of normal duration. (The downslope of the R wave shows a small r' deflection.) Neither P nor P' waves can be seen, so determining a P-R interval or AV relationship is not possible. The rate is generally too rapid for the pacemaker to be the sinus node. Since the QRS duration and shape is normal, the dysrhythmia must have originated above the bifurcation of the His bundle; that is, it is from a supraventricular focus.

4

Rate __60__ /min. Rhythm __irregular__

QRS Duration __0.08__ s. P-R Interval __0.16__ s.

AV Conduction Ratio __1:1__

Interpretation: **SINUS DYSRHYTHMIA.**

Rationale: This tracing shows sinus activity that varies with the phases of ventilation. The ventricular

Pacemaker	P Waves	P-R Interval	QRS Complexes
Sinus	Present	Normal	Narrow
AV junction	Absent or retrograde	Shortened	Narrow
Idioventricular	Absent	Absent	Wide and distorted

Discussion: rhythm is regularly irregular. The R-R interval waxes and wanes regularly. Aside from this disturbance of sinus rhythmicity, everything else appears normal.

Sinus dysrhythmia can be recognized by:

- Normal P-QRS-T cycles
- 1:1 AV conduction
- P-P interval variation.

Discussion: This benign dysrhythmia is frequently observed in children and patients with lung disease. It usually appears more striking at slower rates because the varying R-R intervals are more pronounced.

5

Rate __38__ /min. Rhythm __regular__ P-R Interval __0.16__ s.
QRS Duration __0.12__ s.
AV Conduction Ratio __1:1__

Interpretation: SINUS BRADYCARDIA (40/MINUTE).

Rationale: Ventricular activity is slow but regular. The QRS duration is normal, but the shape is altered by the convex upward sloping of the ST segment. This distorts the ST-T wave segment. Since the rate of 38/min is within the range expected for an idioventricular focus (see discussion), we inspect the area immediately before the QRS to see if atrial activity is present. P waves are indeed seen just prior to the QRS complex at constant P-R intervals, confirming an SA nodal focus. The AV conduction is normal. (A slight amount of movement artifact distorts the baseline.)

Discussion: With bradydysrhythmias, we want to quickly identify the site of pacemaker activity since three areas can be controlling the heart:

6

Rate __140__ /min. Rhythm __grossly irregular__
QRS Duration __0.12__ s. P-R Interval __Absent__
AV Conduction Ratio __variable__

Interpretation: ATRIAL FIBRILLATION WITH A VENTRICULAR RATE OF 120/MINUTE.

Rationale: The QRS complexes occur without a discernible pattern. They are wide, without a bizarre configuration, and reflect supraventricular conduction. Obvious P waves are not found; instead, a flattened baseline between the R waves is observed. The AV relationship is variable. The atria are depolarizing between 350 and 600/minute, but this is not measurable on the ECG. We see only a wavy or flat baseline. Switching to another lead will make the fibrillatory waves more apparent. Despite lacking classical f waves, the interpretation is made based on the tachycardic rate and the irregularly irregular rhythm.

Discussion: The atrial chambers fail to produce effective contractions because of this dysrhythmia. When they are viewed in an open-chested patient, only disorganized quivering is noted. Atrial contraction and its contribution to ventricular filling are lost. This loss is not life-threatening because in a normal cardiac cycle the atria contract late in ventricular diastole when about 75 percent of the blood has already flowed through the AV valves into the lower chambers. Blood returning from the systemic circulation still possesses considerable energy and flows passively into the ventricles. The atria basically serve as passageways from the venae cavae to the lower pumping chambers. As a result of atrial fibrillation, a 25 percent reduction in filling occurs but is tolerated reasonably well by otherwise healthy individuals. Atrial fibrillation will present a more significant problem in patients with preexisting cardiac problems, such as mitral stenosis and congestive heart failure (CHF).

7

Rate ___46___ /min. Rhythm ___regular___
QRS Duration ___0.08___ s. P-R Interval ___absent___
AV Conduction Ratio ___absent___

Interpretation: AN AV JUNCTIONAL RHYTHM AT A RATE OF ABOUT 46/MINUTE. SINUS NODAL DEPRESSION ALLOWS THIS RHYTHM TO EXIST.

Rationale: The ventricular rhythm is regular, and the QRS complexes are narrow. Atrial activity is not present so that an AV relationship cannot be analyzed. The pacemaker exists somewhere in the His bundle at a location before it splits into the bundle branches. This dysrhythmia occurs because the sinus node fails to suppress the AV junction. Normally, the fastest pacemaker will override all slower sites. When sinus activity slows or ceases, the next site in line to pace the heart is the AV junction at a slower inherent rate.

The hallmark findings of an AV junctional rhythm are as follows:

- Missing or altered P waves
- Narrow QRS complexes
- Rate of 40 to 60/minute.

8

Rate ___140___ /min. Rhythm ___regular___
QRS Duration ___0.08___ s. P-R Interval ___0.12___ s.
AV Conduction Ratio ___1:1___

Interpretation: SINUS TACHYCARDIA.

Rationale: The ventricular complexes are narrow and occur at regular intervals. Atrial activity shows regular and upright P waves. The AV relationship shows one P wave for every QRS complex. The only deviation from the criteria for NSR is the sinus rate of greater than 100/min.

Note: Whenever the ventricular rate is between 140 and 160/min and the rhythm is regular, check to see if atrial flutter is present with 2:1 AV conduction. Vagal maneuvers can be used to unmask a hidden F wave. Since the T wave in this tracing is peaked, you should be suspicious of that possibility; however, this was not such a case.

9

Rate ___ventricular 70___/min.
    ___atrial 400___ /min. Rhythm ___regular___
QRS Duration ___0.12___ s. P-R Interval ___absent___
AV Conduction Ratio ___4:1___

Interpretation: ATRIAL FLUTTER WITH A VENTRICULAR RESPONSE OF 70/MIN.

Rationale: Ventricular rhythm is regular. The QRS complexes appear distorted at some points by the rapid atrial waves. The atrial activity is

76

extremely fast. The AV conduction ratio is approximately 4:1, indicating that only one of every four atrial waves gets conducted through the AV node. In other words, three of every four F waves are not being conducted.

10

	A) 60–65 /min.	A) occasionally irregular
Rate	B) 65 /min.	Rhythm B) occasionally irregular
	A) 0.08 s.	A) 0.14 s
QRS Duration	B) 0.08 s.	P-R Interval B) 0.14 s.
	A) 1:1	
AV Conduction Ratio	B) 1:1	

Discussion: The failure of the AV node to conduct all the atrial impulses does **not** reflect a pathologic block. It is due to the long refractory period of the AV node, which prevents the ventricles from being paced too fast. The node functions as a filter and allows a reasonable number (70/ minute in this case) of atrial waves through. The resultant ventricular rate is close to what would be expected in sinus rhythm. Patients who have accessory pathways into the ventricle lose the benefit of the AV node functioning as a "gate keeper." If such patients develop rapid atrial rates, the ventricles will respond in a 1:1 manner until the pathways and myocardium become fatigued.

Interpretation: FREQUENT NONCONDUCTED PACs CAUSE THE PAUSES NOTED IN THIS TRACING.

Rationale: The PACs occur so early in the R-R cycle that they encounter the AV node still refractory from the previous beat. As a result, the PAC is blocked, or not conducted. The clue to this dysrhythmia comes from careful inspection of the T waves that occur just before the pauses. **These T waves are tall and peaked,** displaying a shape that differs from normal T waves. This is because the early P′ waves are buried here. The eighth complex is also a PAC that is conducted but with aberration due to the refractoriness of the AV node and ventricles. See the labeled complexes in Tracing 10 Answer, below.

Remember: The most frequent cause of a pause in sinus activity is a blocked PAC, and not SA blocks!

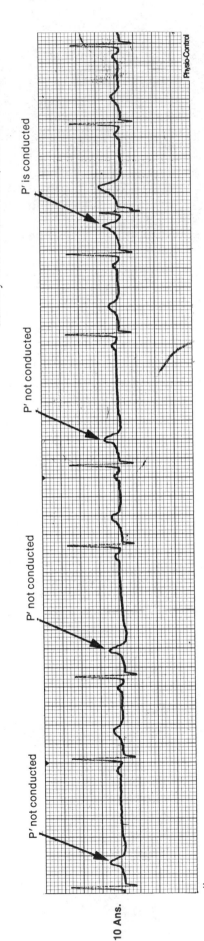

10 Ans.

P′ not conducted

P′ not conducted

P′ not conducted

P′ is conducted

11

	A	B
Rate	75 /min.	40–50 /min.
Rhythm	regular	irregular
QRS Duration	0.08 s.	0.08 s.
P-R Interval	absent	absent
AV Conduction Ratio	see below	see below

Interpretation: STRIP A: ATRIAL FLUTTER WITH A REGULAR VENTRICULAR RESPONSE OF 75/MINUTE. STRIP B: RECORDED A SHORT TIME LATER, SHOWS A MUCH SLOWER CONDUCTION RATIO. THE VENTRICULAR RESPONSE IS BRADYCARDIAC AND AVERAGES 40 TO 50/MINUTE.

Rationale: The sawtooth pattern typical of the flutter waves, immediately catches your eye. Analysis of ventricular activity shows narrow QRS complexes with a regular rhythm. The atrial rate is much faster than the ventricular rate. The ratio of 300 F waves to 75 QRS complexes provides a 4:1 conduction ratio. The refractoriness of the AV node produces a physiologic block that fails to conduct 75 percent of the atrial waves. This is beneficial because it results in a near normal ventricular rate. In strip B, however, the ventricular rate drops significantly owing to increased AV nodal refractoriness. This is usually secondary to medication or carotid sinus massage. Instead of a 4:1 conduction ratio, we see ratios of 8:1, 6:1, and 10:1. This is no longer a physiologic AV block but now represents a pathologic cause of nonconduction. As a result, the ventricular rate is 40 to 50/minute. Since cardiac output is determined to a major extent by heart rate, a high degree of AV refractoriness may result in diminished perfusion.

12

Rate	140 /min.
Rhythm	regular
QRS Duration	0.08 s.
P-R Interval	0.12 s.
AV Conduction Ratio	1:1

Interpretation: SINUS TACHYCARDIA (140/MIN).

Rationale: Ventricular activity appears normal: QRS complexes are sharp and narrow. The P waves are constant in shape, are upright, and precede every QRS complex. The AV conduction is a normal 1:1. The only variation from NSR is the sinus node discharging at a rate greater than 100/minute.

Note: Always check for atrial flutter with 2:1 AV conduction when the rhythm is regular and the rate is between 140 and 160/minute. This is not the case in this tracing, but you should be aware of the possibility.

13

	A	B
Rate	48 /min.	63 /min.
Rhythm	regular	regular
QRS Duration	0.12 s.	0.12 s.
P-R Interval	0.16 s.	0.16 s.
AV Conduction Ratio	1:1	1:1

Interpretation: A IS A SINUS BRADYCARDIA (48/MINUTE), WHICH IS ACCELERATED FOLLOWING ATROPINE ADMINISTRATION. AFTER THERAPY, IN *B*, A REGULAR SINUS RHYTHM IS ESTABLISHED AT 63/MINUTE.

Rationale: A: Aside from the slow rate, the ventricular rhythm is regular with narrow QRS complexes. Atrial activity regularly precedes each QRS complex. The P-R interval is within normal limits, so the AV conduction is 1:1. In *B*, the same general pattern exists but the rate is now more acceptable.

Note: Treatment was required because the patient was hypotensive and lethargic. The majority of cases of sinus bradycardia, however, require no immediate therapy because they are transient and do not compromise cardiac output.

14

Rate __96__ /min. Rhythm __regular__

QRS Duration __0.12__ s. P-R Interval __0.16__ s.

AV Conduction Ratio __1:1__

Interpretation: NORMAL SINUS RHYTHM (NSR) AT 96/MINUTE.

Rationale: Ventricular activity is normal, as is atrial activity. The AV conduction ratio is 1:1. No dysrhythmias are present.

15

Rate __230__ /min. Rhythm __regular__

QRS Duration __0.08__ s. P-R Interval __absent__

AV Conduction Ratio __absent__

Interpretation: SUPRAVENTRICULAR TACHYCARDIA.

Rationale: The dysrhythmia is an SVT because:

- Regular and narrow QRS complexes are present (indicates supraventricular pacemaker site)
- Rate is faster than usual for sinus activity (100–150/min) and within the expected range for this type of dysrhythmia (150–250/min).
- P waves are absent
- Rhythm is perfectly regular.

Note: Atrial tachycardia can occur in paroxysms (bursts) and chronic atrial tachycardia is less common and is usually due to digitalis toxicity.

This dysrhythmia will cease as the offending drug is withdrawn. The bursts may last from several minutes to days, but most often lasts for 20 minutes to an hour, until it is broken by therapy.

16

Rate __56__ /min. Rhythm __regular__

QRS Duration __0.08__ s. P-R Interval __absent__

AV Conduction Ratio __absent__

Interpretation: A SUSTAINED AV JUNCTIONAL RHYTHM EXISTS AT 56/MINUTE. THE CAUSE OF A SUSTAINED AV JUNCTIONAL RHYTHM IS SA NODAL ARREST.

Rationale: The QRS complexes are narrow and normal in shape. Atrial activity is missing; therefore, no AV conduction ratio exists. The rhythm must have originated in the AV junction because the QRS complexes are 0.08 second, the rate is between 40 and 60/minute, and P waves are absent. This dysrhythmia is generally stable, provides an adequate cardiac output, and will subside when the sinus node begins pacing again.

17

Rate __120__ /min. Rhythm grossly irregular

QRS Duration __0.10__ s. P-R Interval __absent__

AV Conduction Ratio __variable__

Interpretation: ATRIAL FIBRILLATION WITH AN UNCONTROLLED (TACHYCARDIAC) VENTRICULAR RESPONSE OF 120/MIN.

Rationale: The ventricular pattern is irregularly irregular and the P waves have been replaced by small fibrillatory f waves. Individual P waves cannot be seen. Instead, a fine, wavy baseline between QRS complexes is present. A fixed AV conduction ratio does not exist. Rather, random conduction of the atrial impulses through the AV node gives the irregular character of the ventricular complexes.

Key Feature: Grossly irregular R-R intervals.

18

Rate A) 84 /min. average B) 30 /min.   Rhythm A and B) irregular

QRS Duration A) 0.20–0.24 s. B) 0.20–0.24 s.   P-R Interval A) 0.20–0.24 s. B) absent

AV Conduction Ratio A) 1:1 B) 1:1

Interpretation: TACHYCARDIA-BRADYCARDIA SYNDROME WITH A 2-SECOND PERIOD OF SINUS ARREST.

Rationale: Strip A shows sinus tachycardia (110/minute), which abruptly begins to slow. The rate further decreases in the early portion of strip B. After the third QRS complex in tracing B the sinus node fails totally for 2 seconds. The fourth and fifth QRS complexes in B emerge to terminate a period of sinus arrest. These two escape pacemaker beats lack P waves but have QRSs that are identical to the earlier sinus complexes. Therefore, they are from an AV junctional site despite their distorted shape.

Discussion: Tachy-brady syndrome is a type of "sick sinus syndrome," but the damage is not confined to a defect in the SA node. The damage involves the tissue in the AV junction as well as the rest of intraventricular paths. The patient is in need of a reliable pacemaker to stabilize cardiac

rhythm. The only source will be an artificial device.

19

Rate 62 /min. Rhythm occasionally irregular

QRS Duration 0.08 s. P-R Interval 0.16 s.

AV Conduction Ratio 1:1

Interpretation: SINUS RHYTHM WITH TWO PREMATURE ATRIAL COMPLEXES (PACs).

Rationale: The rhythm generally looks regular, except for two complexes, which disrupt the rhythm (beats 2 and 11). These two beats occur early, and their QRS complexes do not differ from the other beats. If we block the premature beats from sight with our fingers, the rest of the complexes look like sinus rhythm. Sinus rhythm is confirmed by consistent and upright P waves, each of which is followed by a QRS complex.

Turning our attention to the two premature beats we find narrow QRS complexes; this tells us that they have been conducted normally from a supraventricular focus (that is, from a point proximal to the branching of the His bundle). Now we must decide if they are junctional or atrial beats. Premature atrial beats would be expected to have upright P' waves that differ in shape from the sinus beats. The P-R intervals for PACs usually vary from sinus beats also (they could be greater or lesser, depending on the site of formation and speed of conduction). Indeed, the P-R intervals do differ, and by inspecting the T waves that are deformed by the P' waves, the shape of the atrial complex is also found to be different from the sinus complex.

20

Rate _____80_____ /min. Rhythm _____grossly irregular_____
QRS Duration _____0.08_____ s. P-R Interval _____absent_____
AV Conduction Ratio _____variable_____

Interpretation: **ATRIAL FIBRILLATION WITH A CONTROLLED VENTRICULAR RESPONSE THAT AVERAGES 80/MINUTE.**

Rationale: There is no fixed pattern to the ventricular rhythm. The R-R intervals are irregularly irregular. The QRS complexes are similar in shape and normal in duration. P waves are missing. Fibrillatory (f) waves represent the chaotic atrial activity. The f waves give the baseline a wavy appearance.

21

Rate _____90_____ /min. Rhythm _____regularly irregular_____
QRS Duration _____0.08_____ s.
P-R Interval sinus 0.12 s. PAC 0.10–0.12 s.
AV Conduction Ratio _____1:1_____

Interpretation: **ATRIAL TRIGEMINY. EVERY THIRD BEAT IS A PREMATURE ATRIAL COMPLEX (BEATS 3, 6, 9, AND 12).**

Rationale: The ventricular rhythm is regularly irregular. The R-R intervals vary in a regular pattern. Atrial activity is irregular in the same manner as in the ventricular complexes. The P waves vary in shape and height. The PACs show P' waves that are flatter than P waves. The PACs are labeled in Tracing 21 Answer, below. The QRS complex shapes are the same for the PACs as well as for the sinus beats, confirming that after the premature impulse arrives at the AV node it is conducted normally through the ventricles, just as a sinus impulse.

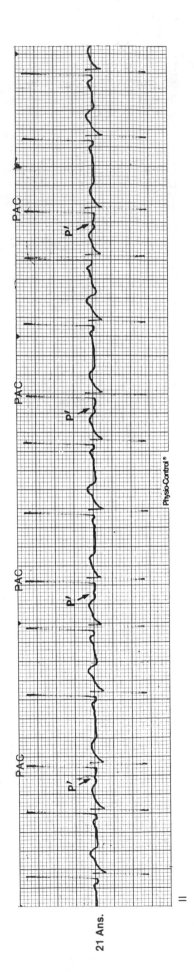

21 Ans.

22

Rate ___40___ /min. Rhythm ___irregular___
QRS Duration ___0.06___ s. P-R Interval ___0.20___ s.
AV Conduction Ratio ___1:1___

Interpretation: **SINUS BRADYCARDIA WITH A SINUS DYSRHYTHMIA.**

Rationale: The ventricular rhythm is irregular (R-R intervals vary). The QRS complexes are normal and identical. The P waves are constant and have a normal shape. The P-R interval is at the upper limit of normal (0.20 second). The P-P intervals are irregular in exactly the same way as the R-R intervals. AV conduction is normal. Therefore, variation in the rate of sinus discharge, which is slow, indicates sinus dysrhythmia. The bradycardia is much more of a concern in evaluating this patient than is the irregular rhythm (which is benign).

23

Rate ___50___ /min. Rhythm ___regular___
QRS Duration ___0.08___ s. P-R Interval ___0.12___ s.
AV Conduction Ratio ___1:1___

Interpretation: **SINUS BRADYCARDIA.**

Rationale: Normal P-QRS-T sequences are present. The ventricular complexes are regular with a normal appearance. The P waves are biphasic and regular. AV conduction is 1:1. The only disorder found here is a slow rate.

24

Rate ___115___ /min. Rhythm ___regular___
QRS Duration ___0.12___ s. P-R Interval ___0.16___ s.
AV Conduction Ratio ___1:1___

Interpretation: **SINUS TACHYCARDIA.**

Rationale: Each cardiac cycle has a sequence of normal P-QRS-T waves. Ventricular activity shows QRS complexes of normal duration that occur regularly. The P waves are upright and show a constant shape. Atrioventricular conduction shows a normal 1:1 relationship. The tracing is normal other than the SA node discharging rapidly.

25

Rate ___ventricular 70___ /min. ___atrial 300___ /min. Rhythm ___regular___
QRS Duration ___0.08___ s. P-R Interval ___absent___
AV Conduction Ratio ___4:1___

Interpretation: **ATRIAL FLUTTER WITH A VENTRICULAR RESPONSE OF 70/MINUTE.**

Rationale: The ventricular rhythm is regular. The QRS complexes appear normal and have a constant shape. P waves are not seen; instead, rapid atrial F waves occur, displaying a flattened sawtooth pattern. The AV conduction ratio is approximately 4:1, that is, four F waves to each QRS complex. By failing to respond to every impulse, the AV node permits the ventricles to be activated within the range that the sinus normally does (60 to 100/minute). The shorter R-R interval of QRS 3 shows a different conduction ratio than 4:1.

26

Rate __63__ /min. Rhythm __regularly irregular__
P-R Interval __Sinus 0.16__ s. __PAC 0.12__ s.
QRS Duration __0.08__ s.
AV Conduction Ratio __1:1__

Interpretation: SINUS RHYTHM WITH ATRIAL TRIGEMINY. EVERY THIRD BEAT IS A PREMATURE ATRIAL COMPLEX (BEATS 2, 5, 8, AND 11).

Rationale: The ventricular and atrial rhythms show a regular irregularity. The third complex of each group happens early in the R-R interval. Sinus beats are recognized by the normal P-QRS-T waves.

The PACs are identified by the following features:

• They are premature.
• The P' waves differ from sinus beats.
• P-R intervals are shorter than sinus beats.
• QRS complexes are identical to sinus beats.

27

Rate __140__ /min. Rhythm __grossly irregular__
P-R Interval __absent__
QRS Duration __0.08__ s.
AV Conduction Ratio __variable__

Interpretation: ATRIAL FIBRILLATION (RATE OF 140/MINUTE).

Rationale: The ventricular rhythm is irregular. P waves are absent. Instead, a wavy baseline is present. The narrow QRS complexes, tachycardic rate and irregularly irregular rhythm are hallmarks of atrial fibrillation.

28

Rate __A) 42__ min. Rhythm __A) regular B) irregular__
__B) 25__ /min.
P-R Interval __A) 0.20__ s. __B) missing__
QRS Duration __A) 0.12__ s. __B) 0.12__ s.
AV Conduction Ratio __A) 1:1__ __B) 1:1__

Interpretation: A: SINUS BRADYCARDIA (40/MIN). B: A PAC (BEAT 2) CAUSES A POST-EXTRASYSTOLIC PAUSE IN SINUS ACTIVITY THAT PERMITS A TWO-BEAT EPISODE OF AV JUNCTIONAL RHYTHM (BEATS 3 AND 4) BEFORE SINUS ACTIVITY RESUMES.

Rationale: The slow rhythm in A consists of regular P-QRS-T cycles. The QRS complexes are of longer duration than normal and have a slightly distorted shape due to an intraventricular conduction abnormality. All are preceded by P waves having a consistant shape and constant P-R intervals, confirming the sinus origin. In B, the rhythm becomes irregular starting with beat 2, yet the QRS complexes are identical to the sinus beats in A. In contrast to A, however, the atrial activity differs markedly. Beat 2 has a notched P' wave, while beats 3 and 4 are not preceded by any signs of atrial activity. The similarity of the QRS complexes to those in A indicates that depolarization follows the same intraventricular conduction pathway even though they arose in different supraventricular sites. Beat 3 occurs late in the R-R interval following the PAC. The pause is caused when the ectopic atrial beat prematurely depolarizes the SA node and "resets" sinus pacemaker mechanism. Then, before the sinus can discharge, a backup focus in the AV junction responds to the pause by pacing the heart.

29

Rate __60__ /min. Rhythm __regular__ P-R Interval __absent__
QRS Duration __0.10–0.12__ s.
AV Conduction Ratio __absent__

Interpretation: **AV JUNCTIONAL RHYTHM SECONDARY TO SA NODAL DEPRESSION.**

Rationale: The ventricular rhythm is regular with narrow QRS complexes. They are not preceded by P waves, indicating an ectopic focus. The rate of complexes is within the range that the AV junction spontaneously depolarizes (40 to 60/minute). Absent P waves and normal appearing QRS complexes are characteristic findings in AV junctional rhythms.

30

Rate __180__ /min. Rhythm __regular__ P-R Interval __absent__
QRS Duration __0.08__ s.
AV Conduction Ratio __absent__

Interpretation: **SUPRAVENTRICULAR TACHYCARDIA.**

Rationale: The ventricular activity is rapid and regular. The narrow QRS complexes indicate a supraventricular focus, but the absence of P waves rule out a sinus origin. Also, the rate of cardiac cycles is too fast to be sinus because the SA node does not usually discharge at rates above 150/minute.

31

Rate __94__ /min. Rhythm __regular__
QRS Duration __0.10__ s. P-R Interval __0.20__ s.
AV Conduction Ratio __1:1__

Interpretation: **REGULAR SINUS RHYTHM.**

Rationale: The QRS complexes have normal shapes and regular R-R intervals. Constant P waves are seen before each QRS complex. A 1:1 AV conduction ratio exists. No dysrhythmias are observed.

32

Rate __53__ /min. Rhythm __regular__
QRS Duration __0.08__ s. P-R Interval __0.16__ s.
AV Conduction Ratio __1:1__

Interpretation: **SINUS BRADYCARDIA.**

Rationale: The R-R intervals are regular and the QRS complexes are regular and linked to each QRS in a normal manner. P waves appear normal. The P-QRS-T sequence is without abnormality. The slow rate (under 60/minute) is the only deviation from RSR.

33

Rate __65__ /min. Rhythm __regular__
QRS Duration __0.10__ s. P-R Interval __absent__
AV Conduction Ratio __absent__

waves. The atrial rate is 280/min while the ventricular rate is 90. The AV relationship is approximately 4:1, that is, four F waves to each QRS.

36

Rate __107__ /min. Rhythm __regularly irregular__

QRS Duration __0.10__ s. P-R Interval __sinus 0.12 s.__ __PAC 0.10 s.__

AV Conduction Ratio: __1:1__

Interpretation: SINUS RHYTHM WITH FREQUENT MULTIFORMED PACs.

Rationale: Beats 3, 6, 13, and 17 are premature and have QRS complexes that are, for the most part, the same as the sinus beats. They differ from sinus beats because they occur early in the R-R cycles. Also, the size, shape, and direction of their P' waves varies from sinus beats. Some of the P' waves are inverted indicating that depolarization is starting low in the atrium and moving retrogradely. The early beats with positive P' waves show P-R intervals and P' waves differing from sinus and other premature beats. This is the reason that they are termed "multi-formed."
The sinus complexes have the following:
- Narrow QRS complexes
- Notched P waves
- Inverted T waves
- 1:1 AV conduction ratio.

Interpretation: AV JUNCTIONAL RHYTHM SECONDARY TO SINUS NODE DEPRESSION.

Rationale: The QRS complexes are narrow and have a normal shape. The rhythm appears regular, but the tracing lacks P waves. This signifies that the sinus node cannot be the pacemaker; however, pacing function must reside somewhere within the atria because the QRS duration is within normal limits (0.10 second or less). The ECG findings are consistent with an AV junctional pacemaker, especially the absent P waves.

34

Rate __110__ /min. Rhythm __regular__ P-R Interval __0.12__ s.

QRS Duration __0.08__ s.

AV Conduction Ratio __1:1__

Interpretation: SINUS TACHYCARDIA.

Rationale: Ventricular activity shows normal QRS complexes and regular R-R intervals. Atrial activity consists of regular upright P waves. In front of each QRS complex is a P wave confirming a normal AV conduction ratio. The discharge of the SA node faster than 100/minute is the basis for its classification as tachycardia.

35

Rate __ventricular 90__ /min.
__atrial 280__ /min

Rhythm __regular__

QRS Duration __0.10–0.12__ s. P-R Interval __absent__

AV Conduction Ratio __4:1__

Interpretation: ATRIAL FLUTTER WITH CONSTANT 4:1 AV CONDUCTION, AND A VENTRICULAR RATE OF 90/MINUTE.

Rationale: Ventricular activity has regular R-R intervals. Atrial activity consists of rapid flutter (F)

37

| Rate | A) 150 /min. |
| | B) 70 /min. |

| Rhythm | A) regular |
| | B) irregular |

| QRS Duration | A) 0.08 s. |
| | B) 0.08 s. |

| P-R Interval | A) absent |
| | B) 0.12 s. |

| AV Conduction Ratio | A) 1:1 |
| | B) 1:1 |

Interpretation: PAROXYSMAL SUPRAVENTRICULAR TACHYCARDIA SUDDENLY CONVERTING TO SINUS RHYTHM.

Rationale: In *A*, the QRS complexes are narrow and occur with a regular rhythm. P waves are not present. Abruptly in *B*, the SVT changes to sinus rhythm, which has sharp, upright P waves. Sudden acceleration and deceleration of rate as the dysrhythmia begins and terminates is typical of an SVT.

Chapter Three
ATRIOVENTRICULAR HEART BLOCKS

IDENTIFYING ATRIOVENTRICULAR BLOCKS

AV heart blocks are delays or failure of one, some, or all sinus impulses to travel through the AV pathway into the ventricles. The AV path can be blocked at several points: lower atrial tissue, AV node, His bundle, or the bundle branches. Based on the type of the lesion, the result is either a prolonged P-R interval or a dropped QRS complex resulting from the nonconducted P waves.

AV blocks have been classified as complete or incomplete. Third degree block is complete interruption of sinus impulses. Incomplete blocks are divided into first degree, in which none of the impulses are blocked, only delayed, and second degree, in which one or more of the QRS complexes are not conducted. Second degree heart block is further characterized as type 1 (Wenckebach) or type 2, based on whether the P-R interval increases or is fixed. Figure 3–1 classifies the different types of AV block.

First degree AV block, the most benign, has P-R intervals in excess of 0.20 sec, but after this delay **all** the P waves are conducted. Since none of the QRS complexes are dropped, the ECG will not show any pauses in ventricular activity and the conduction ratio will be 1:1. Note that the criteria for first degree block apply only when the patient is in sinus rhythm with a rate of 60/minute or greater. The P-R interval is a function of the rate, and a P-R interval greater than 0.20 sec associated with a bradycardia may not be abnormal.

Second degree block occurs when some, but not all, of the P waves are blocked. Second degree AV block **Mobitz type 1 (Wenckebach)** shows a **progressive lengthening** of the P-R intervals before the dropped beat. As a result, the ECG shows cycles of grouped beats separated by a pause caused by the nonconducted P wave. The P-P intervals are constant because the sinus node regularly discharges. However, the R-R intervals change as the AV node becomes more refractory and the impulse takes longer to reach the ventricles.

Second degree AV block **Mobitz type 2** shows **constant** P-R intervals before the dropped beats occur. The nonconducted P waves may exist in a regular fixed ratio (such as every third or fourth P wave with 3:2 and 4:3 AV conduction) or may be an occasional event such as one or two per minute. A summary of ECG findings is presented in Figure 3–2.

Third degree block, the most serious, exists when **no** sinus impulses are conducted. The complete interruption of AV conduction causes an independent ventricular pacemaker to emerge. Complete AV dissociation is reflected on the ECG as independent P waves and QRS complexes. Since the rates of the two pacemakers differ, the P-P intervals will be regular as well as the R-R intervals, but **they are not related to each other.**

The primary consideration in managing any type of AV block is the rate of ventricular complexes. This will depend on the sinus rate and the conduction ratio. A 3:2 conduction ratio when the sinus rate is 100/minute will still provide an adequate pulse rate, whereas the same ratio in a patient with a sinus rate of 60/minute will usually cause a marked fall in cardiac output. For this reason, the complete interpretation should include the conduction ratio as well as the average ventricular rate.

INCOMPLETE ATRIOVENTRICULAR BLOCKS

1. First degree: All P waves are conducted, fixed P-R intervals

2. Second degree: Some P waves are not conducted; every QRS complex is preceded by a P wave, but not all are followed by a QRS
    A. Mobitz type 1 (Wenckebach): Increasing P-R intervals for at least two consecutively conducted impulses until dropped beat occurs
    B. Mobitz type 2: Fixed P-R intervals for consecutively conducted beats before dropped beat occurs
        (1) Fixed ratio (2:1, 3:2, 4:3), that is, every other, every third, or every fourth beat is dropped
        (2) Occasional beats are dropped
        Note: In second degree AV blocks with 2:1 AV conduction, it is not possible to tell if it is type 1 or type 2

COMPLETE ATRIOVENTRICULAR BLOCKS

1. Third degree: No P waves are conducted, no fixed P-R intervals

FIGURE 3–1. Classification of atrioventricular blocks.

ECG FINDING	CONCLUSION
1. More P waves than QRS complexes are present	A second or third degree heart block exists.
2. Some P waves are followed by dropped QRS complexes	A second degree heart block exists.
3. The P waves have no relationship to the QRS complexes	Complete AV dissociation exists.
4. All the P waves are followed by QRS complexes, and all the QRS complexes follow P waves	The only type of heart block with 1:1 conduction is first degree.
5. A fixed P-R interval exists before some of the QRS complexes are dropped	The second degree must be a Mobitz type 2.
6. A progressive increase in the P-R interval is noted before some of the QRS complexes are dropped	A Wenckebach (Mobitz type 1) form of second degree heart block is present.

FIGURE 3–2. Differentiation of heart blocks.

During heart blocks when a pause in ventricular activity occurs following a nonconducted P wave, patients often lose consciousness because of a fall in cerebral perfusion (Stokes-Adams syndrome). The syncopal episodes are transient since the rhythm may revert spontaneously, or an idioventricular or junctional escape pacemaker focus may take over.

FIRST DEGREE AV HEART BLOCK

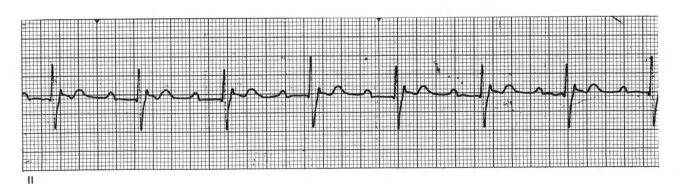

II

FIGURE 3–3. First degree AV block (P-R interval is 0.32 sec).

Ventricular Rate:	Normal.
Ventricular Rhythm:	Regular R-R intervals.
QRS Shape:	Normal.
QRS Duration:	Normal.
Atrial Rate:	Normal.
Atrial Rhythm:	Regular P-P intervals.
P Wave Configuration:	Normal.
P-R Interval:	Prolonged beyond 0.20 second.
Conduction Ratio:	1:1 AV relationship.
Significance:	Prolonged P-R intervals result from a delayed conduction of the sinus impulse within the AV node. The node has the greatest degree of refractoriness of the entire conduction system. This causes a slight pause following atrial stimulation before the ventricles are activated. As a result, the atria are able to contract and fill the ventricles before the lower chambers are depolarized. Since none of the sinus impulses are actually blocked, this dysrhythmia is not dangerous in itself.
	If it develops acutely in the setting of a myocardial infarction, it may be due to injury to or swelling of the node or the tissue surrounding it. In some patients who develop more advanced blocks, a prolonged P-R interval may be one of the earliest findings. Digitalis and other drugs that depress conduction velocity, as well as conditions with high degrees of vagal stimulation, can cause first degree block.
Acute Drug Therapy:	No therapy is indicated if this is the only abnormality.
Concepts about This Dysrhythmia:	• A first degree heart block will have **no** adverse effects on cardiac output provided that the sinus rate is acceptable.
	• In sinus bradycardia as a consequence of increased parasympathetic tone, an associated increase in the P-R interval often occurs.
	• Of the four major types of AV block, this is the only one in which **no** QRS complexes are dropped. Therefore, the atrial and ventricular rhythms are constant in relationship to each other. Again, this is the only AV heart block in which the AV ratio remains 1:1, as in NSR.
	• The location of the delay is within the AV node proper.

SECOND DEGREE AV HEART BLOCK—MOBITZ TYPE 1 (WENCKEBACH TYPE)

The pattern of grouped beating, P-R intervals progressively increasing until a dropped beat occurs, and shortening of the R-R intervals, is due to the AV node becoming increasingly refractory. As a result, the conduction velocity decreases and the last P wave of each cycle never makes it completely through the AV node. This is reflected by a dropped QRS complex and a pause in ECG activity. Following the pause, during which the node recovers, the next P-R interval is shortest, and the cycle begins again.

Ventricular Rate:	Depends on ratio of block, but is always **less** than the atrial rate.
Ventricular Rhythm:	Irregular with shortening of the R-R intervals.

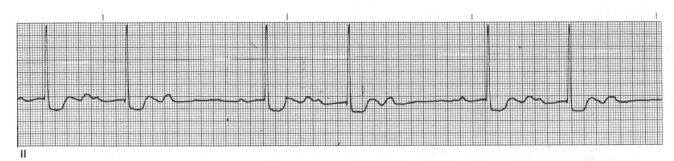

FIGURE 3–4. Second degree AV block; Mobitz type 1 (Wenckebach); 3:2 AV conduction ratio.

QRS Configuration:	Normal.
QRS Duration:	Normal.
Atrial Rhythm:	Normal P-P intervals.
P Wave Configuration:	Normal.
P-R Interval:	Progressive increase until one P wave is not conducted.
Conduction Ratio:	Greater than 1:1. The ratio depends on the frequency with which the AV junction fails to conduct a sinus impulse. The common ratios are 3:2 (three P waves to two QRS complexes) and 4:3 (four P waves to three QRS complexes). The ratios are usually constant but may vary.
Etiology:	This relatively benign dysrhythmia is due to increased AV nodal refractoriness, which is commonly caused by high vagal tone or drugs such as digitalis or propranolol. It is not uncommon in athletes and often accompanies a resting bradycardia.
Acute Drug Therapy:	No therapy is needed unless the ventricular rate is so slow as to cause symptoms of inadequate perfusion. In such rare cases, consult the bradycardia treatment flowchart (see Fig. 2-4).
Concepts about This Dysrhythmia:	• The hallmark signs of Wenckebach are grouped beating, dropped beats, and progressively increasing P-R intervals.
	• The first conducted P-R interval of a cycle may be normal or a first degree block (duration greater than 0.20 second).
	• The Wenckebach type is **more common** than Mobitz type 2, and is usually transient and benign unless there is progression to Mobitz type 2 or to third degree block.
	• The QRSs are usually narrow and normal, in contrast to Mobitz type 2.
	• The site of the block is usually within the AV node (**intranodal**) but may exist distal to the node.
	• The pauses, which include the dropped beats, are **less** than twice the shortest R-R cycle. This is a helpful sign even when the P-R intervals can't be measured.
	• The R-R intervals shorten because the initial increment in the P-R interval is shortest. As a result, the subsequent R-R intervals will be less.
	• In **2:1 AV conducted rhythms**, it is *not* possible to determine whether Mobitz 1 or 2 second degree block exists. Wencke-

bach can only be identified if **at least two consecutively** conducted P waves are examined. The term Mobitz type: "nonspecific" should be used for 2:1 blocks.

SECOND DEGREE AV HEART BLOCK—MOBITZ TYPE 2

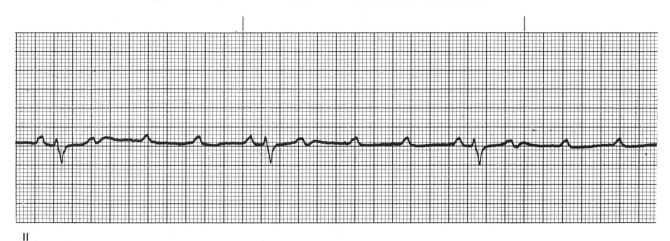

II

FIGURE 3–5. Second degree AV block; Mobitz type 2; 4:1 AV conduction ratio. This is a high grade form of AV block because two or more consecutive P waves are blocked.

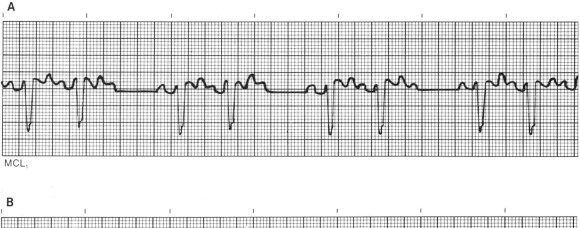

MCL₁

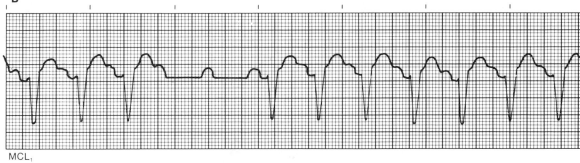

MCL₁

FIGURE 3–6. Second degree AV blocks. *A*, Mobitz type 2, with 3:2 AV conduction. *B*, High grade Mobitz type 2.

There is a fixed or intermittent blockage of some impulses. The conducted beats have **constant** P-R intervals. The blocked beats have normal P waves but no associated QRS complexes. The blocked beats usually occur in fixed ratios (4:3, 3:2, 4:1) but may occur in mixed ratios, or as occasionally dropped beats. The AV junction typically fails to respond to every third or fourth atrial impulse.

Ventricular Rate: Depends on ratio of block, but is always less than atrial rate.

Ventricular Rhythm: Irregular R-R intervals.

QRS Shape: Usually wide (see Significance).

Atrial Rate: Normal.

Atrial Rhythm: Regular P-P intervals.

P-Wave Configuration: Normal.

P-R Interval: Constant.

Conduction Ratio: Greater than 1:1, that is, there are more P waves than QRS complexes. Usually a fixed block, such as 3:2, 4:3, or 3:1, exists.

Significance: Of the two types of second degree block, type 2 is much **less common** but also **more serious.** Whereas, type 1 often requires no treatment and subsides spontaneously, Mobitz type 2 patients are likely to progress to third degree (complete) heart block. This is because the site of blockage is **infranodal,** that is, involving the bundle branches, branch fasicles, or AV bundle. As a consequence of the abnormal intraventricular conduction, the QRS tends to be wide and distorted.

How this dysrhythmia affects cardiac output and blood pressure is dependent on the sinus rate and the AV conduction ratio. The key concern in managing these patients centers on the ventricular rate; for example, a sinus rate of 100/minute with 2:1 conduction ratio provides an adequate number of beats per minute, but a sinus rate of 60/minute with the same block would cause a drastic fall in output.

Acute Drug Therapy: See Figure 2–4 for bradycardia treatment protocol. In some situations **no** therapy will be needed, only careful monitoring. When the patient is hemodynamically unstable or this dysrhythmia occurs in the setting of an acute myocardial infarction, therapy is indicated. Pacemaker insertion for standby or pacing is treatment of choice. Atropine may be useful as temporary measure but use with caution as it may paradoxically increase level of block and slow ventricular rate.

Concepts about This Dysrhythmia:
- Unlike Wenckebach, this dysrhythmia usually signifies significant organic disease of the conduction system.
- Atrial rhythm is regular, but the ventricular rhythm is regularly irregular.
- The pause caused by the dropped QRS may be terminated by an escape complex.
- In the high degree (advanced) forms of Mobitz type 2, two or more consecutive P waves are blocked. In such situations, third degree heart block may be imminent.
- Many times a second degree heart block with 2:1 conduction will be termed Mobitz type 2 in the mistaken belief that since no lengthening of the P-R interval is observed, it must be a fixed P-R interval. This is incorrect; 2:1 AV conduction is really a type "nonspecific," meaning that we cannot be sure which type exists. The reason for this is because we need **at least two consecutively conducted P waves** in order to assess the P-R intervals.

• In 2:1 AV block there are clues that may help to distinguish type 1 from type 2. Since Wenckebach is usually due to an intranodal block, we observe a normal QRS complex but a prolonged P-R interval. In contrast, Mobitz 2 shows a wide QRS complex but a normal P-R interval.

Mobitz Type	P-R Interval	QRS Duration
Wenckebach	Prolonged	Normal
Mobitz type 2	Normal	Wide

THIRD DEGREE AV HEART BLOCK (COMPLETE HEART BLOCK)

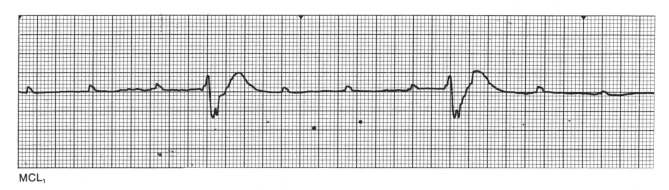

MCL₁

FIGURE 3–7. Third degree (complete) AV block.

In third degree heart block there is complete disruption of the conduction of sinus impulses to the ventricles. This is the most serious type of AV block. A lower, backup pacemaker in the ventricles begins to fire at a slower rate, while the atria are independently paced by the sinus node. A state of atrioventricular dissociation exists, in which none of the P waves are associated with QRS complexes. The site of blockage may be within the AV node itself, in the AV bundle, or in the bundle branches or fasicles, but is most commonly infranodal.

Ventricular Rate: Usually below 50/minute.

Ventricular Rhythm: Regular R-R intervals.

QRS Shape: Depends on the site of escape pacemaker. If it arises from the AV junction it will be narrow (0.10 second) with a normal shape. If it arises lower in the His-Purkinje system, it will be wider (greater than 0.12 second) and distorted.

QRS Duration: Variable.

Atrial Rate: Depends on sinus rate, but will be faster than ventricular rate.

Atrial Rhythm: Regular P-P intervals (occasionally atrial fibrillation or flutter).

P Wave Configuration: Normal.

P-R Interval: No constant relationship.

Conduction Ratio: None. The atria and ventricles beat independently.

Etiology: This dysrhythmia occurs due to advanced organic disease. Fibrosis of the conduction system as part of the aging process is a frequent cause. An acute myocardial infarction can involve the conduction system causing third degree block, but the disorder may be temporary, resolving as the tissue swelling subsides.

Significance: How the patient tolerates this dysrhythmia is based on the rate of the escape pacemaker. Sites located relatively high in the ventricle generally pace the heart at rates between 50–60/min, which are well tolerated. Rates below 40/min that are generated by low-lying sites are much less well tolerated.

Acute Drug Therapy: Treatment is indicated only when the bradycardia is associated with unstable vital signs or signs of inadequate perfusion. See Figure 2–4 for bradycardia treatment flow chart.

1. Isoproterenol infusion (1 mg diluted in 250 ml of 5 percent dextrose in water), titrating the rate in order to maintain blood pressure
2. Atropine, 0.5 to 1 mg IV
3. Emergency transvenous pacing

Concepts about This Dysrhythmia:

- The most common blockages are those located below the His bundle, as in simultaneous blockages in the left and right bundle branches, or a combination of the right bundle branch in addition to both divisions (anterior and posterior fasicles) of the left.
- P waves appear to "march through" the QRS complexes. In some cycles the P waves are first noted before the QRS complexes, then merged in the complex, then following (in the ST-T waves), and so forth. There is no order to where the P waves are in relation to the QRS complex.
- Although usually regular, P-P intervals may be irregular if a sinus dysrhythmia is present.
- The shape and rate of the QRS complexes indicates the site of the escape pacemaker: If they are narrow and occur at a rate of 40 to 60/minute, they probably arise in the AV junction; if they are wide or distorted and slow (below 40/minute), the focus is low in the ventricle (His-Purkinje fibers).
- AV junctional escape pacemakers are associated with a better cardiac output than ventricular escape rhythms.
- A frequent source of confusion is the difference between the terms AV dissociation and complete or third degree heart block. AV dissociation exists whenever there is independent atrial and ventricular activity. Third degree AV block is only one subset of AV dissociation, which can exist in the absence of block.

  An example of this is accelerated idioventricular rhythm, in which there is independent atrial and ventricular activity. Thus, AV dissociation is caused by the rapid ventricular rate. However, there are occasions when a P wave will be conducted through to the ventricle, and thus, heart block does not exist. In other words, all cases of third degree block involve AV dissociation, but not all cases of AV dissociation are due to heart block.

TABLE 3–1. Dysrhythmia Synopsis: AV Heart Blocks

	P Waves	QRS Complexes	AV Relationship	Key Features
1. First degree	Normal **All** P waves are conducted	Normal **No QRS** complexes are dropped	P-R interval over 0.20 second **Only** AV block wtih 1:1 AV conduction	Long P-R interval Site of block: within AV node
2. Second degree				
A. Wenckebach type	Normal **Some** P waves are not conducted	Normal **Some** QRS complexes are dropped	**Progressive** increase in P-R intervals followed by dropped QRS complex Ratio typically 3:2, 4:3, etc. P-R interval of first beat in each cycle often greater than 0.20 second	Grouped beating Increasing P-R intervals The longest R-R interval is equal to **less** than twice the shortest one Site of blocks: intranodal
B. Mobitz type 2	Normal **Some** P waves are not conducted	Wide **Some** QRS complexes are dropped	**Fixed** P-R interval prior to dropped beats Ratio may be 3:2, 4:3 or higher degrees (4:2, 5:3, etc.) P-R interval usually normal	Fixed P-R intervals Site of block: infranodal
3. Third degree	Normal shape, regular intervals **No** P waves are conducted **More** P waves than QRS complexes	Escape rhythm depends on level of block Usually wide and distorted if low in ventricle Narrow if high in ventricle Regular R-R intervals Rate slower than atrial (usually below 50/minute)	Complete dissociation They are independent of one another	Site of block: infranodal AV dissociation

Note: Not all second degree blocks with 2:1 AV conduction are type 2 blocks.

EXERCISE B: SELF-ASSESSMENT ECG TRACINGS 38 TO 54

The following ECGs show a variety of atrioventricular block dysrhythmias. Analyze each tracing according to the systematic approach outlined in Chapter One and formulate an interpretation. Check your answer with the suggested interpretations beginning on page 106.

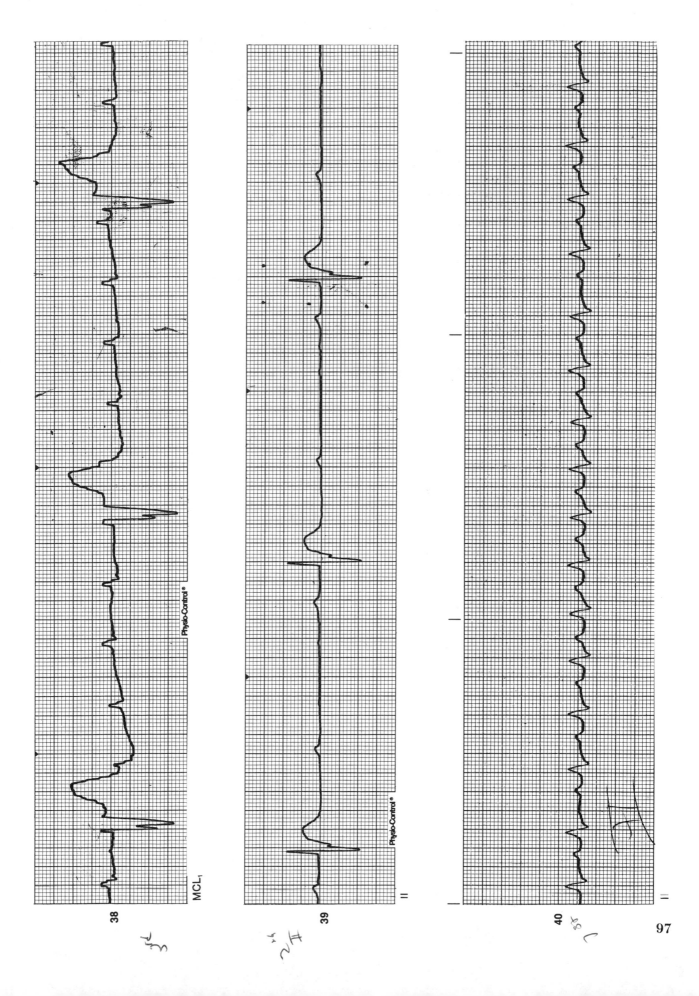

MCL₁

II

II

38

39

40

97

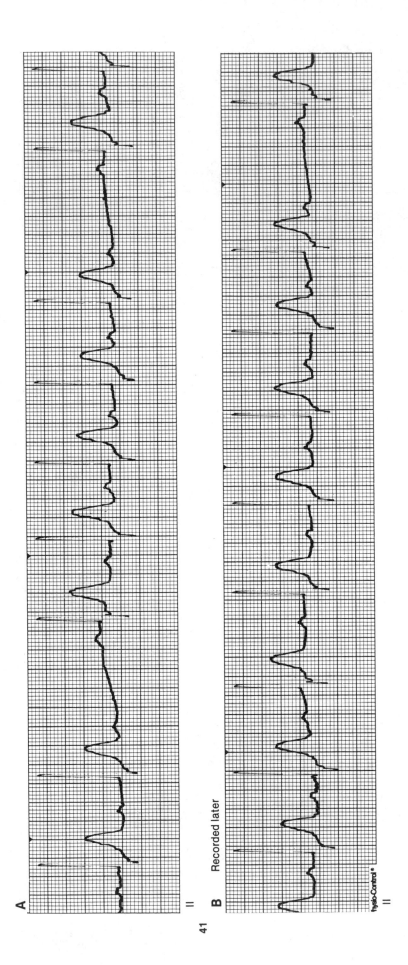

A

II

B

Recorded later

II

41

98

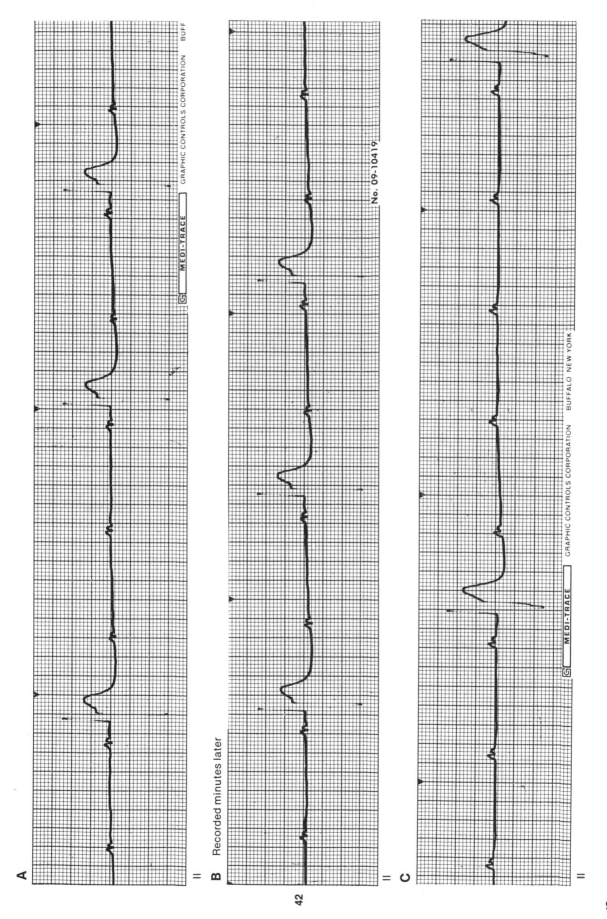

A

B Recorded minutes later

C

42

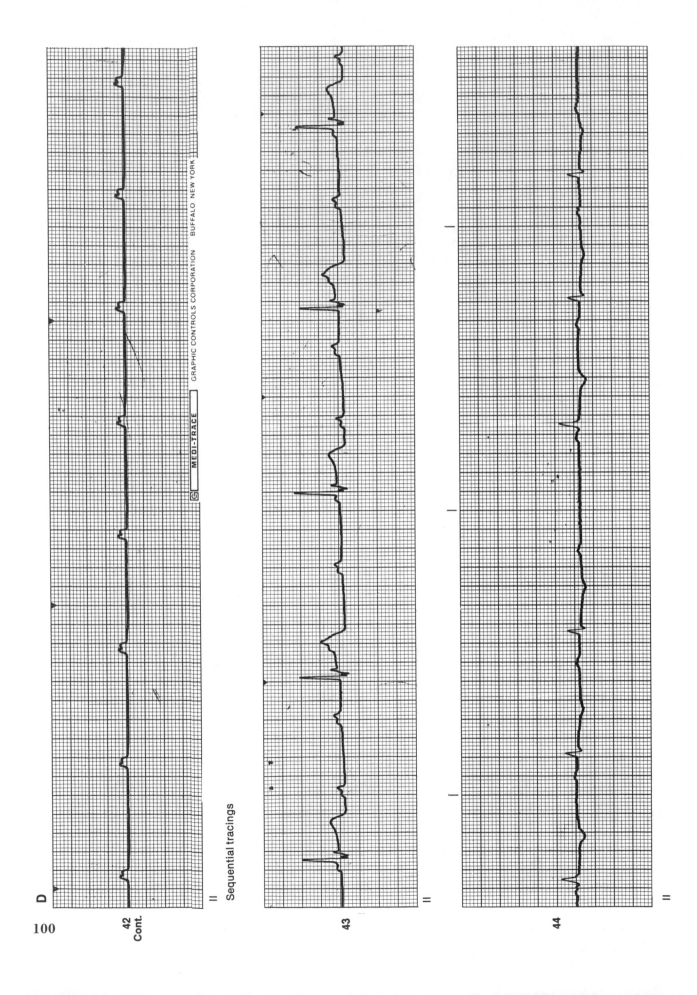

D

100

42
Cont.

II

Sequential tracings

43

II

44

II

Continuous recording

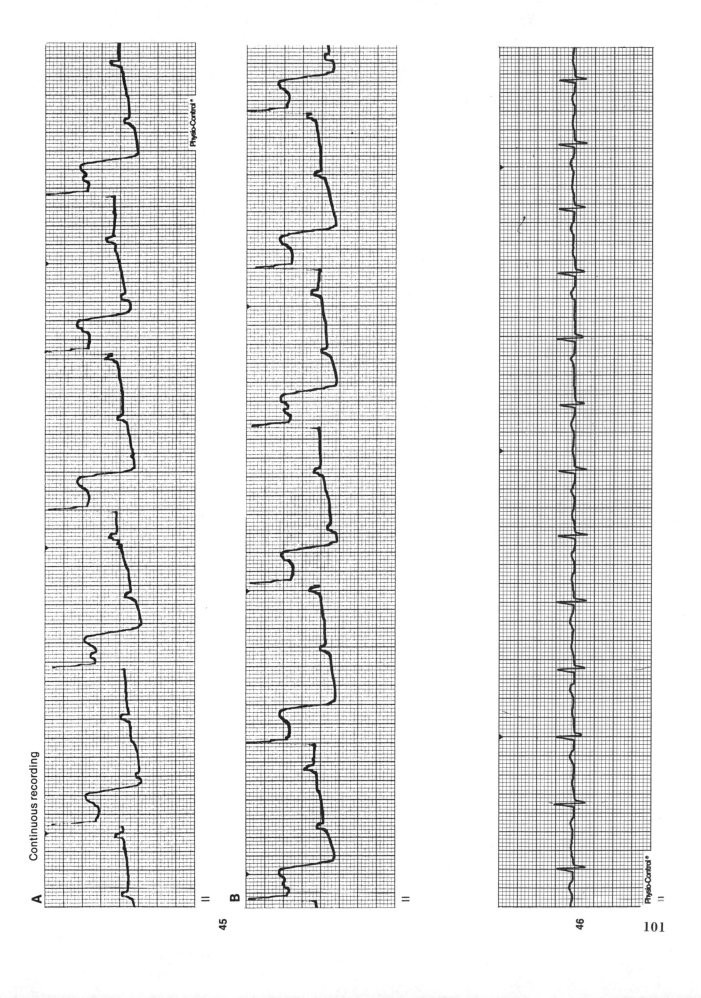

A

II

B

II

45

II

46

101

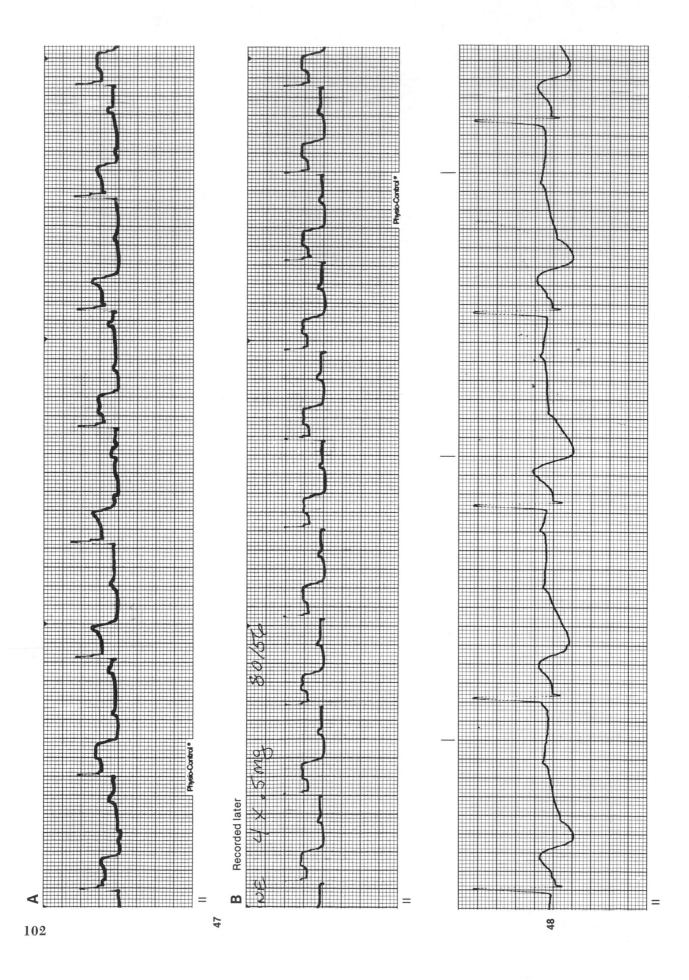

A

102

47

B Recorded later

of 4 x .5mg   8.0 /5.0

48

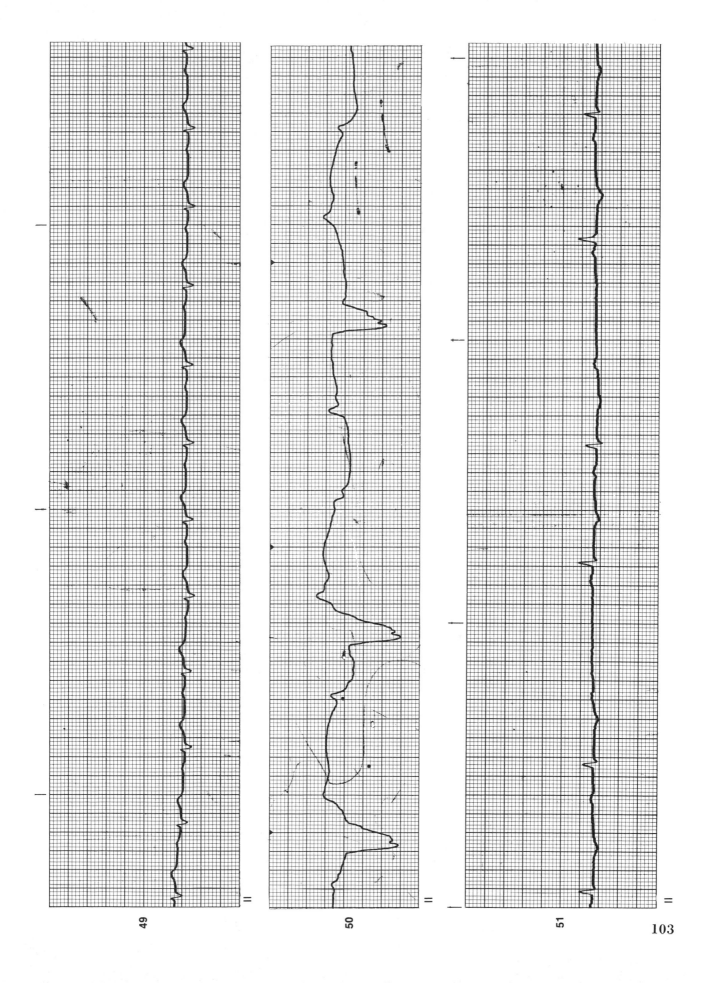

49

50

51

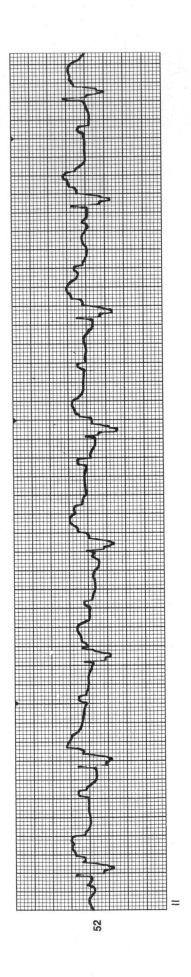

52

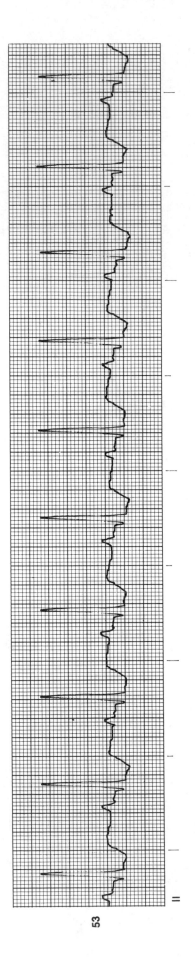

53

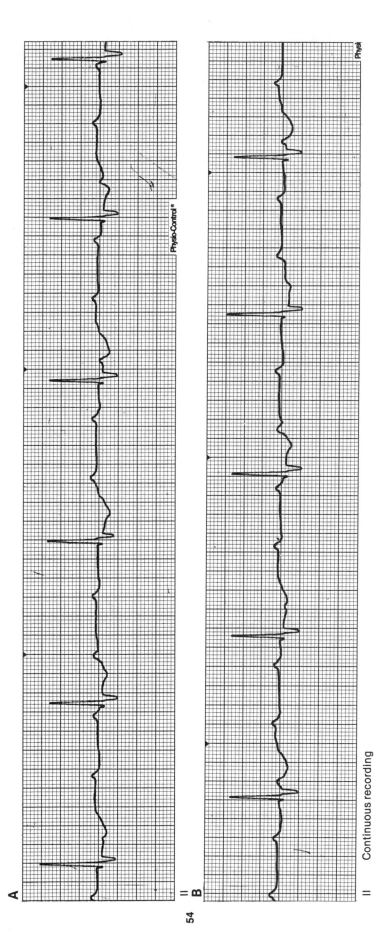

A

II

B

II

Continuous recording

54

105

ANSWERS TO PRACTICE ECG TRACINGS 38 TO 54

38

Rate: ventricular 20/min. sinus 92 /min. Rhythm regular QRS Duration 0.20 s. P-R Interval absent AV Conduction Ratio absent

Interpretation: Sinus rhythm with complete (third degree) AV block.

Rationale: The QRS complexes are slow, wide, and bizarre, reflecting a low ventricular pacemaker. The atrial activity is more rapid and regular. P waves appear pointed and tall. The P waves do not have a fixed relationship to the QRS complexes. Complete interruption of AV transmission is characterized by the following:

• regular R-R intervals
• regular P-P intervals
• absence of atrioventricular conduction

Discussion: The slow ventricular rate is not compatible with life. The slow discharge of this escape pacemaker reflects failure of higher escape pacemakers in the AV junction and His bundle to discharge. It is therefore unreliable and unable to sustain a reasonable cardiac output.

39

Rate: ventricular 20/min. sinus 40/min. Rhythm regular QRS Duration 0.10 s. P-R Interval 0.40 s. AV Conduction Ratio 2:1

Interpretation: Sinus bradycardia with first and second degree AV heart block (2:1 AV conduction).

Rationale: The slow ventricular rhythm consists of surprisingly narrow QRS complexes. The atrial rhythm shows twice as many P waves as QRS complexes. The P-R intervals for the conducted P waves (1, 3, 5, 7) show a fixed delay of 0.40 second. The second P wave of each cycle is blocked, and the QRS complex is absent.

Because the AV conduction ratio is 2:1, it is not possible to determine with certainty whether it is a Mobitz type 1 or 2 form of second degree block. We would have to examine the P-R intervals for at least two **consecutively** conducted P waves in order to determine if the P-R interval increases or is fixed prior to the dropped beat. Even though we cannot be absolutely certain, there is a clue that indicates that this is probably type 1 (Wenckebach). The P-R interval is prolonged and the QRS complex is narrow, suggesting an **intranodal** delay. In type 2, the P-R interval is usually normal, while the QRS complex is wider. In the latter case, an **infranodal** delay is usually the cause.

40

Rate 100 /min. Rhythm irregular QRS Duration 0.16 s. P-R Interval 0.24 s. AV Conduction Ratio 1:1

Interpretation: Sinus dysrhythmia with a first degree AV heart block.

Rationale: Ventricular activity is regularly irregular; most likely due to sinus alteration caused by respirations, a normal variation of NSR. All the QRS complexes have the same configuration with a duration beyond 0.10 second. Atrial activity corresponds to the ventricular pattern, and P wave shapes are constant. The P-R interval shows a duration of 0.24 second and constitutes a first degree block. The AV relationship is 1:1.

Note: Even though this dysrhythmia is a form of heart block, **no sinus impulses are actually prevented** from reaching the ventricles. Rather, a **delay** in the onset of ventricular activity exists.

Discussion: Ventricular activation should occur within 0.10 second while delays of 0.12 second or greater indicates that the spread of depolarization is delayed owing to either a slowed velocity of conduction or a block in the bundle branches or because the impulse follows an aberrant route. A delay in the start of ventricular activation is present. Most likely, this signifies an obstruction of the atrial impulse in traversing the AV node.

Mobitz type 2, in which case a constant P-R interval is found prior to the blocked beats.

42

Rate ___ A & B) 30 ___ /min. ___ C) occasional ___ D) absent
atrial: A-D) regular

Rhythm ___ ventricular: A-D) irregular
QRS Duration ___ A-C) 0.08–0.12 s. ___ D) absent
P-R Interval ___ A & B 0.28s. ___ C) 0.32 s. ___ D) absent
A-C varies: 3:1, 2:1, 4:1, 5:1

AV Conduction Ratio ___ D) absent

This sequence of tracings shows the lethal progression of second degree heart block (Mobitz type 2) into third degree AV block. Owing to the failure of an escape idioventricular rhythm to develop, ventricular standstill results.

Tracings A and B

Interpretation: High degree second degree AV block, Mobitz type 2; ventricular response averages about 20 to 30/minute. (Of lesser significance is the first degree block with a P-R interval of 0.28 second for conducted beats.)

Rationale: The QRS activity is irregular with unusually narrow complexes for such a slow rhythm. The atrial activity is composed of notched P waves at a regular frequency of 60/minute. The AV relationship shows more P waves than QRS complexes and a prolonged P-R interval for conducted beats. Every QRS complex is preceded by a P wave at a fixed interval, but not every P wave is followed by a QRS. This is the main feature of an AV block. The conduction ratio varies between 2:1 and 3:1. It is classified as high degree because more than one P wave is blocked consecutively.

Tracing C

Tracing C was recorded a few minutes following A and B.

41

Rate ___ 55–65 ___ /min. Rhythm ___ irregular
QRS Duration ___ 0.08 ___ s.
P-R Interval ___ (progressively increases)
AV Conduction Ratio ___ varies (see below)

Interpretation: Sinus rhythm with a second degree AV block; Mobitz type 1 (Wenckebach), with an average ventricular rate between 55 and 65/minute.

Rationale: The ventricular rhythm is irregular at the two points where the pauses are noted. It appears as if a QRS complex has been dropped after beats 2 and 7. Atrial activity is regular and demonstrates constant P-P intervals. Atrial depolarization is occurring as expected. The AV conduction ratio is not 1:1, meaning that some of the P waves are not conducted. Therefore, we know that some type of second degree block is present. Next we examine the P-R intervals to determine if it is type 1 or 2. The P-R intervals are not constant; they gradually increase until one P wave is not associated with a QRS complex. In the first cycle we see an AV conduction ratio of 3:2 and for the second group, it is 6:5.

Note: The most common AV ratio in Mobitz type 1 is 3:2. Avoid confusing this dysrhythmia with

Interpretation: Advanced second degree AV block, Mobitz type 2, 4:1, 5:1 AV conduction.

Tracing *D*

Two minutes after C, this final tracing was obtained.

Interpretation: Third degree AV block with ventricular standstill. No escape pacemakers develop.

Rationale: Ventricular activity is completely absent. Atrial activity is regular at a rate of 50/minute. Since none of the notched P waves are conducted, third degree (complete) AV block exists.

43

Rate $\underline{\text{ventricular 30}}$/min. $\underline{\text{sinus 75}}$ /min. Rhythm $\underline{\text{regular}}$ P-R Interval $\underline{\text{absent}}$
QRS Duration $\underline{\text{0.12}}$ s.
AV Conduction Ratio $\underline{\text{absent}}$

Interpretation: Sinus rhythm with complete (third degree) AV heart block.

Rationale: Ventricular activity is slow with regularly occurring QRS complexes that are 0.12 second in duration. The QRS complexes look close to normal in shape and signify a focus relatively high in the AV bundle.

The P waves are notched and widened indicating that a conduction disturbance exists in the atrial activation as well as AV conduction. P waves are hidden in the T wave of the second and fourth QRS complexes, distorting their shapes (see Tracing 43, Answer).

No AV relationship exists, and complete dissociation is evident by the appearance of P waves "marching through" the QRS complexes. The atria are paced at a fast rate while the ventricles are plodding along at a much slower rate set by an independent pacemaker. This tracing shows the key features of third degree AV block:
- Regular P-P intervals
- Regular R-R intervals
- No relationship between the Ps and the QRSs.

44

Rate $\underline{\text{ventricular 48}}$/min. $\underline{\text{sinus 36}}$ /min. Rhythm $\underline{\text{regularly irregular}}$
QRS Duration $\underline{\text{0.10}}$ s.
P-R Interval $\underline{\text{0.16, 0.24, 0.36 s.,}}$ $\underline{\text{dropped beat}}$
AV Conduction Ratio $\underline{\text{4:3}}$

Interpretation: Sinus bradycardia with a second degree AV heart block Mobitz type 1 (4:3 conduction ratio).

Rationale:
- Grouped QRS beating ("periods")
- P-R interval increments

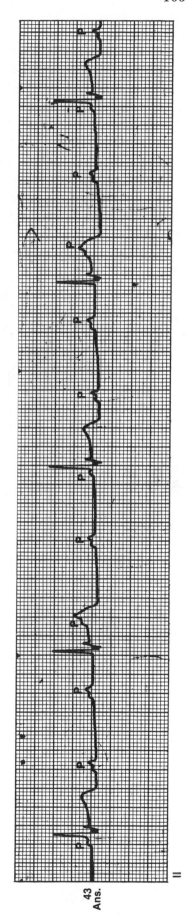

43 Ans.

110

- Pause associated with the dropped beat is less than twice the length of the last cycle of the group
- Rate of P waves less than 60/minute (bradycardia)

45

Rate   ventricular 36/min.   sinus 100 /min.   Rhythm   regular
QRS Duration   0.10   s.   P-R Interval   absent
AV Conduction Ratio   absent

Interpretation: Sinus rhythm with third degree (complete) AV heart block.

Rationale: There is no fixed relationship between the P waves and the ventricular activity. The P waves appear to march through the QRS complexes. The rate for the atria is 100/minute while the ventricles are beating at a much slower rate of 36/minute. The QRS pattern is regular but with distorted ventricular complexes.

46

Rate   84   /min.   Rhythm   regular
QRS Duration   0.08   s.   P-R Interval   0.24   s.
AV Conduction Ratio   1:1

Interpretation: Sinus rhythm with a first degree AV block.

Rationale: Normal ventricular and atrial activity is found. A 1:1 conduction ratio exists, but the P-R interval is beyond 0.20 second. Prolongation of the P-R interval indicates a delay in the start of ventricular activation following atrial stimulation.

47

Rate   A) sinus 136, ventricular 48/min.   B) sinus 115, ventricular 58/min.
Rhythm   regular
QRS Duration   A) 0.08   s.   A) absent   B) 0.08   s.   P-R Interval   B) 0.32   s.
AV Conduction Ratio   A) absent   B) 2:1

Interpretation: A: Sinus rhythm with third degree AV block. B: Sinus rhythm (first degree AV block) with second degree AV block and 2:1 AV conduction ratio.

Rationale: In A, both the atrial and ventricular rhythms are regular but they lack any fixed relationship.

Recorded later

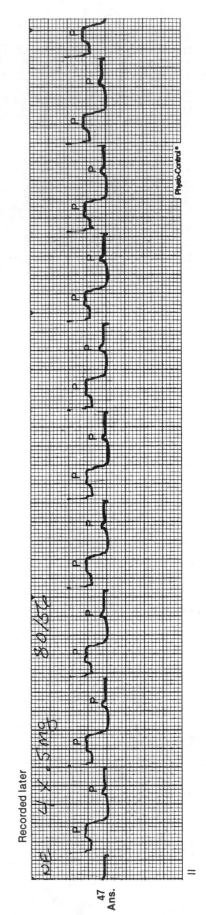

47
Ans.

In *B*, the ventricular rhythm is regular and there are two P waves for every QRS complex. Many of the P waves are hidden in the ST segments and have been labeled in Tracing 47, Answer.

48

Rate ventricular 25 /min.
sinus 100 /min. Rhythm __regular__ P-R Interval __absent__
QRS Duration __0.10__ s.
AV Conduction Ratio __absent__

Interpretation: **Sinus rhythm with complete (third degree) heart block.**

Rationale: The ventricular rate is extremely bradycardic, yet the QRS complexes look remarkably normal. The R-R intervals are regular. The atrial rate is faster, with many of the P waves hidden in the QRS-ST complexes. There is no fixed relationship between the P waves and the QRS complexes, indicating complete atrioventricular dissociation. The P waves are labeled in Tracing 48, Answer, and they can be seen "marching through" the QRS complexes.

49

Rate __7.5__ /min. Rhythm __regular__
QRS Duration __0.08__ s. P-R Interval __0.24__ s.
AV Conduction Ratio __1:1__

Interpretation: **Sinus rhythm with a first degree AV block. (The voltage is low.)**

Rationale: The QRS complexes and P waves are normal. One P wave exists for every QRS complex. AV conduction shows that every P wave is conducted through the AV node but only after a delay (0.24 second).

50

Rate ventricular 25 /min.
sinus 60 /min. atrial: regular Rhythm ventricular: regular
QRS Duration __0.36__ s. P-R interval __absent__
AV Conduction Ratio __absent__

Interpretation: **Sinus rhythm with third degree AV block.**

Rationale: The ventricular activity is very slow with wide and bizarre QRS complexes. P waves occur at a much more rapid rate than ventricular activity.

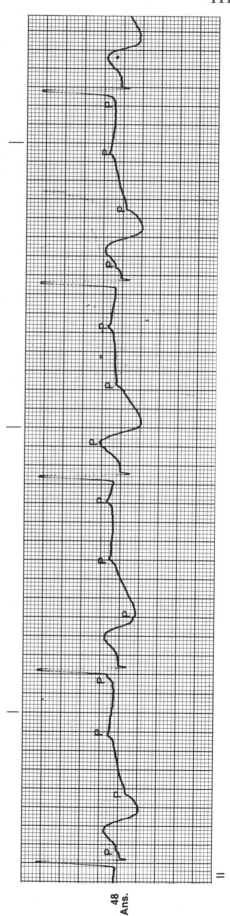

48
Ans.

112

There is no association between the atrial and ventricular activity. Complete interruption of the AV pathway exists and the sinus impulses are blocked from reaching the ventricles. The distorted ventricular complexes hardly resemble QRS complexes. They are irregular and slow—indicative of an unreliable pacemaker low in the His-Purkinje system.

51

Rate: sinus 50 /min., ventricular 38/min. Rhythm: sinus: regular, ventricular: regularly irregular
QRS Duration 0.10 s.
P-R Interval 0.20, 0.40 s., dropped beat
AV Conduction Ratio 3:2

Interpretation: Sinus bradycardia (50/min) with a second degree AV block Mobitz type 1 (Wenckebach); 3:2 AV conduction. The ventricular rate is about 30 to 40/minute.

Rationale: The ventricular rhythm shows grouped beating: two QRS complexes followed by a pause. The atrial rhythm shows regular P-P intervals at a rate of 50/minute. Complicating the slow rate is that only two of each three P waves are conducted. Every third QRS complex is dropped because the P wave is blocked. The hallmark finding is the progressive increase in the P-R intervals until the dropped QRS complex occurs. Then, the cycle begins anew.

52

Rate: sinus 120 /min., ventricular 52/min. Rhythm: sinus: regular, ventricular: regular P-R Interval absent s.
QRS Duration 0.16 s. P-R Interval absent
AV Conduction Ratio absent

Interpretation: Sinus rhythm with third degree AV block exists.

Rationale: The atria are being paced at 120/min by the sinus node while an escape focus in the ventricles beats at about 52/minute. This dysrhythmia is recognized by the P waves marching through the ventricular complexes. This occurs because the upper and lower chambers of the heart are being paced independently. The atrial and ventricular activities bear no fixed relationship to one another; hence, the P waves are not related to the QRS complexes. The atrial pacemaker is more rapid so the ECG shows more P waves than QRS complexes. In this strip, the atrial rate is almost two and one half times that of the ventricles.

53

Rate 64 /min. Rhythm regular
QRS Duration 0.12 s. P-R Interval 0.24 s.
AV Conduction Ratio 1:1

Interpretation: Sinus rhythm with first degree AV block.

Rationale: Ventricular activity is normal, as is atrial activation. The AV conduction ratio is 1:1. The only disturbance in conduction is an extended period before ventricular activity occurs (P-R interval equals 0.24 second).

54

Rate $\dfrac{\text{ventricular } 35}{\text{sinus } 94}$/min. Rhythm $\dfrac{\text{atrial: regular}}{\text{ventricular: regular}}$

QRS Duration ___0.16___ s. P-R Interval ___absent___

AV Conduction Ratio ___absent___

Interpretation: **Sinus rhythm with third degree complete AV heart block.**

Rationale: The ventricular rhythm is regular, as is the atrial rhythm. However, no fixed relationship between the waves and the QRS complexes exists. This is a case of complete AV dissociation.

Chapter Four
VENTRICULAR DYSRHYTHMIAS

The characteristics shared by all ventricular dysrhythmias include: missing P waves and an altered sequence of ventricular depolarization, resulting in widened QRS complexes. The repolarization sequence is also altered, resulting in ST-segment and T-wave changes.

PREMATURE VENTRICULAR COMPLEXES (PVCs)

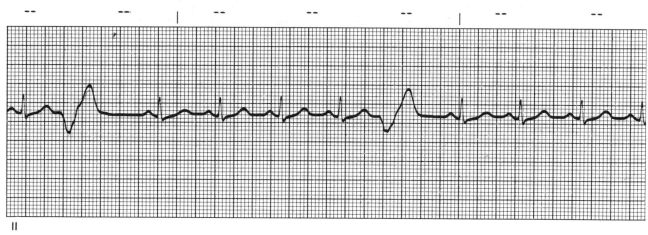

FIGURE 4–1. Two uniformed PVCs (beats 2 and 7).

Ventricular Rate:	Equal to rate of sinus beats plus PVCs.
Ventricular Rhythm:	Irregular at points that PVCs occur.
QRS Shape:	Abnormally shaped, wide, bizarre.
QRS Duration:	0.12 second or greater.
Atrial Rate:	The atrial rate can be computed by assessing the P-P interval when no PVC is present.
Atrial Rhythm:	Irregular; premature beat occurs before next P wave is expected.
P Wave Shape:	Usually absent. Because ventricular depolarization proceeds in a reverse direction along the normal pathway (retrograde), the atria may be depolarized by the PVC and this may cause a P wave to occur **after** the QRS complex.
P-R Interval:	Absent.

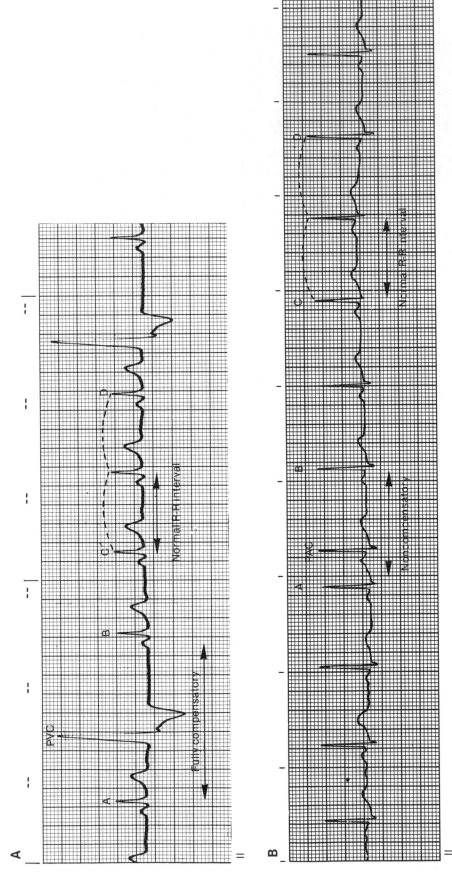

FIGURE 4–2. Postextrasystolic pauses. *A*, PVC with fully compensatory pause. The interval from the sinus beat before the PVC to the one following equals two normal R-R intervals. Thus, A → B is equal to C → D. *B*, PAC with noncompensatory pause. The interval from the sinus beat preceding the PAC to the one following is less than two R-R intervals. Thus, A → B is shorter than C → D.

116

Conduction Ratio:	Absent.
Other Significant Findings:	Commonly, the ectopic QRS complex is of a higher voltage (taller) than the normal beats, and the T wave is in the opposite direction of the bizarre QRS complex. The PVC is commonly followed by a **compensatory pause.** The shortened R-R interval preceding the PVC and the longer R-R interval following the PVC are equal to **two** normal R-R intervals (Fig. 4–2). A PVC can also be **interpolated,** that is, occurring between two normal R waves without interrupting the rhythmicity. This occurs when the PVC occurs early enough in the R-R interval when the cells are repolarized and ready to accept the next normal sinus impulse.
Regularly Occurring PVCs:	When the PVCs occur with regularity and in fixed ratios with normal beats, they are termed coupled PVCs. Based on the ratio of normal beats to PVCs, the following terms apply (Figs. 4–3 to 4–5): • Ventricular **bigeminy.** Every other beat is PVC. The VPCs are normally unifocal and occur at the same point following the normal QRS. • Ventricular **trigeminy.** One PVC occurs after every two normal beats. • Ventricular **quadrigeminy.** One PVC occurs after every three normal beats.
Etiology:	Premature depolarization of the ventricles is due to a reentry impulse or caused by an irritable focus (increased automaticity) in the His-Purkinje system.

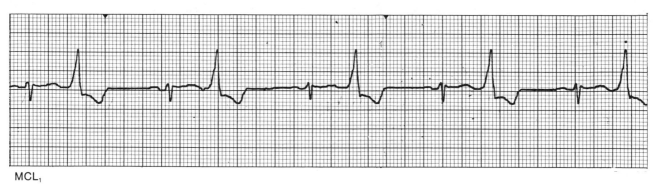

MCL₁

FIGURE 4–3. Ventricular bigeminy.

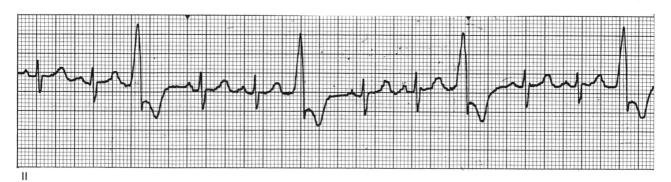

II

FIGURE 4–4. Ventricular trigeminy.

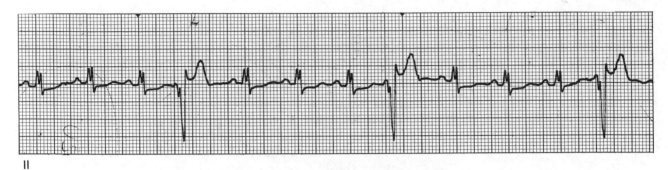

II

FIGURE 4–5. Ventricular quadrigeminy.

Significance: Varies greatly, depending on the patient's clinical situation and the frequency of occurrence. Benign PVCs occur in most healthy persons, but the frequent occurrence in an acute myocardial infarction patient may be a warning of more serious life-threatening dysrhythmias, such as ventricular tachycardia or ventricular fibrillation. More serious types of PVCs are:

1. Five or more unifocal PVCs per minute
2. Those that occur in salvos, or "runs" of consecutive PVCs (three or more consecutive PVCs are termed ventricular tachycardia) (see Fig. 4–6 *A* and *B*)
3. Those that strike close to the vulnerable T wave of the preceding normal beat (R-on-T, may precipitate ventricular fibrillation) (see Fig. 4–7)

A

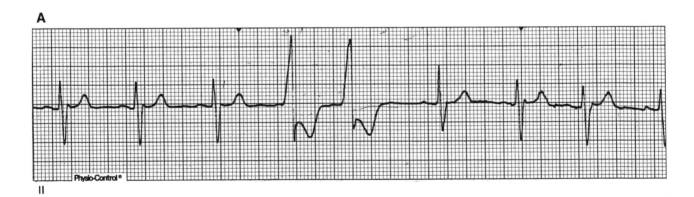

II

B

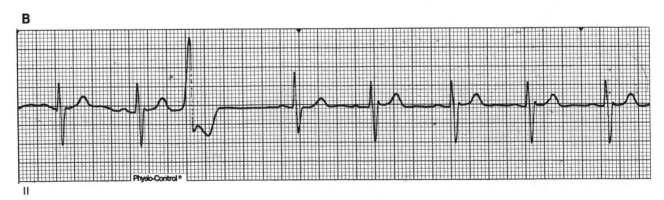

II

FIGURE 4–6. Consecutive PVCs (beats 4 and 5).

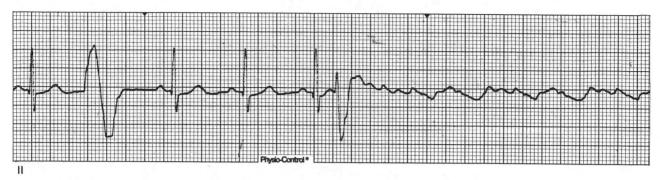

FIGURE 4–7. A PVC during the vulnerable period (T wave) causes ventricular fibrillation.

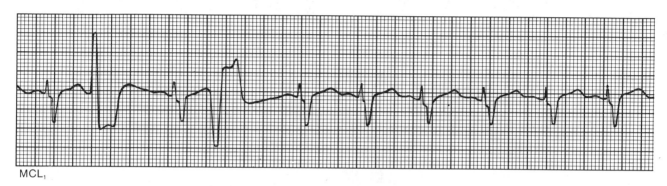

FIGURE 4–8. Multiformed PVCs (beats 2 and 4).

4. Those having a multifocal or multiformed appearance (see Fig. 4–8)

Acute Drug Therapy:

The majority of PVCs do not require pharmacologic intervention. Treatment should be implemented only when the patient is at risk for sudden death, such as acute myocardial infarction, unstable angina, unexplained syncope, or when the rate of VPCs results in decreasing cardiac output to the point of hypotension. Other relative indications for treatment include: multifocal PVCs, where PVCs fall on preceding T waves or for PVCs in couplets or short runs of ventricular tachycardia until significance of these beats are established by hospitalization. (See Fig. 4-9 for treatment flow chart.)

Hallmark Findings:

- Occur early in the R-R interval.
- Do not have P waves preceding the ectopic QRS complex.
- Have bizarrely shaped QRS complexes.
- Are usually followed by a compensatory pause.
- The T wave of the ectopic complex often occurs in the opposite direction of the QRS deflection.

Concepts about PVCs:

- When two PVCs occur in succession, they are called a couplet or paired PVCs, and may portend degeneration into a more life-threatening ventricular dysrhythmia.
- PVCs with the same shape are termed **uniformed** or **unifocal**, signifying that they probably arose from the same site. PVCs with varied QRS shapes are termed **multiformed** or **multifocal**. Multiformed PVCs may arise from more than one site,

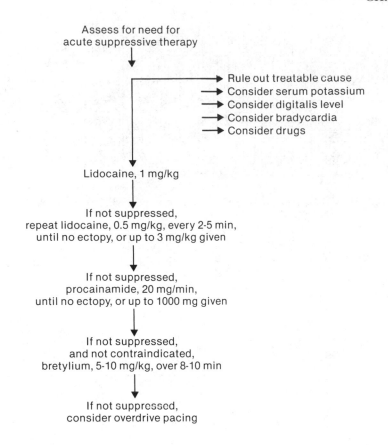

Assess for need for
acute suppressive therapy

→ Rule out treatable cause
→ Consider serum potassium
→ Consider digitalis level
→ Consider bradycardia
→ Consider drugs

Lidocaine, 1 mg/kg

If not suppressed,
repeat lidocaine, 0.5 mg/kg, every 2-5 min,
until no ectopy, or up to 3 mg/kg given

If not suppressed,
procainamide, 20 mg/min,
until no ectopy, or up to 1000 mg given

If not suppressed,
and not contraindicated,
bretylium, 5-10 mg/kg, over 8-10 min

If not suppressed,
consider overdrive pacing

Once ectopy resolved, maintain as follows:

After lidocaine, 1 mg/kg ... lidocaine drip, 2 mg/min
After lidocaine, 1-2 mg/kg ... lidocaine drip, 3 mg/min
After lidocaine, 2-3 mg/kg ... lidocaine drip, 4 mg/min
After procainamide ... procainamide drip, 1–4 mg/min (check blood level)
After bretylium ... bretylium drip, 2 mg/min

FIGURE 4–9. Acute suppressive therapy for ventricular ectopy. This sequence was developed to assist in teaching how to treat a broad range of patients, although some may require therapy not specified here.

but they also can develop in the identical site and take different conduction pathways.

- PVCs are also termed ventricular extrasystoles and ventricular premature beats (VPBs).
- Ventricular tachycardia or fibrillation may be precipitated by a PVC striking the T wave of the previous beats.
- The coupling intervals of the PVC to the previous beat is usually fixed.
- Stroke volume is less for PVCs because the ventricles are activated sequentially instead of simultaneously and the atrial kick contribution to ventricular filling is lost.
- PVCs occur frequently in young people and in the absence of intrinsic heart disease. Thus, their significance is related to the associated clinical features of the case. Blanket attempts at suppression of all PVCs by protocol are not indicated.

Escape Ventricular Beats:

In bradycardiac rates, lower ventricular pacemakers may occur that resemble PVCs but are escape ectopic beats that are beneficial. Ventricular escape beats can be distinguished from PVCs because they occur *late* in the R-R interval rather than prematurely. These backup pacemakers, occurring when the sinus node slows or ceases to discharge, provide additional cardiac output and should **not** be suppressed with lidocaine. In such cases, the ectopic beats will subside when the rate is increased.

PVCS VERSUS PACS WITH ABERRANT CONDUCTION

The wide, bizarre looking complex on the ECG monitor that we generally associate with PVCs can be mimicked by a supraventricular premature beat that cannot be conducted normally by the ventricular conducting system, either because it occurred too early after the last normal beat so the conducting system did not have a chance to fully recover and be ready to conduct the next beat, or because there is intrinsic disease (usually due to coronary atherosclerosis) of the conducting system itself, making it incapable of conducting any premature beat normally. There are certain things we look for to try to differentiate a true PVC from an aberrantly conducted PAC. The presence of some form of **P′ wave** preceding the QRS complex, whether it be an atrial or a junctional P wave, is probably the best proof that we can find that we are dealing with a PAC. Employing different leads, doubling the speed of the printer, and doubling the amplitude of the complexes can sometimes reveal such P waves.

If this is unsuccessful, then we can apply certain **general** criteria to try to differentiate the two (this is based on the *Advanced Cardiac Life Support* text). Aberrant PACs often have:

1. An early P′ wave.
2. A QRS complex that is "splintered, notched, or slurred in configuration."
3. A QRS complex with an r-s-R′ configuration in lead MCL, or lead V_1 (similar to the "rabbit ears" of a RBBB).
4. A QRS complex with a q-R-s configuration in lead MCL_6 or lead V_6.
5. The initial deflection of the QRS complex the same as that of the flanking normal beats.

These may be helpful guidelines, but unless we are **certain** we are dealing with PACs and not PVCs, they don't always help us to know what to do in the specific situations in which they may appear. When uncertain, it is probably best to treat for the most serious possibility and try to figure it out later. In the case of PACs versus PVCs, this would mean that, in the patient presenting with active myocardial ischemia, recent syncopal episode, digitalis toxicity, etc. (situations in which **not** treating PVCs could lead to more serious consequences), it would be best to try treating the complexes **as though they were PVCs** and do the detailed analysis of the ECG or monitor strip at a later time.

This also applies to sustained dysrhythmias in which a supraventricular tachydysrhythmia with aberrant conduction may be difficult or impossible to differentiate from a ventricular dysrhythmia. Probably the classic example of this is PSVT with aberrancy versus ventricular tachycardia. Again, it's possible to pore over the ECG or monitor strip for long periods of time, looking for P waves, looking for fusion beats, or looking for some of the characteristics of the QRS complexes mentioned above. However, as was mentioned earlier, it is the status of the patient that should determine what we do. If the underlying circumstances of the dysrhythmia (e.g., patient is having ischemic chest pain) or the hemodynamic consequences (e.g., patient is in shock) are serious enough, then—whatever it is—the dysrhythmia **must** be stopped immediately. Whether that means a trial of drug therapy, use of vagal maneuvers, or immediate cardioversion will depend on the circumstances and not just what is being observed on the monitor.

VENTRICULAR TACHYCARDIA

Defined as three or more consecutive PVCs occuring at a rate greater than 100/minute, ventricular tachycardia is a grave dysrhythmia. This highly unstable ventricular dysrhythmia precipitates acute heart failure and frequently degenerates into ventricular fibrillation. This rhythm disturbance resembles a series

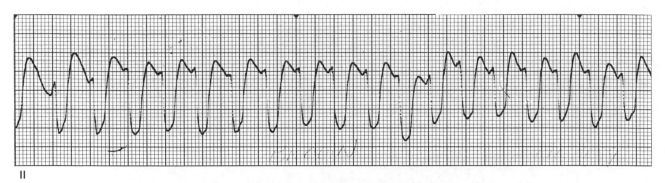

II

FIGURE 4–10. Ventricular tachycardia (160/min).

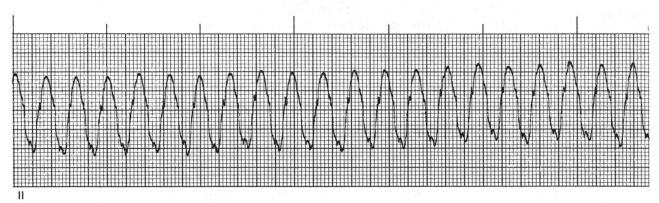

II

FIGURE 4–11. This figure shows the difficulty in distinguishing between ventricular tachycardia and supraventricular tachycardia with aberrent ventricular conduction.

of PVCs coupled together and is indicative of an irritable ventricle. Ventricular tachycardia may predispose the patient to sudden death.

Ventricular Rhythm:	Regular or slightly irregular R-R intervals.
Ventricular Rate:	100 to 200/minute (usually around 150/minute).
QRS Shape:	Wide and bizarre (similar to a PVC).
QRS Duration:	Prolonged (0.12 second or greater).
Artrial Rate, Rhythm, Shape:	Usually not seen.
P-R Interval:	Absent.
Conduction Ratio:	Absent.
Other Significant Findings:	Atrial rhythm usually continues independently of ventricular activity, and thus, P waves may coexist. However, P waves are observed only sporadically. Sometimes the P wave can be conducted through a polarized AV junction and "capture" the ventricles.
Etiology:	A rapidly discharging ectopic ventricular focus or a reentry pattern in the His-Purkinje system.
Acute Drug Therapy:	Figure 4–12 shows a treatment flow chart.
Concepts about This Dysrhythmia:	• Ventricular tachycardia is much more serious than supraventricular tachycardia.

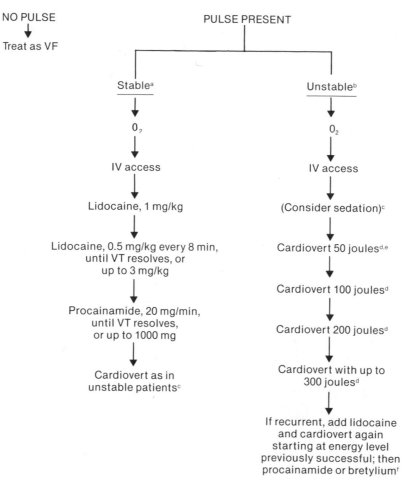

NO PULSE   PULSE PRESENT
↓
Treat as VF

Stable[a]   Unstable[b]

O₂   O₂

IV access   IV access

Lidocaine, 1 mg/kg   (Consider sedation)[c]

Lidocaine, 0.5 mg/kg every 8 min,   Cardiovert 50 joules[d,e]
until VT resolves, or
up to 3 mg/kg

                                    Cardiovert 100 joules[d]

Procainamide, 20 mg/min,   Cardiovert 200 joules[d]
until VT resolves,
or up to 1000 mg

                                    Cardiovert with up to
                                    300 joules[d]

Cardiovert as in
unstable patients[c]

                                    If recurrent, add lidocaine
                                    and cardiovert again
                                    starting at energy level
                                    previously successful; then
                                    procainamide or bretylium[f]

FIGURE 4–12. Sustained ventricular tachycardia (VT). This sequence was developed to assist in teaching how to treat a broad range of patients with sustained VT. Some patients may require care not specified herein. This algorithm should not be construed as prohibiting such flexibility. Flow of algorithm presumes that VT is continuing. VF indicates ventricular fibrillation.

[a]If patient becomes unstable (see footnote b for definition) at any time, move to "Unstable" arm of algorithm.   [b]Unstable indicates symptoms (e.g., chest pain or dyspnea), hypotension (systolic blood pressure <90 mm Hg), congestive heart failure, ischemia, or infarction.   [c]Sedation should be considered for all patients, including those defined in footnote b as unstable, except those who are hemodynamically unstable (e.g., hypotensive, in pulmonary edema, or unconscious).   [d]If hypotension, pulmonary edema, or unconsciousness is present, unsynchronized cardioversion should be done to avoid delay associated with synchronization.   [e]In the absence of hypotension, pulmonary edema, or unconsciousness, a precordial thump may be employed prior to cardioversion.   [f]Once VT has resolved, begin intravenous (IV) infusion of antiarrhythmic agent that has aided resolution of VT. If hypotension, pulmonary edema, or unconsciousness is present, use lidocaine if cardioversion alone is unsuccessful, followed by bretylium. In all other patients, recommended order of therapy is lidocaine, procainamide, and then bretylium.

- Patients may be stable and tolerate this rhythm well, while others may be in shock.
- This dysrhythmia may exist with or without a pulse.
- It may be difficult or impossible to tell this dysrhythmia apart from SVT if aberrant intraventricular conduction exists. Characteristics that help identify ventricular tachycardia include AV dissociation and a right bundle branch block pattern in V_1.
- **Accelerated idioventricular rhythms,** at rates above 40 to 100/min, have a different significance. Such rhythms are better tolerated because the rate is within a normal range. Accelerated idioventricular rhythms are more stable than

either ventricular tachycardia or slower rhythms, both of which may degenerate into ventricular fibrillation. The misnomer "slow ventricular tachycardia" is sometimes applied, but the term should be avoided because of its ambiguity. Typically, it develops suddenly without precipitation and subsides spontaneously without treatment. The cause and significance are unknown.

TORSADE DE POINTES

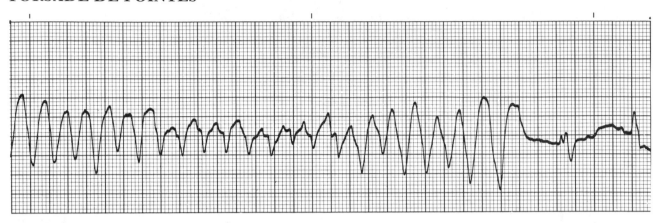

FIGURE 4–13. Torsade de pointes variation of ventricular tachycardia converting spontaneously to sinus rhythm.

Torsade de pointes is a variant of ventricular tachycardia in which the polarity of the wide QRS complexes rhythmically changes between positive and negative. The French term means "twisiting of points"—an apt description of its ECG appearance. In contrast to the uniform shape and rhythm in the classical form of ventricular tachycardia, torsade de pointes shows a waxing and waning in the size of ventricular complexes as the QRS apices swing above and below the baseline. This peculiarity has given rise to several other terms: polymorphous ventricular tachycardia, paroxysmal ventricular fibrillation, and atypical ventricular tachycardia.

Torsade de pointes arises in settings where ventricular repolarization is delayed. This is manifest by prolongation of the Q-T interval, which increases the likelihood of reentry. Circumstances in which this occurs includes electrolyte disorders, such as hypocalcemia and hypomagnesemia, congenital Q-T prolongation, and use of drugs that delay repolarization, including lidocaine, procainamide, amidarone, quinidine, disopyramide, phenothiazines, and tricyclic antidepressants.

Torsade de pointes is often interspaced with normal QRS complexes and fortunately reverts spontaneously to NSR (as shown in Fig. 4–13). It may, however, degenerate into ventricular fibrillation as with the classical form of ventricular tachycardia. Correct identification of torsade de pointes is crucial because many of the traditional antidysrhythmic agents for ventricular tachycardia prolong repolarization and may, therefore, be ineffective or even worsen the problem.

Acute Drug Therapy: Phenytoin, propranolol, bretylium, and overdrive ventricular pacing to reduce dispersion of refractory periods. Theoretically, atropine and isoproterenol can be given to increase the rate and shorten the Q-T interval, but this is risky in the setting of ischemia.

VENTRICULAR FLUTTER

Ventricular flutter is an advanced form of ventricular tachycardia and therefore is not truly a distinct type of dysrhythmia. Ventricular flutter is a transitional dysrhythmia that is sometimes observed briefly following ventricular tachycardia just before it degenerates into ventricular fibrillation. It is a serious

A

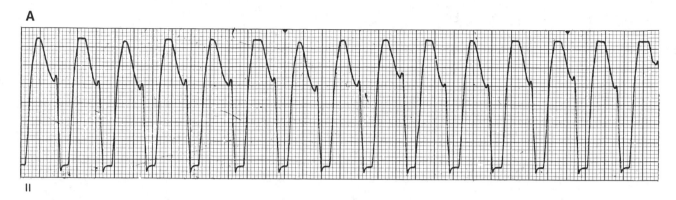

II

B

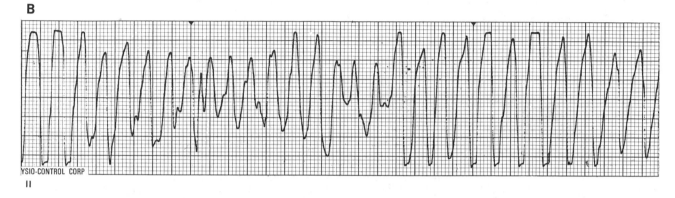

YSIO-CONTROL CORP

II

C

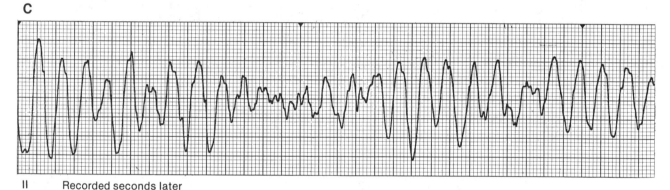

II   Recorded seconds later

FIGURE 4–14. This tracing shows the fatal progression of ventricular tachycardia through periods of flutter and fibrillation.

dysrhythmia, lasts for a few seconds, and has the appearance of a sine wave (regular, smooth, rounded ventricular waves) at a rate of 150 to 300/minute. There is usually no pulse associated with ventricular flutter and in that case defibrillation should be performed.

Etiology and significance are the same as for pulseless ventricular tachycardia.

Acute Drug Therapy: If pulse is present (rare), treat as malignant ventricular tachycardia. If there is no evidence of hemodynamics, treat as ventricular fibrillation with immediate defibrillation.

IDIOVENTRICULAR RHYTHM

Idioventricular rhythm is a general term used when there is an unstable, slow, and deteriorating ventricular focus. This dysrhythmia is seen frequently following defibrillation of ventricular fibrillation before

A

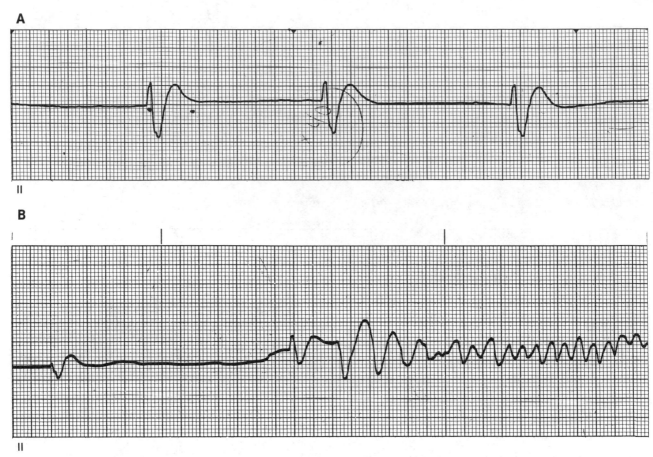

B

FIGURE 4–15. *A*, Idioventricular rhythm (30/min). *B*, The highly unreliable nature of an idioventricular pacemaker is illustrated by this tracing. The slowly discharging focus (20/min) degenerates into ventricular fibrillation.

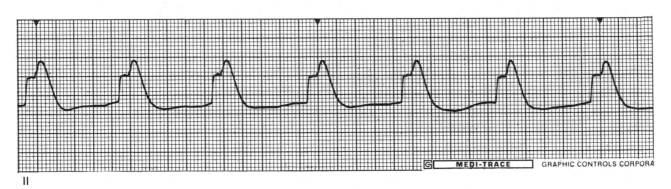

FIGURE 4–16. Idioventricular rhythm (accelerated at 60/min).

a higher focus takes over, and also as a deteriorating situation in a dying heart. Often, it occurs as a pulse-less rhythm during resuscitation efforts.

Idioventricular impulse formation is indicative of spontaneous depolarization of the Purkinje fibers or myocardial tissue. The rate of automaticity is approximately 20 to 40/minute, although it can be even slower. Sporadic idioventricular complexes are termed agonal rhythm.

Ventricular Rhythm: Regular or irregular.

Ventricular Rate: Escape: 20 to 40/minute.
                                        Accelerated: 40 to 100/minute.

QRS Shape:	Wide, bizarre; similar to a series of PVCs.
QRS Duration:	0.12 second or beyond.
Atrial Rate:	None.
Atrial Rhythm:	None.
P-R Interval:	None.
Conduction Ratio:	None.
Etiology:	This dysrhythmia develops when higher pacemakers (that is, atrial, SA, and AV nodes) fail to discharge. Since the rhythm originates from within the ventricles, the QRS complexes have a wide and bizarre appearance. The lack of atrial depolarization is the reason that P waves are lacking. The bradycardia and lack of atrial contractions causes cardiac output to fall. The pacemaker site is unstable and cannot be relied upon to generate a rhythm indefinitely. The spontaneous discharge of the Purkinje fibers is an escape rhythm and will subside if higher pacemakers return or artificial pacing is successful.

Dysrhythmia	Rates/Minute
Idioventricular rhythm	20 to 40
Accelerated idioventricular rhythm	Greater than 40 to 100
Ventricular tachycardia	Greater than 100

Acute Drug Therapy:	If associated with a pulse, isoproterenol or artificial pacing. If electromechanical dissociation exists, institute resuscitation measures.

VENTRICULAR FIBRILLATION

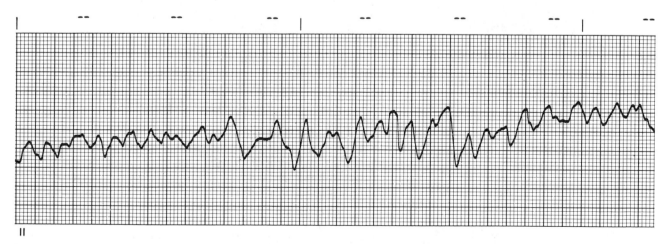

FIGURE 4–17. Coarse ventricular fibrillation.

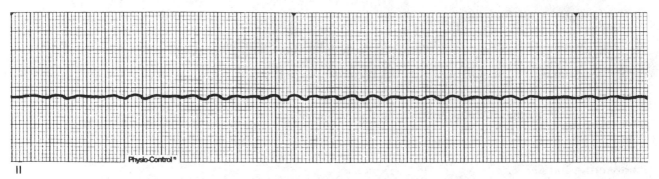

FIGURE 4–18. Fine amplitude ventricular fibrillation.

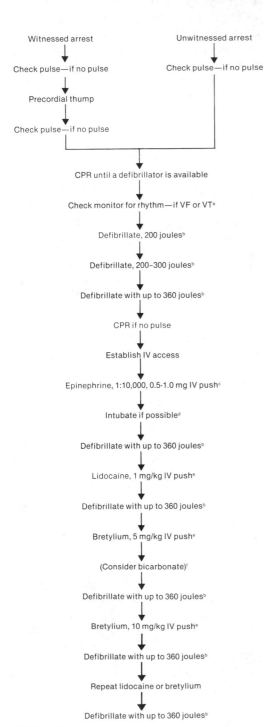

FIGURE 4–19. Ventricular fibrillation (and pulseless ventricular tachycardia). This sequence was developed to assist in teaching how to treat a broad range of patients with ventricular fibrillation (VF) or pulseless ventricular tachycardia (VT). Some patients may require care not specified herein. This algorithm should not be construed as prohibiting such flexibility. Flow of algorithm presumes that VF is continuing. CPR indicates cardiopulmonary resuscitation.
[a]Pulseless VT should be treated identically to VF. [b]Check pulse and rhythm after each shock. If VF recurs after transiently converting (rather than persists without ever converting), use whatever energy level has previously been successful for defibrillation. [c]Epinephrine should be repeated every 5 min. [d]Intubation is preferable. If it can be accomplished simultaneously with other techniques, then the earlier the better. However, defibrillation and epinephrine are more important initially if the patient can be ventilated without intubation. [e]Some may prefer repeated doses of lidocaine, which may be given in 0.5 mg/kg boluses every 8 min to a total dose of 3 mg/kg. [f]Value of sodium bicarbonate is questionable during cardiac arrest, and it is not recommended for routine cardiac arrest sequence. Consideration of its use in a dose of 1 mEq/kg is appropriate at this point. Half of original dose may be repeated every 10 min if it is used.

Ventricular fibrillation is characterized by chaotic electrical activity and totally disorganized myocardial activity in which there is no cardiac output. Often the myocardium is salvageable if the electrical rhythm can be corrected. The bizarre appearance of this dysrhythmia is easy to recognize because no organized pattern or complexes can be observed. This dysrhythmia can be mimicked by a loose electrode; therefore, it is essential to palpate a carotid pulse and ascertain if cardiac output is present. Patients in ventricular fibrillation will lose consciousness within 10 seconds. Ventricular fibrillation is a life-threatening dysrhythmia and the leading cause of sudden death due to coronary artery disease.

Ventricular Rate:	Absent.
Ventricular Rhythm:	Absent.
QRS Configuration:	Absent.
QRS Duration:	Absent.
Atrial Rate:	Absent.
Atrial Rhythm:	Absent.
P-R Interval:	None.
Conduction Ratio:	None.
Other Significant Findings:	Ventricular fibrillation may be coarse (high amplitude) with complexes greater than 3 mm in height, or fine (low amplitude) with complexes of 3 mm or less.
Etiology:	Results from a ventricular reentry rhythm. Often caused by an ectopic premature ventricular beat occurring during the vulnerable T-wave (R-on-T phenomenon).
Clinical Significance:	Life-threatening dysrhythmia that must be corrected by immediate defibrillation and resuscitative measures.
Acute Drug Therapy:	See Figure 4–19 for treatment flow chart.

ASYSTOLE (COMPLETE CARDIAC STANDSTILL)

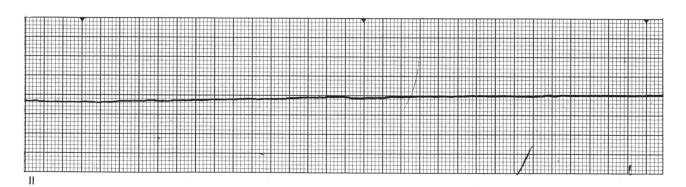

II

FIGURE 4–20. Asystole.

Asystole is the complete absence of electrical and mechanical activity. The SA node is not firing, nor are any other backup pacemakers. As a result, cardiac output ceases and the heart is silent.

The ECG appears as a flat line and indicates extensive damage to the heart's electrical conduction system. The absence of impulse formation makes resuscitation very difficult in the cardiac patient. In trauma patients with asystole restoration of blood volume may restore electrical activity. (Make sure that straight line ECG is not really low voltage ventricular fibrillation by moving the lead selector to a perpendicular lead and ensuring the amplitude gain is maximum.

Ventricular Rhythm and Rate:	Absent.
Conduction Ratio:	Absent.
Atrial Rhythm and Rate:	Absent.
Acute Drug Treatment:	See Figure 4–21 for the treatment flow chart.

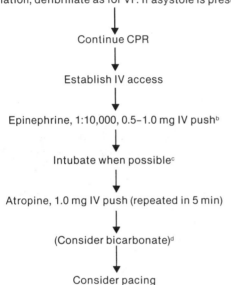

FIGURE 4–21. Asystole (cardiac standstill). This sequence was developed to assist in teaching how to treat a broad range of patients with asystole. Some patients may require care not specified herein. This algorithm should not be construed to prohibit such flexibility. Flow of algorithm presumes asystole is continuing. VF indicates ventricular fibrillation; IV, intravenous.

[a]Asystole should be confirmed in two leads. [b]Epinephrine should be repeated every 5 min. [c]Intubation is preferable; if it can be accomplished simultaneously with other techniques, then the earlier the better. However, cardiopulmonary resuscitation (CPR) and use of epinephrine are more important initially if patient can be ventilated without intubation. (Endotracheal epinephrine may be used.) [d]Value of sodium bicarbonate is questionable during cardiac arrest, and it is not recommended for the routine cardiac arrest sequence. Consideration of its use in a dose of 1 mEq/kg is appropriate at this point. Half of original dose may be repeated every 10 min if it is used.

TABLE 4–1. Dysrhythmia Synopsis: Ventricular Rhythms

	P Waves	QRS Complexes	AV Relationship	Other Features
1. Escape idioventricular rhythm	Absent	Depends on level of escape focus High in ventricle are narrow and 40–50/min Low in ventricle are wide and 20–40/min	Absent	Life-sustaining in event of sinus arrest and third degree heart block
2. Accelerated idioventricular rhythm	Absent	Wide, distorted Rate 50–100/minute	Absent or AV dissociation Occasional ventricular capture complexes	Originally thought to be benign; now considered pathologic
3. Ventricular tachycardia	Absent or sporadically present	Wide and bizarre Rate: above 100/minute (commonly about 150/minute)	Absent	Resembles a string of PVCs

TABLE 4–1. *continued*

	P Waves	QRS Complexes	AV Relationship	Other Features
4. Torsade de pointes (variation of ventricular tachycardia)	Absent	Wide and slurred QRS axis constantly changing in the same lead	Absent	Prolonged Q-T interval in NSR prior to or following episode of ventricular tachycardia
5. Ventricular fibrillation	Absent	No defined pattern	Absent	Chaotic tracing with complexes of varying heights and shapes
6. Asystole	Absent	Absent	Absent	Flat line

TABLE 4–2. Dysrhythmia Synopsis: Ectopic Complexes

	P Waves	QRS Complexes	AV Relationship	Key Features
1. Premature Complexes				
A. PAC/atrial	Premature ectopic P′ wave	Normal if conducted. May be blocked or aberrantly conducted	1:1 AV conduction P-R interval differs from sinus complexes	Noncompensatory pause Normal T waves
B. PJC/junctional	Retrograde P′ wave just before or after QRS complex Often P′ wave missing	Normal	May be 1:1 or missing P-R interval often shortened	Noncompensatory pause Normal T waves
C. PVC/ventricular	Absent	Wide, bizarre	Absent	Compensatory pause Abnormal T waves (slope opposite aberrant QRS)
2. Escape Complexes:				
A. Atrial	P′ wave	Normal	Variable	Occur in cases of sinus depression
B. Junctional	Retrograde P′ wave or missing	Normal Sustained rhythm at rate of 40–60/min	Variable	Occur when sinus node is depressed
C. Ventricular	Missing	Wide, bizarre Sustained rhythm at rate of 20–40/min	Missing	Occur when sinus and AV junction fail as pacemaker

Notes: Premature beats occur early in the R-R interval while escape beats occur late. Premature beats compete with sinus node for pacemaker role (interrupt R-R cycles of dominant rhythm); escape beats "reluctantly" assume pacemaker role when SA node fails (end R-R cycles longer than dominant rhythm.

EXERCISE C: SELF-ASSESSMENT ECG TRACINGS 55 TO 81

The following ECGs show a variety of ventricular dysrhythmias. Analyze each tracing according to the systematic approach outlined in Chapter One and formulate an interpretation. Check your answer with the suggested interpretations beginning on page 142.

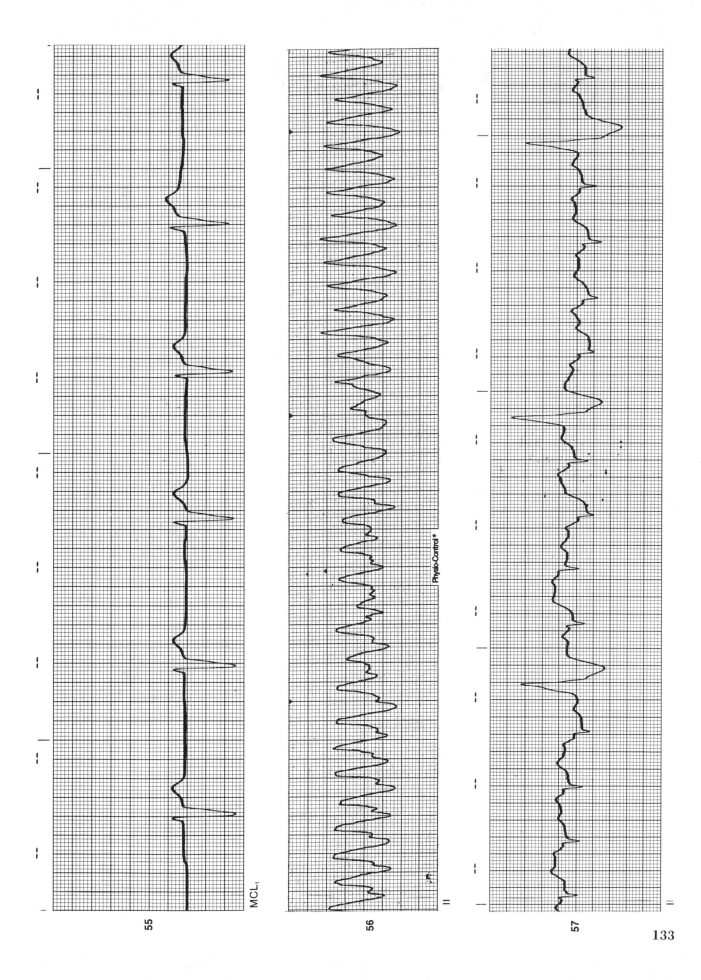

MCL₁

55

56

Physio-Control®

57

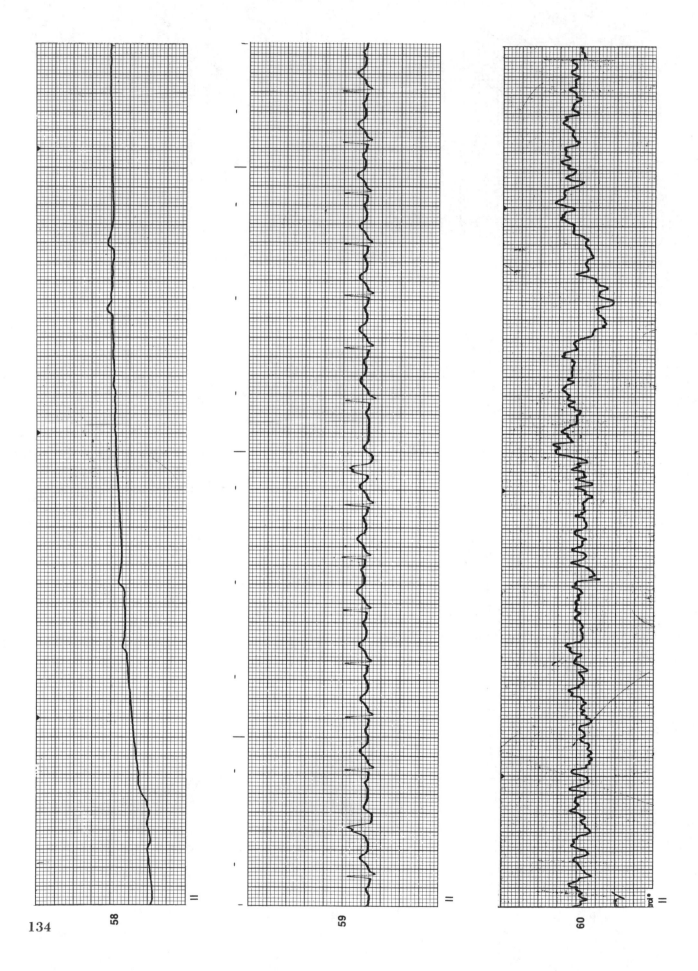

58

59

60

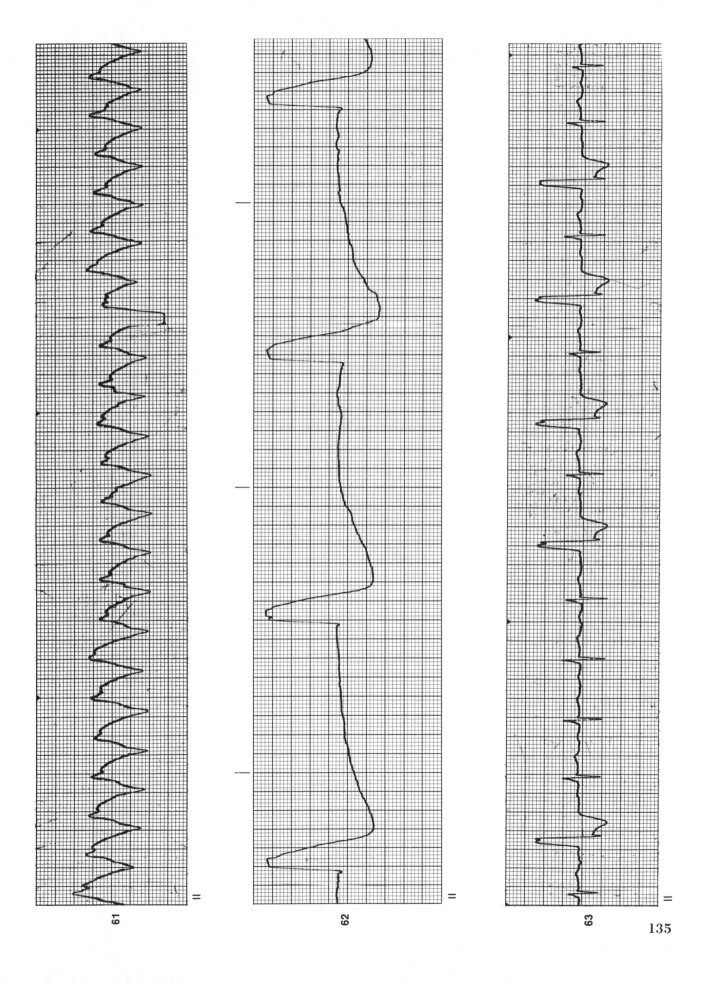

61

62

63

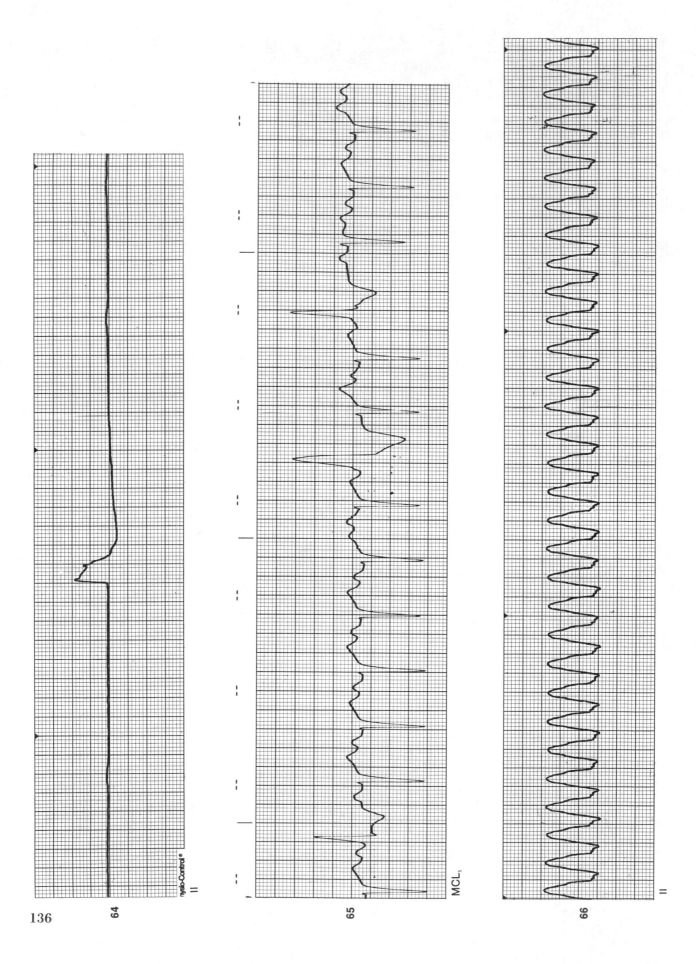

64

nysio-Control®

II

65

MCL₁

66

II

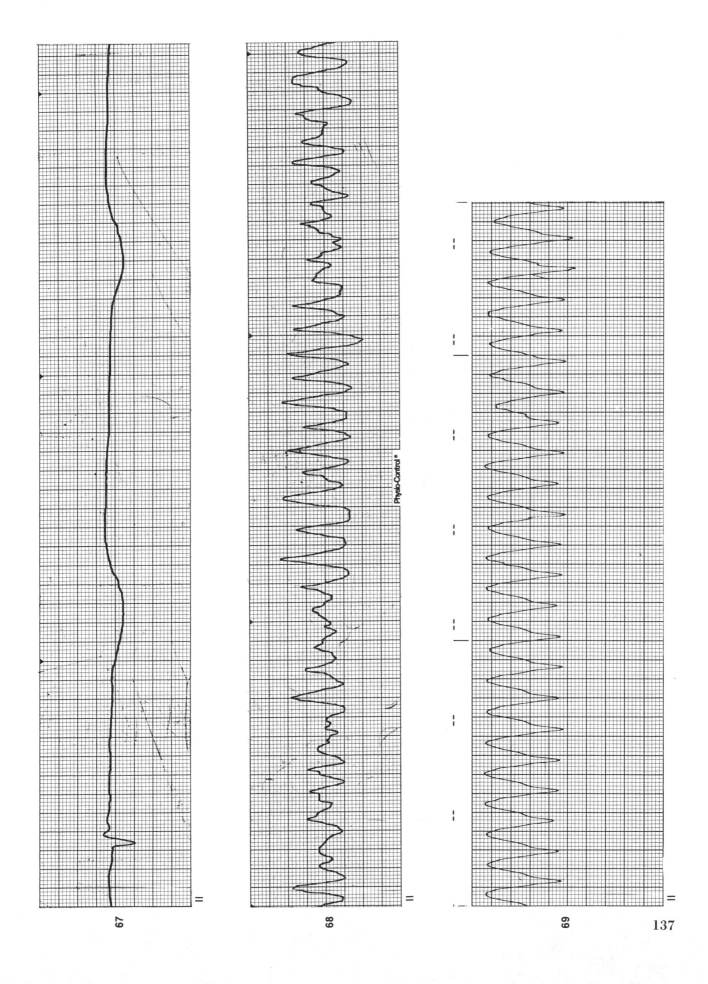

67

68

Physio-Control®

69

137

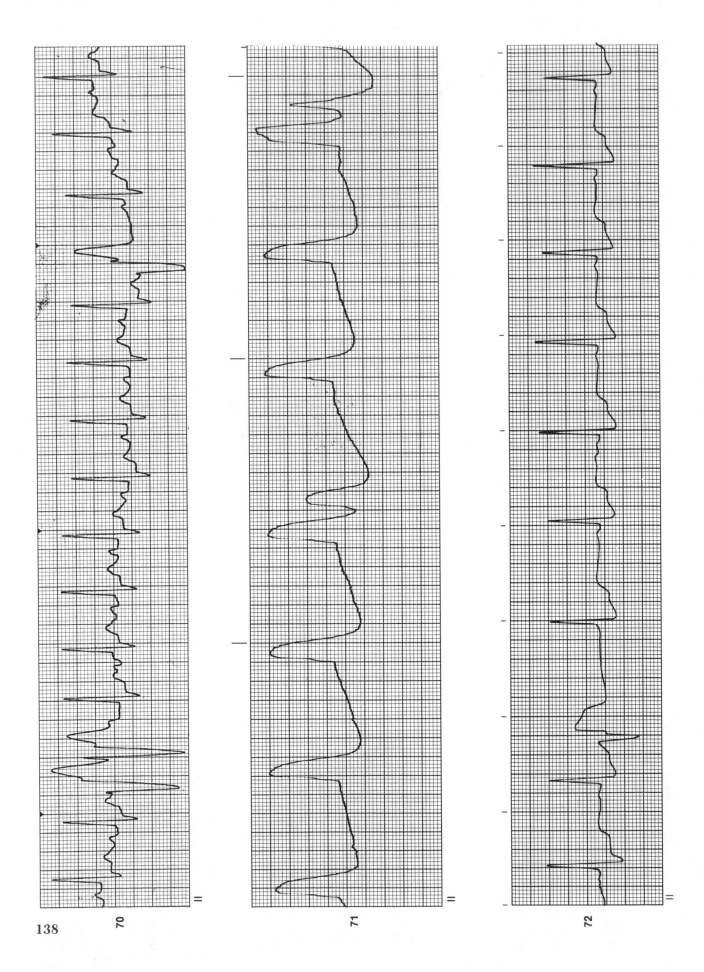

70

71

72

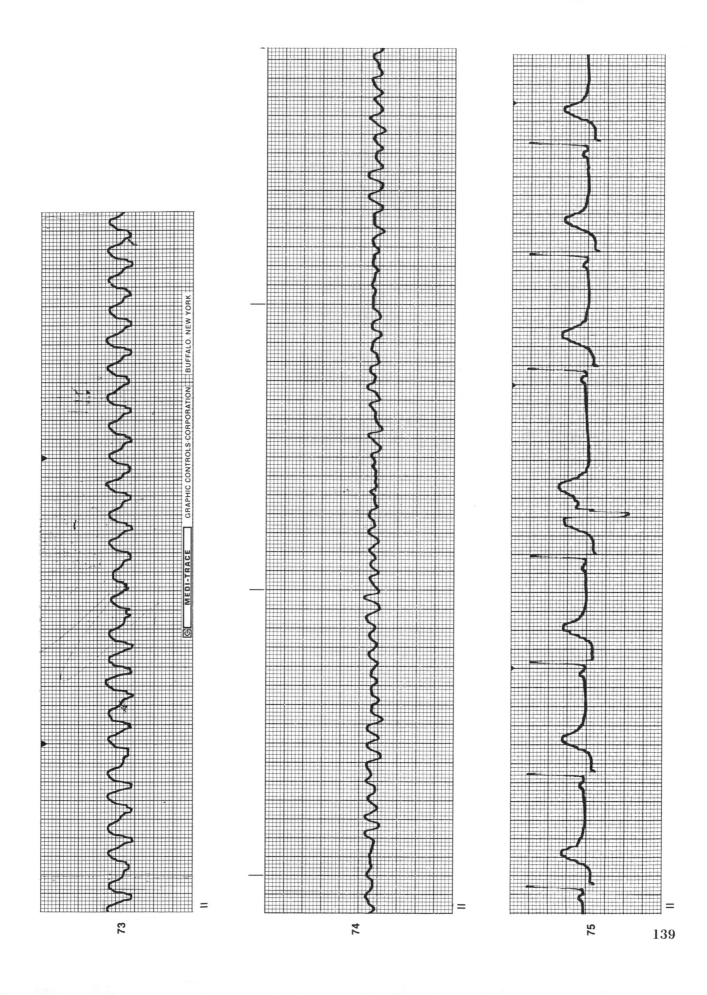

73

74

75

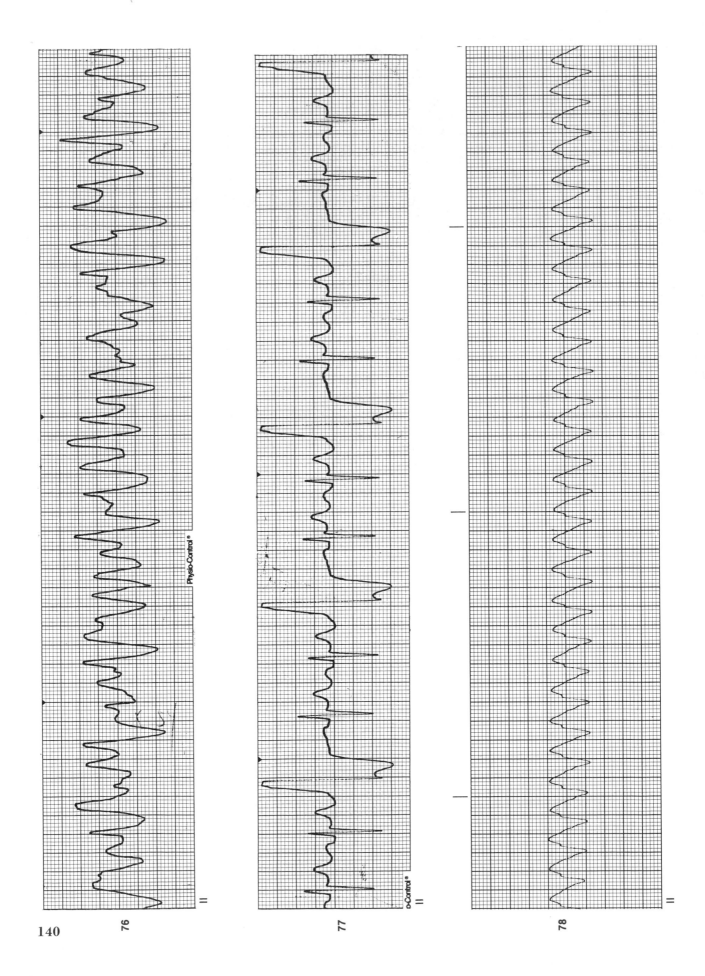

140

76

77

78

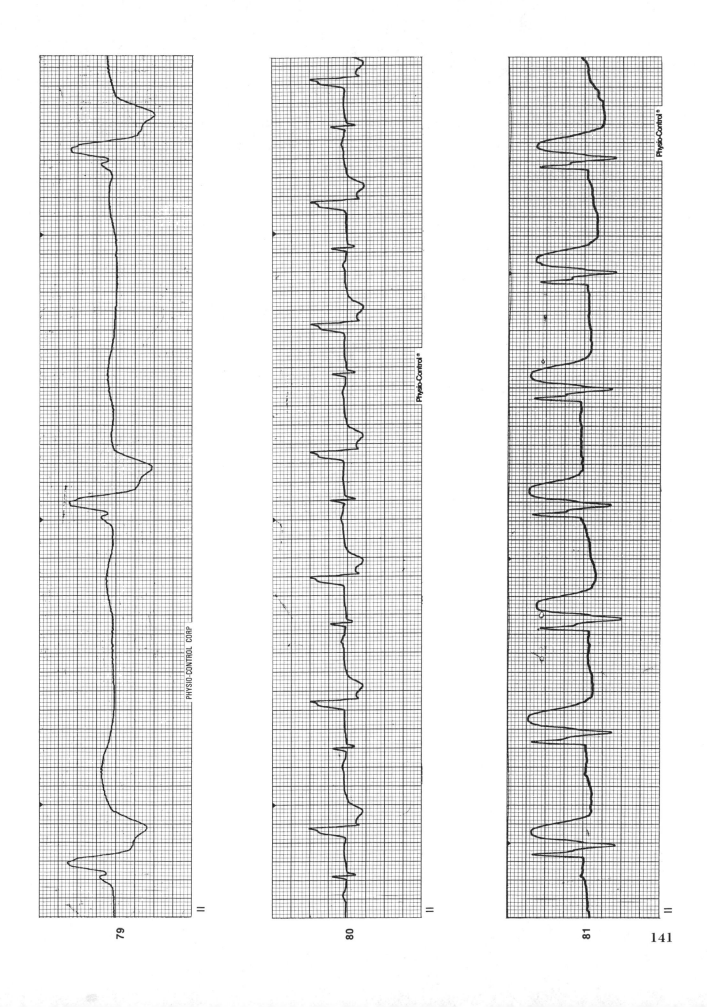

79

PHYSIO-CONTROL CORP

80

Physio-Control®

81

Physio-Control®

141

ANSWERS TO PRACTICE ECG TRACINGS 55 TO 81

PVCs. The individual QRS complexes are identical to PVCs. If left untreated, this dysrhythmia usually degenerates into ventricular fibrillation.

55

Rate __40__ /min.   Rhythm __regular__
QRS Duration __0.20__ s.   P-R Interval __absent__
AV Conduction Ratio __absent__

Interpretation: Escape idioventricular ventricular rhythm.

Rationale: The aberrant QRS complexes are wide and occur regularly. Atrial activity is absent, indicated by missing P waves. Therefore, an AV relationship is absent. The slow rate is within the range expected for spontaneous discharge of an idioventricular focus (20 to 40/minute).

Discussion: The wide QRS complexes indicate abnormal ventricular activation. Only QRS durations of 0.10 sec or less are certain to be supraventricular, that is, to have originated above the His bundle branch point. Impulses formed below this site cause distorted QRS complexes because the activation follows an abnormal route. In such cases the impulse arises in one ventricle and activates the other ventricle sequentially—rather than simultaneously—across the septum via the muscular fibers. The conduction velocity is slower than normal, and the QRS duration increases. Both factors cause the wide and distorted QRS complexes seen in ventricular beats and rhythms.

56

Rate __180__ /min.   Rhythm __irregular__
QRS Duration __0.16–0.24__ s.   P-R Interval __absent__
AV Conduction Ratio __absent__

Interpretation: Ventricular tachycardia.

Rationale: The ventricular complexes are aberrantly shaped, have a variable R-R interval, and occur at a rate greatly exceeding 100/minute. Atrial action is missing; therefore, no AV relationship exists. This dysrhythmia consists of a string of

57

Rate __94__ /min.   Rhythm __regularly irregular__
PVC 0.16 s.
QRS Duration __sinus 0.8__ s.   P-R Interval __sinus 0.16__ s.
AV Conduction Ratio __1:1__

Interpretation: Sinus rhythm disrupted by frequent unifocal PVCs occurring about every fifth complex (ventricular quintigeminy).

Rationale: The sinus beats have ST segments that are displaced downward, and this distorts the QRS-T complexes. The PVCs can be recognized by the following:
• Wide and distorted QRS complexes
• Prematurity (early in R-R interval)
• Missing P waves
• T waves that are opposite in direction to abnormal R wave
• The coupling intervals of the PVCs to the preceding sinus beats are fixed

58

Rate __absent__ /min.   Rhythm __absent__
QRS Duration __absent__   P-R Interval __absent__
AV Conduction Ratio __absent__

Interpretation: Asystole with several low voltage complexes, possibly isolated P waves. Ventricular standstill exists.

Rationale: Except for the few positive deflections noted, asystole exists. The flat baseline is recorded because electrical activity fails to produce P-QRS-T wave complexes.

144

61

Rate __140__ /min. Rhythm __regular__
QRS Duration __0.34__ s. P-R Interval __absent__ s.
AV Conduction Ratio __absent__

Interpretation: **Ventricular tachycardia.**

Rationale: Regular ventricular activity is present with very wide (0.34 second) and bizarre QRS complexes. Atrial activity is missing. The dysrhythmia originates within the His-Purkinje system.

62

Rate __10__ /min. Rhythm __regular__
QRS Duration __0.36__ s. P-R Interval __absent__
AV Conduction Ratio __absent__

Interpretation: **Idioventricular (agonal) rhythm.**

Rationale: The ventricular activity shows large, bizarre, and very slow QRS complexes. Atrial activity is lacking. The rate of 20/minute is within the range expected for a ventricular focus (20 to 40). The bizarre QRS complex and prolonged duration attest to the abnormal ventricular activation. The lack of P waves eliminates the sinus node as pacemaker. Such low ectopic pacemakers are notoriously unstable and cannot generate an adequate cardiac output. The term agonal is applied to such dysrhythmias because they often degenerate in asystole within a short time.

59

Rate __106__ /min. Rhythm __irregular__
QRS Duration PVC 0.16 s. P-R Interval __0.16__ s.
AV Conduction Ratio __1:1__

Interpretation: **Sinus tachycardia with two uniformed PVCs.**

Rationale: The rhythm is regular except for the two early and wide QRS complexes. The remainder of the tracing is sinus because of the regular occurrence of normal P-QRS-T complexes. The two ectopic beats have wide and distorted QRS complexes. They occur early in the R-R interval. They lack P waves and are followed by compensatory pauses. They differ from typical PVCs in two ways: the T waves are not opposite the deflection of the QRS complexes, and their size is not taller than the normal beats.

60

Rate __absent__ /min. Rhythm __absent__
QRS Duration __absent__ P-R interval __absent__
AV Conduction Ratio __absent__

Interpretation: **Coarse ventricular fibrillation.**

Rationale: The waves have an amplitude of at least 5 mm. The findings are as follows:

- Ventricular activity is chaotic.
- Atrial activity is absent.
- AV conduction is absent.
- Pacemaker site: A reentry pattern has been established in the ventricular system.
- Mechanical activity is absent. Effective cardiac contraction can take place only when it is preceded by an orderly sequence of electrical stimulation.

145

63

Rate ___94___ /min. Rhythm ___irregular___
QRS Duration sinus 0.08 s. PVC 0.16 s. P-R Interval ___0.20___ s.
AV Conduction Ratio ___sinus: 1:1___

Interpretation: Sinus rhythm with frequent uniformed PVCs, which occur in a bigeminal pattern for a brief period (beats 7, 9, 11, and 13).

Rationale: The large and distorted aberrant beats (2, 7, 9, 11, 13) stick out during initial viewing of the strip. The PVCs disrupt the otherwise regular rhythm of the sinus complexes. The ectopic ventricular beats show wide QRS complexes, T waves that slope away from the abnormal QRS, absent P waves, and compensatory pauses. Each of the last four PVCs alternates with a sinus beat. Because all the PVCs have the same shape, they are called uniformed (or unifocal). Sinus rhythm is found in all other complexes. They have normal P-QRS-T waves and regular cycles.

64

Rate ___occasional___ /min. Rhythm ___absent___
QRS Duration ___0.28___ s. P-R Interval ___absent___
AV Conduction Ratio ___absent___

Interpretation: Asystole with a single agonal idioventricular complex.

Rationale: Ventricular activity is missing except for a single wide and distorted QRS complex that lacks a P wave. The rest of the tracing shows no electrical activity, reflected by an isoelectric baseline.

65

Rate ___100___ /min. Rhythm ___irregular___
QRS Duration sinus 0.10 s. PVC 0.12–0.20 s. P-R Interval ___0.16___ s.
AV Conduction Ratio ___1:1___

Interpretation: Sinus rhythm with multiformed PVCs. The first PVC is a fusion complex.

Rationale: Aside from the PVCs, the sinus rhythm is regular and shows normal P-QRS-T waves. The three premature beats (1, 8, and 11) have distorted QRS complexes, which differ from each other. The PVCs lack P waves except for beat 1, which is a fusion complex. **Fusion complexes** show characteristics of two pacemakers: P waves plus aberrant QRS complexes. A fusion complex results because the PVC occurs late in the R-R interval when the sinus node has already been able to depolarize the atria. The impulses from the sinus node and the retrograde depolarizing wave from the ventricles meet and cause the QRS to be narrower than ordinary PVCs. The pauses following the PVCs 1 and 3 are fully compensatory, but PVC 2 shows less than a complete pause.

Discussion: Even though most PVCs do show a compensatory pause, the pause may be less than or even greater than compensatory. A compensatory pause happens because a PVC makes the atrial tissue refractory without disturbing sinus rhythmicity. Thus, when the next sinus discharge occurs, it cannot be transmitted to the atrial tissue. When this occurs, the sinus node will wait until its next scheduled time to discharge. PVCs that show the atypical (less than compensatory) period happen because the retrograde conduction from the PVC is able to depolarize the SA node and this "resets" it. The sinus node will then fire in the time equivalent to one R-R cycle, causing a less than compensatory pause.

66

Rate __190__ /min. Rhythm __regular__
QRS Duration __0.24__ s. P-R Interval __absent__
AV Conduction Ratio __absent__

Interpretation: **Ventricular tachycardia.**

Rationale: The ventricular activity is rapid and is composed of wide and bizarre QRS complexes. Atrial activity is hidden among the QRSs.

Discussion: This rhythm resembles a string of PVCs because this is exactly what we have. The rapid ectopic rhythm is due to either enhanced automaticity of a ventricular focus or a reentry pattern leading to repetitive activation.

Terminology: This tracing is one example of a group of related disturbances termed **tachydysrhythmias** or **tachyarrhythmias**. It pertains to those rhythms, regardless of where the pacemaker is, occurring at ventricular rates over 100/min. For instance, it includes sinus, AV junctional, PSVTs, atrial fibrillation, and atrial flutter, as well as those of ventricular origin.

67

Rate __occasional__ /min. Rhythm __absent__
QRS Duration __0.20__ s. P-R Interval __absent__
AV Conduction Ratio __absent__

Interpretation: **A single agonal idioventricular beat is followed by asystole.**

Rationale: Ventricular activity consists of one wide, bizarrely shaped QRS. P waves are missing.

68

Rate __absent__ /min. Rhythm __absent__
QRS Duration __Absent__ P-R Interval __absent__
AV Conduction Ratio __absent__

Interpretation: **Coarse ventricular fibrillation.**

Rationale: No QRS complexes, P waves, or P-R intervals exist. Only a wavy distorted baseline appears.

69

Rate __180__ /min. Rhythm __regular__
QRS Duration __0.24__ s. P-R Interval __absent__
AV Conduction Ratio __absent__

Interpretation: **Ventricular tachycardia.**

Rationale: We find wide, distorted QRS complexes occurring at a rapid rate. The regular ventricular activity appears similar to a string of PVCs; this is characteristic of this ventricular dysrhythmia. Atrial activity is absent, as P waves are not seen. Ventricular tachycardias occur in a range of 100 to 200/minute, usually averaging around 150/minute.

70

Rate __100__ /min. Rhythm __irregular__
QRS Duration sinus 0.12 s. PVC 0.16 s. P-R Interval __0.20__ s.
AV Conduction Ratio __1:1__

Interpretation: **Sinus rhythm with frequent uniformed PVCs, two occurring in a couplet.**

Rationale: The rhythmicity of sinus rhythm is disordered by the PVCs. Beats 3 and 4 show two consecutive (back to back) PVCs, an ominous warning that more malignant dysrhythmias may follow.

The third PVC is beat 13. PVCs have wide and distorted QRS complexes, while those of sinus origin are narrow. Atrial activity is absent in PVCs and is present just before the QRS complexes of the sinus beats. The conduction ratio is 1:1 for the sinus and absent for PVCs.

Discussion: Salvos of PVCs cause much more concern than isolated PVCs because they are considered potentially more harmful. Such bursts often precipitate ventricular tachycardia, which is a sustained rhythm of PVCs. Salvos are often considered warning signs of potential life-threatening dysrhythmias. In contrast to occasional PVCs, which are often found in healthy individuals, salvos occur when there is underlying disease.

71

Rate 47 /min. Rhythm irregular
QRS Duration 0.28 s. P-R Interval absent
AV Conduction Ratio absent

Interpretation: **Idioventricular rhythm.**

Rationale: The rhythm of ventricular activity is irregular. The QRS complexes are wide and distorted, hardly resembling the tall and pointed ventricular activation complex. T waves are missing because the ST segment and T waves have merged with the QRS complexes to form the wide complexes. Because P waves are missing, the pacemaker cannot be in the SA node. Heart activity is controlled by a pacemaker originating low in the ventricles. It is emerging from within the His-Purkinje fibers to stimulate a dying heart. Notoriously unreliable, the idioventricular focus usually fails and asystole follows.

72

Rate 63 /min. Rhythm irregular
QRS Duration sinus 0.08 s. / PVC 0.16 s. P-R Interval 0.16 s.
AV Conduction Ratio 1:1

Interpretation: **Sinus rhythm with a PVC (beat 3). A postextrasystolic pause follows the PVC, which is terminated by a junctional complex. The PVC strikes during the preceding T wave, the so-called "R-on-T" phenomenon.**

Rationale: The ventricular rhythm is disturbed by the early, wide QRS complex. The sinus activity consists of normal P-QRS-T complexes. The junctional complex is missing a P wave and has a QRS similar to the sinus beats.

Discussion: **R-on-T premature complexes** have been associated with an increased risk of ventricular fibrillation. The upstroke of the T wave is called the vulnerable period because a stimulus may cause life-threatening dysrhythmias. The ventricular fibers are in different states of repolarization during the vulnerable phase. A full compensatory pause is not observed because the long R-R intervals from the low heart rate allows a junctional escape complex to occur.

73

Rate 190 /min. Rhythm irregular
QRS Duration 0.16–0.24 s. P-R Interval absent
AV Conduction Ratio absent

Interpretation: **Ventricular tachycardia.**

Rationale: The rapid rate of QRS complexes shows slightly irregular R-R intervals. The QRS complexes are wide and bizarre. Several isolated P waves are scattered among the QRS complexes.

74

Rate __absent__ /min. Rhythm __absent__ P-R Interval __absent__
QRS Duration __absent__ AV Conduction Ratio __absent__

Interpretation: **Coarse ventricular fibrillation.**

Rationale: No organized electrical activity exists, only a distorted zigzag of the baseline.

75

Rate __50__ /min. Rhythm __irregular__
                sinus 0.08 s.
QRS Duration __PVC 0.16__ s. P-R Interval __0.16__ s.
AV Conduction Ratio __1:1__

Interpretation: **Sinus bradycardia with one PVC striking the T wave, termed an "R-on-T" phenomenon.**

Rationale: The sinus rhythm occurs at a bradycardiac rate. Sinus beats have normal P-QRS-T configurations. The PVC (beat 5) occurs prematurely—so early that it lands on the T wave of the prior sinus beat. This happens during the so-called "vulnerable period," meaning that a PVC has greater likelihood of initiating ventricular fibrillation than if it occurred after the T wave. The PVC has a wide QRS complex and T wave, having an opposite deflection than the abnormal QRS complex.

76

Rate __absent__ /min. Rhythm __absent__ P-R Interval __absent__
QRS Duration __absent__ AV Conduction Ratio __absent__

Interpretation: **Coarse ventricular fibrillation.**

Rationale:
- Ventricular activity is absent.
- Atrial activity is absent.
- Atrioventricular relationship does not exist.
- Chaotic baseline movement.

77

Rate __94__ /min. Rhythm __irregular__
                sinus 0.10 s.
QRS Duration __PVC 0.24__ s. P-R Interval __0.20__ s.
AV Conduction Ratio __1:1__

Interpretation: **Sinus rhythm with ventricular trigeminy. (Every third beat is a PVC.)**

Rationale: The PVCs show the characteristic wide, distorted QRS complexes, absent P waves, and T waves sloping opposite to the QRS complex. The regular occurrence of a PVC after two sinus beats causes the grouped beating. The sinus beats have normal P-QRS-T waves and 1:1 AV conduction.

78

Rate __180__ /min. Rhythm __regular__
QRS Duration __0.20–0.28__ s. P-R Interval __absent__
AV Conduction Ratio __absent__

Interpretation: **Ventricular tachycardia.**

Rationale: This rapid regular rhythm looks like a string of PVCs. The QRS complexes are wide and distorted. P waves are not visible.

148

79

Rate **20** /min. Rhythm **regular** P-R Interval **absent**

QRS Duration **0.40** s.

AV Conduction Ratio **absent**

Interpretation: **Idioventricular rhythm.**

Rationale: The QRS complexes are distorted and occur at a very slow rate. Their bizarre shapes do not resemble the sharp deflections typical of ventricular complexes. P waves are absent. The small positive deflections just before the Q waves are the initial portions of the QRS complex.

80

Rate **84** /min. Rhythm **regularly irregular**

QRS Duration **PVC 0.16** s. P-R Interval **0.20** s. sinus 0.08 s.

AV Conduction Ratio **1:1**

Interpretation: **Sinus rhythm with ventricular bigeminy. (Every other beat is a PVC.)**

Rationale: The ventricular rhythm is regularly irregular with grouped beating. The R-R intervals show a pattern of long-short, long-short, etc. This is due to the early PVC coupled to the compensatory pause. The QRS complexes of the sinus beats are narrow, while those of the PVCs are wide. Sinus beats have P waves before the QRS complexes with fixed P-R intervals. The PVCs lack P waves because they originate in the ventricles.

81

Rate **50** /min. Rhythm **regular** P-R Interval **absent**

QRS Duration **0.24–0.28** s.

AV Conduction Ratio **absent**

Interpretation: **Idioventricular rhythm.**

Rationale: The ventricular activity is characterized by wide and bizarre QRS complexes occurring at a slow rate. The ST-T waves merge and distort the complex. Regular P waves are missing; however, the deflections between the first three QRS complexes may represent some isolated atrial activity. Idioventricular fibers usually depolarize at rates between 20 to 40/minute; this tracing shows an accelerated rate.

Chapter Five
ARTIFICIAL PACEMAKERS, ARTIFACTS, AND RESUSCITATION RHYTHMS

ARTIFICIAL PACEMAKERS AND PACEMAKER-RELATED ECG RHYTHMS

Pacemakers are usually utilized to prevent undue pauses or slowing of the ventricular rate. All use a generator/power pack, inserted at a distance from the heart (usually subcutaneously), and connecting electrode leads to the heart which stimulate the chambers and may serve to sense the underlying cardiac rhythm. Over the past 20 years we have seen dramatic improvements in battery life, electrode durability, programming capabilities of the generator, miniaturization of the components, and dependability.

TYPES OF PACEMAKER SYSTEMS

The early pacemaker systems used in the 1950s were crude by today's standards; electrode leads were placed externally across the chest, and the heart was stimulated by uncomfortable, even painful electrical discharges. During the 1960s, electrode leads were attached to the epicardium directly and were stimulated by an external power pack, with the leads passing percutaneously. Later, the battery/generator was miniaturized and placed subcutaneously with no external wiring visible. Also in the 1960s, the transvenous lead system was developed, utilizing electrode leads that were inserted into a peripheral vein, such as the antecubital, subclavian, or femoral. The electrode was then advanced into the right ventricle, where it became fixed among the muscular trabeculae at the apex and stimulated the endocardium. This transvenous lead could be powered by an external generator, as a temporary pacing system, or could be attached to a subcutaneous generator for long term pacing. Nowadays, most permanent pacing is accomplished by the latter transvenous lead system, with the generator implanted under the skin in the pectoral region, and with the venous system entered via the subclavian or jugular veins (Figs. 5–1 and 5–2).

COMMON VENTRICULAR STIMULATING SYSTEMS

Basic Characteristics of Paced Complexes

Typically, one sees (1) a spike, (2) ectopic QRS-T complex, and (3) independence from atrial activity (Fig. 5–3).

1. **The spike is a narrow deflection,** due to the electronic stimulus delivered. Its amplitude is variable. All are less than 5 mm with bipolar pacemaker electrodes. Some are large, between 5 and 50 mm, in unipolar systems, although particular leads may show a small amplitude spike.
2. **The QRS-T complex is ectopic-like.** It is wide and bizarre, resembling a PVC, which is also a depolarization originating in the ventricle. There is usually a left bundle branch block (LBBB) pattern,

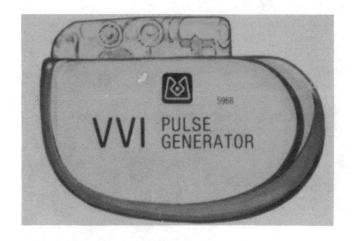

FIGURE 5–1. Programmable pulse generator. (Courtesy of Medtronic, Inc.)

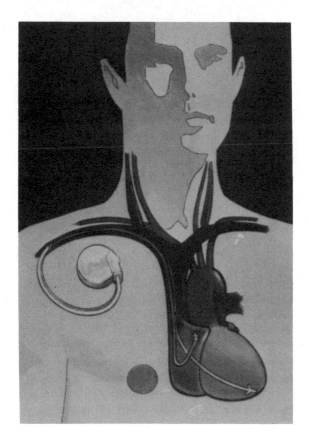

FIGURE 5–2. Cardiac leads in both the atrium and ventricle enable a dual chamber pacemaker to sense and pace in both heart chambers. (Courtesy of Medtronic, Inc.)

for the following reason: The majority of pacemaker electrode systems are transvenous and terminate within the right ventricle. When stimulated, the depolarization wave propagates from the right ventricle to the left ventricle, producing a LBBB-like complex. Sometimes, if an electrode tip stimulates the left ventricle first, as with the leads affixed to the heart during cardiac surgery, the QRS pattern is right bundle branch block (RBBB).

3. **The stimulated ventricular activity is usually independent from atrial activity,** that is, AV dissociation is produced. The atria are cued by the sinus node, or by other ectopic foci, such as atrial fibrillation or atrial flutter, while the ventricles are cued by the pacemaker—not related to the atrial activity. The cardiac output is usually adequate, even without proper synchronization between atrial and ventricular activity, although there are conditions in which the cardiac output improves with the usual AV sequential relationship (see Figs. 5–4 and 5–5).

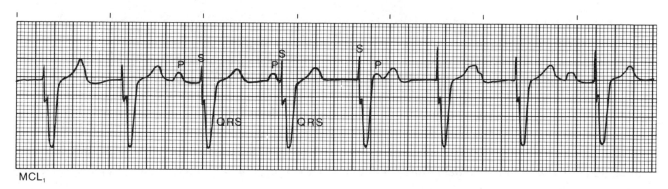

MCL₁

FIGURE 5–3. Pacemaker-induced ventricular rhythm at 72 beats per minute with underlying complete heart block. Each QRS complex is preceded by a pacemaker spike (S). The atrial depolarizations (P) occur at 58/min, march through the QRS complexes, and are not associated with the ventricular depolarizations.

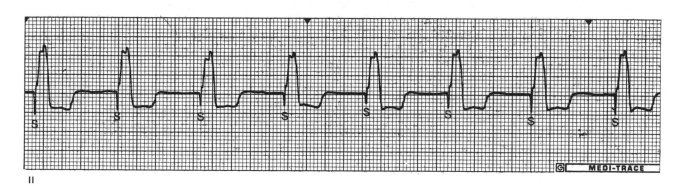

II

FIGURE 5–4. Artificially paced rhythm. S is pacer spike.

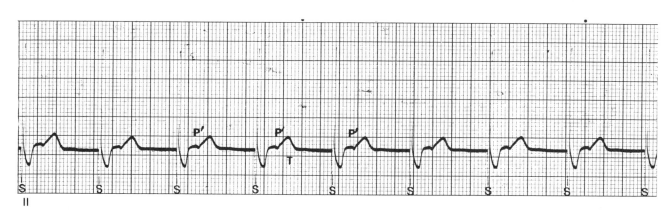

II

FIGURE 5–5. Artificially paced rhythm. S is pacer spike, and P′ is the retrogradely conducted atrial depolarization.

THE CODING SYSTEM

Technologic advances have led to the development of an assortment of pacemaker systems, due to improved ventricular and atrial electrodes, microchip circuitry, and long lasting power sources, usually made of lithium. Demand pacemakers may be triggered as well as inhibited; atria may be paced; ventricular pacing can be cued to the atrial rate; and both atria and ventricles can be sequentially paced. In addition, pacemaker generators can be programmed at different rates, sensing thresholds, power outputs, and the mode of operation can be changed at will—all noninvasively, via radio frequency signals!

A three-letter code has been developed to briefly describe the various combinations available:

First letter—**chamber paced:** V (ventricle), A (atrium), D (double)
Second letter—**chamber sensed:** V (ventricle), A (atrium), D (double), 0 (none)
Third letter—**mode of response** to sensing: T (triggered), I (inhibited), D (double) (both responses), 0 (none)

According to this code, fixed-rate ventricular pacing would be coded V-0-0; and demand, noncompetitive ventricular pacing, with output inhibited by sensed ventricular signals, would be coded V-V-I.

Pacing Modes: Fixed Rate/Asynchronous (V-0-0) and Demand/Noncompetitive (V-I-I) Pacing

The preceding examples demonstrate totally paced ventricular rhythms. No conducted or spontaneous ectopic ventricular activity is occurring. In **asynchronous or fixed rate pacing** (V-0-0 coded) the patient's ventricle is stimulated at a preset fixed rate, usually between 70 and 80/min. This is a very basic configuration and by and large has been supplemented by more sophisticated devices. It is still used occasionally in elderly patients with chronic complete heart block.

Often, in fact usually, patients with complete AV heart block or profound sinus bradycardia will have only intermittent ventricular bradycardia. At other times, they show the capacity to produce and conduct atrial impulses to ventricles or to have spontaneous ventricular ectopic activity. This can lead to competition with the pacemaker-induced ventricular rhythm, as shown in Figure 5–6, and is why they have been replaced by the more complex demand pacing systems.

Such competition is undesirable, as pacemaker stimuli firing during the T wave of a prior QRS-T complex may produce ventricular tachycardia or fibrillation. There is a vulnerable period for certain hearts when certain stimuli occurring during the repolarization period will provoke sustained ventricular tachycardia or ventricular fibrillation. This is a special threat during ischemia, electrolyte imbalance, and digitalis toxicity.

To prevent this disastrous event, **demand pacemaker systems** (coded V-V-I) were developed. The intrinsic electrical activity of the ventricles is sensed. The generator fires at predetermined intervals unless inhibited by a QRS complex sensed during that interval, and this then resets the timing interval. The pacemaker may thus be on "standby" status when the ventricular rate is adequate—i.e., during NSR or atrial fibrillation with normal ventricular rate. It will "fire"—stimulating the ventricle—only when a pause occurs that exceeds the limits of the set interval. Function in the standby, demand mode may extend battery life, as little electrical energy is required for the sensing and inhibition operations.

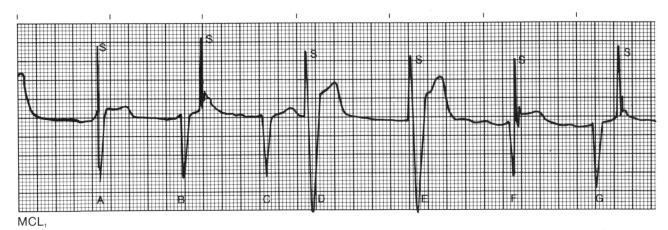

MCL₁

FIGURE 5–6. Fixed rate pacemaker competing with normal sinus rhythm. Complexes A, B, and C represent normal sinus rhythm with first degree AV block at a rate of 70/min. Pacemaker stimuli (S) are firing at 57/min. No QRS is provoked by the stimulus firing during beat A. The stimulus after beat B provokes a small afterpotential but no significant depolarization. The stimulus after beat C occurs after the absolute refractory period, and does provoke a QRS complex D. Beat E is also a QRS complex stimulated by a pacemaker spike. Beats F and G represent normal sinus rhythm, each followed by a pacemaker spike ineffectively occurring during its absolute refractory period.

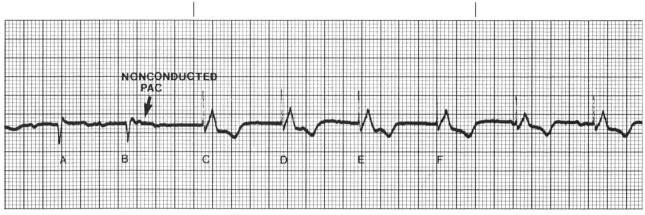

MCL₁

FIGURE 5–7. A nonconducted PAC disrupts normal sinus rhythm and is followed by a pause that is long enough to allow the demand pacemaker to fire. Complexes A and B represent normal sinus rhythm with first degree AV block. Beat B is followed by a nonconducted PAC, which produces a pause after which complexes C, D, E, and F are stimulated by the demand pacemaker at 72/min, which was inhibited by faster rates of conducted ventricular depolarization.

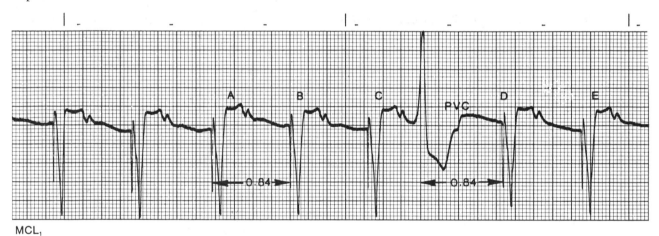

MCL₁

FIGURE 5–8. Sinus suppression and demand pacemaker discharge. A PVC inhibits and resets the pacemaker. Complexes A, B, and C are paced, following pacemaker spikes at 72/min, with an interval of 0.84 sec between spikes. A PVC occurs after complex C, which inhibits the pacemaker, resetting it to fire 0.84 sec later, stimulating beat D.

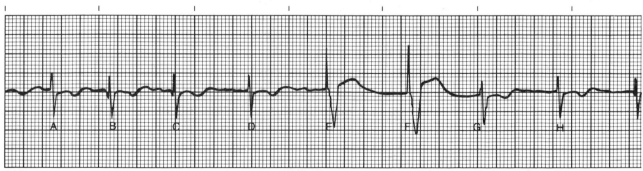

MCL₁

FIGURE 5–9. Demand pacemaker at 72/min with underlying atrial fibrillation. Beats A, B, C, and D are conducted from the atrial fibrillation. A pause occurs after beat D and is terminated by pacemaker-induced beats E and F at 72/min. Beats G and H are intrinsically conducted ventricular complexes occurring at a rate faster than 72/min, inhibiting the pacemaker.

Demand (V-V-I) pacemakers are by and large the most commonly implanted. They are used in patients who have Stokes-Adams attacks (loss of consciousness due to intermittent heart block) or intermittent sinus node dysfunction. These units pace from the right ventricle, sense from the right ventricle, and are inhibited by the patient's intrinsic electrical activity if the patient's rate exceeds a preset escape rate. When the patient's heart rate falls below the preset rate the pacemaker turns on and artificially stimulates the ventricle at a preset rate. For example, the pacemaker may be set to begin pacing when the patient's heart rate falls below 60 beats/min. The most advanced pacemaker systems can now change the preset rate to meet the patient's physiologic demands. They react to body motion, pectoral muscle discharges, blood pH, or body temperature, increasing the minimum rate as needed (see Figs. 5-7, 5-8, and 5-9).

LESS COMMONLY EMPLOYED PACING SYSTEMS

Atrial Timed Ventricular Pacing (V-A-T)

Some patients require a properly timed atrial contraction before ventricular contraction for optimal cardiac output; they may also need to vary the ventricular rate to meet the body's hemodynamic needs. Atrial timed ventricular pacing provides these advantages for patients in heart block.

One electrode terminates in the right atrium, sensing atrial activity (P waves). Another electrode has its distal lead in the right ventricle, stimulating that chamber about 20 msec (0.20 sec) after the atrial depolarization is sensed. Thus, the usual sequence of P→QRS-T is maintained (Fig. 5-10). This program has a lower rate limit, at which the ventricle will be paced if the atrial rate declines markedly. It also has an upper rate limit, above which it will stimulate the ventricle to follow every other P wave in case an atrial tachycardia develops.

Atrial Demand Pacing (A-A-I)

Some patients have a sick sinus syndrome, with episodic slowing of the sinus node, pauses, and syncope. If AV conduction is intact, then an atrial demand pacing system may be utilized. Here the lead is fixed in the right atrium, sensing atrial depolarizations, which inhibit pacing discharges—unless the sinoatrial rate falls below a lower rate limit, at which rate atrial pacing will occur.

Although sensible in theory, this program has several practical drawbacks. Atrial electrodes have until recently been unstable, often slipping out of contact with the atrial endocardium, resulting in failure to sense and failure to pace. Modern atrial electrode design incorporates a spring-like "J" design, tensing the tip in the atrial appendage. It also includes a flanged or tined tip, which entraps itself in the atrial wall. Both modifications minimize atrial lead displacement. There is also the relatively common problem of undependable AV conduction, found in 30 to 50 percent of patients with sick sinus syndrome, in whom pure atrial pacing is inadequate. For these reasons, atrial demand pacing is used much less frequently than ventricular demand pacing (Fig. 5-11).

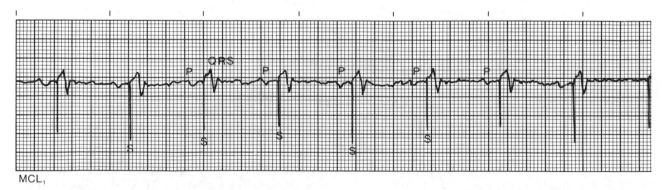

MCL₁

FIGURE 5-10. Atrial triggered ventricular pacing. The atrium is intrinsically depolarized (P waves) at 77/min. Each P wave is followed 0.20 sec later by a pacemaker spike (S), which stimulates ventricular depolarization (QRS).

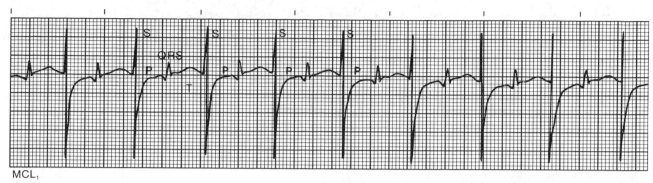

FIGURE 5–11. Atrial pacing. The large spikes (S) are unipolar pacemaker spikes stimulating the atrium, resulting in P waves (P). These then conduct to the ventricle in the normal fashion, producing QRS-T complexes.

Atrioventricular Sequential Dual-Chamber Pacing: (D-D-D)

The most sophisticated of the modern pacemakers has leads in both the right atrium and the right ventricle. Both leads can sense and pace, with pacing inhibited or triggered by sensed impulses. Usually this system is programmed to sense atrial depolarizations and to stimulate the ventricles after an appropriate "atrioventricular (AV) interval." However, if the sinoatrial rate slows excessively, then the atrium is paced, following the "AV interval," by ventricular pacing. Upper and lower rate limits can be established. This pacing system has greater energy drain, more complexity, greater likelihood of lead displacement, and higher cost than the traditional ventricular demand pacemaker systems (Fig. 5–12).

Emergency Pacemaker Systems

Transvenous pacemaker. This system consists of a long pacemaking cable lead which can be passed through a large bore needle into a central or peripheral vein. The usual site is via the left subclavian or the right internal jugular vein. The leads are connected to an external pulse generator, which can be programmed to function as a V-0-0 or V-V-I pacemaker. Because the electrode is floated into position in the apex of the right ventricle, blind passage requires adequate cardiac output to float the catheter downstream to the proper location.

Transthoracic pacing electrode. In cardiac arrest situations a transthoracic pacemaker may be the only route by which emergency pacing can be established. This system consists of a catheter electrode system that is passed into the right ventricle through a cardiac needle. Cardiac puncture is performed via the subxiphoid approach into the right ventricle. The catheter is connected to the same external pulse generator used in the transvenous pacemaker system. This system allows rapid institution of pacing in the cardiac arrest situation but entails the hazards of cardiac puncture.

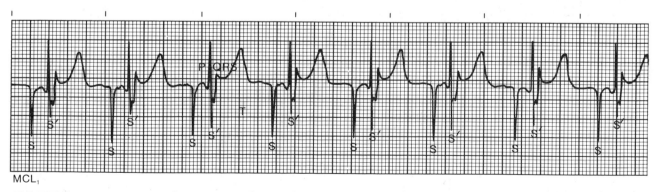

FIGURE 5–12. AV sequential pacing. S is the atrial pacemaker spike, followed by atrial depolarization (P). There is then a spike (S′) fired into the ventricle, producing a QRS ventricular depolarization.

Transcutaneous pacing systems. The original external pacing electrodes and pulse generator for external application to the chest wall were abandoned because they caused painful shocks that were intolerable to the awake patient and because these systems wcrc unreliable pacing systems. Recently this external pacing system has been redesigned to improve its effectiveness and to reduce the discomfort to the patient. The system, termed a transcutaneous pacemaker, is currently available from a number of manufacturers. Some models are designed to only pace asynchronously while others have a demand mode. In some devices the transcutaneous pacemaker is combined with a monitor defibrillator. These devices have been used both in prehospital care and in hospitalized patients. The device is remarkably simple to use and appears to be effective in temporary pacing of patients with life-threatening bradycardias. It, unfortunately, is of minimal utility in patients who are in cardiac arrest due to unconvertible ventricular fibrillation or asystole.

EVALUATION AND MANAGEMENT OF A PATIENT WITH A PACEMAKER

The presence of a pacemaker does not change any of the basic resuscitation guidelines or protocols. Thus, defibrillation should be performed in the same manner and for the same criteria as that used for patients without an implanted pacemaker. Many patients who have had pacemakers implanted have cardiovascular disease and can present with an acute myocardial infarction or with an anginal attack. Their treatment is also identical to that for patients with similar presenting complaints who do not have an implanted pacemaker. In addition, patients with pacemaker implants can present with specific problems related to pacemaker dysfunction. A frequent clinical problem is the evaluation of a syncopal episode in a patient with a pacemaker to determine whether it is due to pacemaker failure or another intercurrent process.

Every patient with a pacemaker implant is given an information card upon discharge from the hospital. The card identifies the implanted unit, gives the date of insertion, and notes the parameters of sensing and pacing. It also provides a hot-line telephone number for emergency consultation with the manufacturer of the devices. The patient should carry this card at all times. Patients with pacemakers are followed by periodic telephone telemetry monitoring of the patient's ECG—usually at 1 month intervals.

PACEMAKER DYSFUNCTION AND MAGNET PATTERNS

An intact pacemaker system is complex, including the power source, sensing circuits, stimulating circuits, reprogramming circuits, the electrode leads, and the myocardial characteristics at the site of electrical contact. In addition, the system is affected by electromagnetic interference from nearby generators, such as large microwave ovens or motors, and also by skeletal myopotentials in the active or tremulous patient. Pacing failure can occur at any site, and is reflected in the ECG rhythm pattern.

Interpretation is confused by some of the peculiarities of normal functioning of particular varieties of pacemakers, which can mislead inexperienced observers. Sometimes the pacemaker activity is not evident in demand systems, when the patient's "own" conducted ventricular rate exceeds the pacemaker rate and inhibits its firing. In order to provide testing, a reed switch is employed which can be activated by a magnet held over the pacemaker outside the chest. This switch then temporarily converts the pacer system to another mode, which reveals the pacing activity.

Conversion of Demand System to Fixed Rate Pacing

Most often, the magnet converts the pacemaker from a demand, QRS-inhibited system, to a fixed rate pacemaker. This reverts back to the demand mode when the magnet is removed. The ECG during the magnet phase shows three sorts of QRS complexes:

- The patient's own conducted QRS complex
- Pacemaker stimulated QRS complexes
- Hybrids—fusion beats—due to the simultaneous occurrence of the patient's own conducted beats plus a pacemaker spike and its stimulated QRS

After 4 to 7 years, as the battery becomes depleted, the pacing rate in the free running and magnet modes slows down, thereby signaling the need for generator replacement (Fig. 5–13A and B).

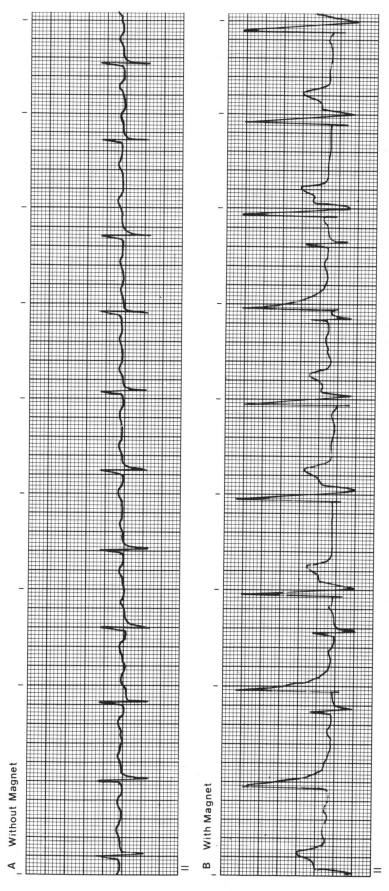

A Without Magnet

B With Magnet

FIGURE 5–13. The function of the QRS-inhibited ventricular pacemaker is tested by application of a magnet. The intrinsic normal sinus rhythm of the 75/min prevails in the QRS-inhibited mode. On application of the magnet, a paced rhythm emerges at 60/min, in competition with the intrinsic sinus rhythm for ventricular capture. (From Morse, D, Steiner, RM, Parsonnet, V (eds): A Guide to Cardiac Pacemakers. FA Davis, Philadelphia, 1983.)

Conversion of Demand System to Faster Demand Pacing

Some brands of demand pacemakers respond to the magnet by increasing the demand pacing rate, for example, from the usual 72/minute to 100/minute. Although the pacemaker might still be inhibited by the patient's own ventricular rate, it is unlikely that the patient will have a tachycardia—over 100/minute—at rest (see Fig. 5–14A and B).

Pacemaker Dysfunction—Failure to Stimulate

In this condition, pacemaker spikes are seen **not** to be followed by ectopic-appearing complexes. The patient's underlying rhythm can be recognized as well. Causes of failure to capture are:

- Depletion, but not total absence, of battery energy
- Fractured lead wire
- Displaced lead wire (out of the ventricle or, with atrial leads, out of the atrium)
- Myocardial fibrosis at the electrode contact site, raising the threshold for electrical stimulation

It can sometimes be treated by increasing the generator current output by noninvasive programming (Fig. 5–15).

Pacemaker Dysfunction—Failure to Sense

A pacing system may fail to sense a conducted or spontaneous complex, although it maintains normal stimulating function. In the most commonly employed system, the ventricular inhibited, demand system

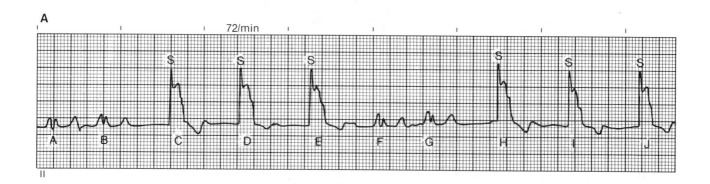

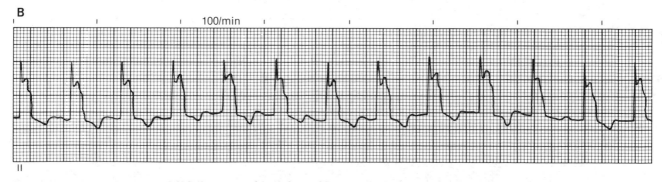

FIGURE 5–14. A, Note atrial fibrillation, with conducted beats in A, B, F, and G. After pauses, the demand pacemaker is activated, producing beats C, D, E, H, I, and J at a rate of 72/min. B, With the magnet applied, the pacing rate is now 100. This is an acceleration of the demand mode (V-V-I) and if any spontaneously conducted or ectopic QRS complexes were noted, the pacemaker would have sensed them and then recycled.

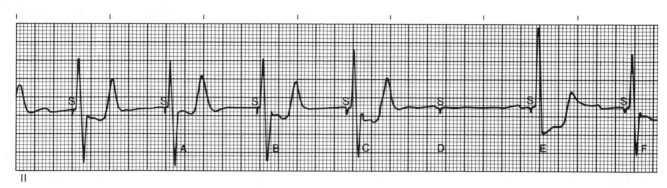

FIGURE 5–15. Failure to stimulate. Note the pacemaker spikes (S) at 62/min. QRS complexes A, B, C, and F are stimulated by the pacemaker spike. At site D, the spike is not followed by a QRS-T complex, representing failure to stimulate. Beat E has a different QRS complex and, although following a pacemaker spike, it is probably an escape, not a paced, beat.

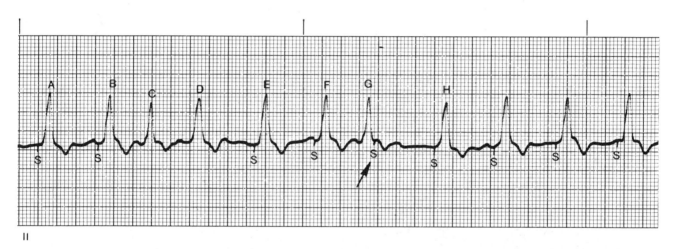

FIGURE 5–16. Sensing failure. Complexes A, B, E, F, H, and thereafter are all paced beats, each QRS complex following a small pacemaker spike. Beats C, D, and G are conducted, probably from atrial fibrillation, with a QRS configuration slightly different from the paced ventricular complexes. Note that the pacemaker spike is inhibited by beats C and D. However, beat G shows the pacemaker spike (↑) after the R wave, clearly not inhibited by the QRS that should have been sensed. The next pacemaker spike at H is on time.

(V-V-I), this appears as failure of the pacemaker to be inhibited by a QRS complex. The pacemaker behaves like a fixed rate system, not aware of the patient's own ventricular activity (Fig. 5–16). This state can be caused by

- Myocardial damage or fibrosis, with the production of very small QRS complexes—too small to be sensed
- Circuitry dysfunction—with inability to process the QRS signal in the generator

Sometimes, the pacemaker can be reprogrammed to lower the sensing threshold to correct the problem.

Pacemaker Dysfunction—Runaway Pacemaker

One variety of pacemaker dysfunction encountered 20 years ago but now fortunately very uncommon is runaway pacemaker (Fig. 5–17). Breakdowns in the circuitry led to rapid firing of the pacemaker—up to 250 to 300 beats/minute—with resultant cardiovascular collapse. Design improvements with secure rate limits have subsequently eliminated this potential disaster.

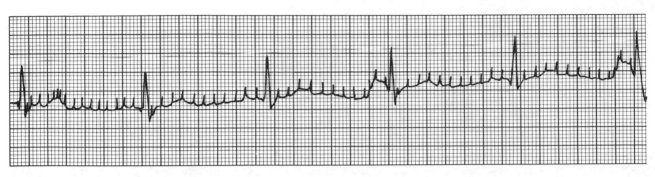

FIGURE 5–17. Pacemaker "runaway." Shows very rapid pacer spikes with no ventricular capture. (From Morse, D, Steiner, RM, and Parsonnet, V (eds): A Guide to Cardiac Pacemakers. FA Davis, Philadelphia, 1983.)

Pacemaker System Dysfunction—Endless Loop Tachycardia

A final example of dysfunction is the consequence of mistiming in atrial-ventricular sequential, dual channel pacemakers. It is usually precipitated by a PVC with retrograde conduction up the His bundle/ AV node structures to depolarize the atrium. Such a retrograde P wave is then sensed by the atrial sensing circuit and results in ventricular stimulation (after the AV sequencing delay). The stimulated ventricular depolarization again travels retrogradely to the atrium, where it is again sensed and triggers a ventricular stimuli. This perpetuation of impulses results in an endless loop tachycardia. Luckily, it can be interrupted and prevented readily by noninvasive reprogramming measures (Fig. 5–18).

AUTOMATIC IMPLANTED CARDIOVERTER-DEFIBRILLATORS

While pacemakers are traditionally employed to treat episodic or sustained bradycardias, sophisticated models may also be used to manage tachydysrhythmias. One variety can sense tachycardias exceeding a predetermined rate, and automatically fire a burst of rapid pacing stimuli, which can interrupt the ectopic focus. Another can be activated by the patient sensing his or her own rapid heart action, via a radio-induction coil positioned over the implanted unit, triggered by a switch in the patient's pocket. Here, too, a burst of pacing can terminate the dysrhythmia.

The most dramatic pacing modification is the automatic implantable cardioverter-defibrillator (AICD) unit that consists of a pulse generator sealed in titanium and implanted subcutaneously in the periumbilical area. Three leads are employed: one positioned transvenously in the low superior vena cava near the right atrium; one in the right ventricle; and a flexible rectangular patch electrode sewn over the apex. A thoracotomy is necessary for installation. Ventricular tachycardia or fibrillation is identified by a double system, recognizing both rapid rate and abnormal shape. Then the capacitor is charged to 720 volts and a 25 joule pulse is delivered to the patient. The second, third, and fourth pulses can be delivered approximately every 30 seconds if needed. Hundreds of successful reversions have been documented and the mortality rate of patients with refractory life-threatening ventricular tachyarrhythmias has been improved. Of course, complications of thoracotomy, infections, lead displacement, and spurious discharges (especially during atrial dysrhythmias) have all been encountered.

ECG ARTIFACTS

It is important to be able to recognize artifacts, which are manmade sources of ECG interference, because several of them closely resemble dysrhythmias. In the sample tracings (Figs. 5–19 to 5–22) for example, the artifact caused by loose or displaced electrodes closely mimics ventricular fibrillation. The example showing the effects of patient movement caused by parkinsonian tremors distorts the NSR and makes it seem like atrial fibrillation exists. Most of the sources of artifact alter the normally flat (isoelec-

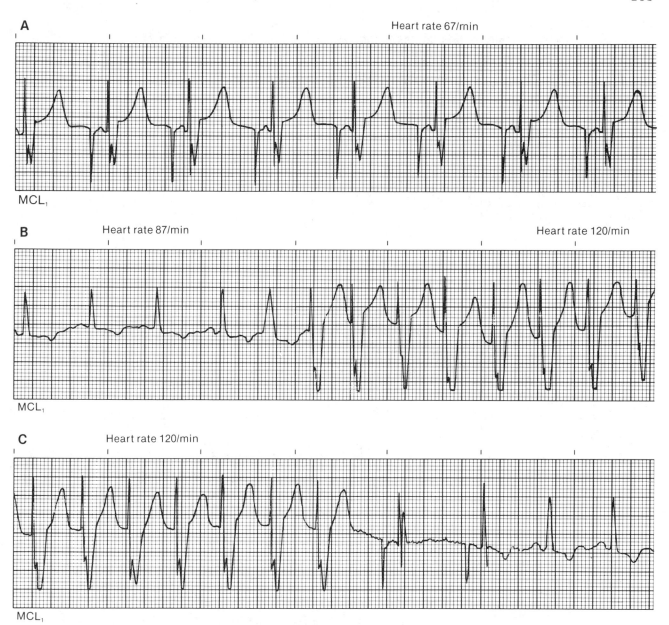

FIGURE 5–18. Endless loop tachycardia. Strip *A* shows AV sequential pacing at a heart rate of 67/min. There are pacemaker spikes before each P wave and each QRS complex. In strip *B*, the initial rhythm is normal sinus rhythm at 87/min. The fifth beat is a PVC with retrograde conduction to the atrium, which is then sensed by the atrial sensing electrode, followed by a ventricular spike and QRS complex. This, in turn, is associated with a retrograde atrial depolarization, not evident on the surface ECG recording, that is sensed by the atrial lead and is followed by another ventricular complex, producing a regular tachycardia at the rate of 120/min. Finally, in strip *C*, the tachycardia terminates, either because of failure to produce or failure to sense a retrograde atrial activation, and the rhythm returns to AV sequential pacing for two beats and then to normal sinus rhythm.

tric) baseline between cardiac cycles and make interpretation difficult. The following list describes common sources of artifact:

1. Improper grounding—stray electrical currents create 60 cycles/second interference.
2. Patient or cable movement (shivering, seizures, etc.).
3. Dried out or inadequate conducting jelly.
4. Cracked electrode/lead cable.

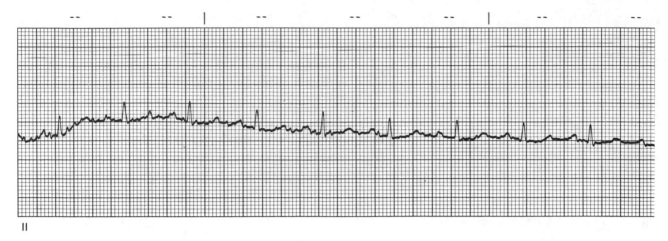

FIGURE 5–19. Regular sinus rhythm distorted by musical tremor artifact.

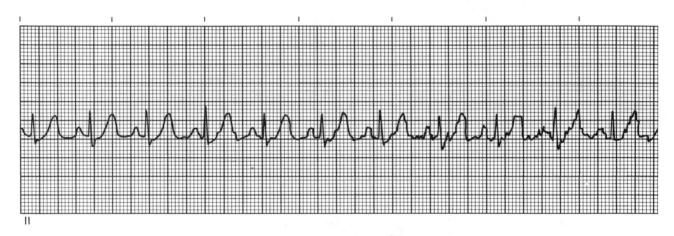

FIGURE 5–20. Movement artifact superimposed on NSR.

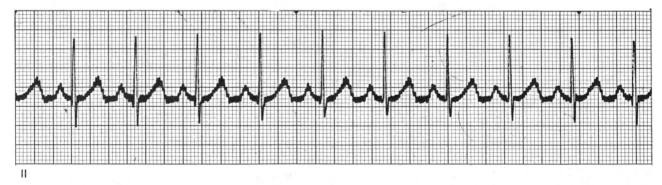

FIGURE 5–21. Artifact caused by electrical interference from an improperly grounded ECG machine.

5. Standardization/calibration signal.
6. Artificial pacemaker signals—ventricular impulse generators have spikes before the QRS complexes, atrial impulse generators have spikes before the P waves, and AV sequential impulse generators have a spike before the P wave and the QRS complex. (See discussion of artificial pacemakers later in this chapter for examples.)

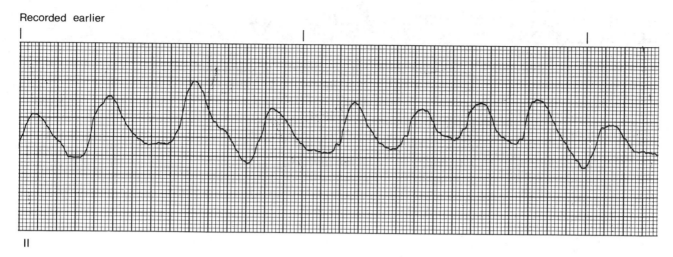

FIGURE 5–22. The bizarre complexes are due to cardiac compression artifact. Intrinsic heart activity can be assessed by briefly stopping CPR.

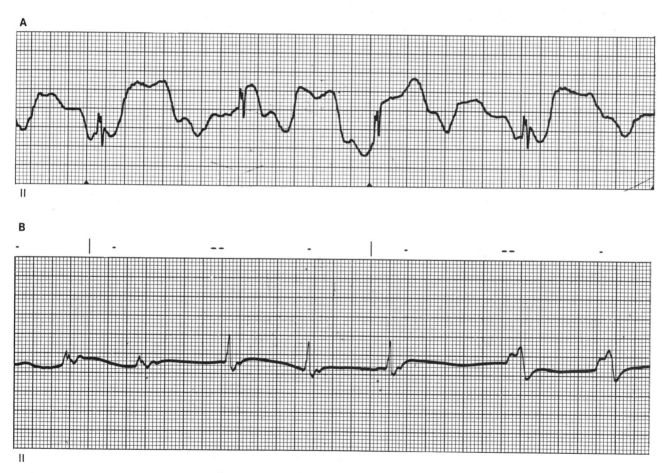

FIGURE 5–23. *A,* This tracing was obtained during cardiopulmonary resuscitation from a patient in electromechanical dissociation; that is, the QRS activity did not cause myocardial contraction. The external cardiac compressions cause ECG artifact, which distorts the baseline and QRS activity. In order to assess the intrinsic heart activity, CPR should be briefly interrupted. *B,* This ECG shows how rapidly cardiac rhythms can change during cardiac resuscitation. In the span of 6 sec, at least three totally different QRS complexes appear. The shape, QRS duration, and R-R intervals vary considerably. These beats are of ventricular origin because they lack P waves and have bizarre shapes.

DYSRHYTHMIAS ENCOUNTERED DURING CARDIAC RESUSCITATIONS

Cardiopulmonary resuscitation efforts are common in critical care areas. The ECG usually shows disorganized electrical activity while the heart has stopped beating. There are only three basic dysrhythmias encountered: asystole, ventricular fibrillation, and pulseless ventricular tachycardia. Electromechanical dissociation (EMD), in which an organized rhythm exists but without associated pulses is also seen. The most common forms of EMD are bradydysrhythmias, primarily of idioventricular origin but less commonly sinus, junctional, or AV block rhythms.

These tracings were encountered previously in individual chapters but are grouped together here because they frequently occur in combined forms, yielding distorted complexes, and abruptly change back and forth during a code. Complicating the patterns are artifacts caused by CPR and artificial pacemaker spikes as illustrated in Figure 5–23A.

The tracings will usually show more than one dysrhythmia as well as beats with different shapes (Fig. 5–23B). The goal is to become familiar with the large variability in the appearance of ECG patterns that is common during a cardiac resuscitation. For a discussion of treatment the reader is directed to *Advanced Cardiac Life Support*, a text published by the American Heart Association.

EXERCISE D: SELF-ASSESSMENT ECG TRACINGS 82 TO 109

The following ECGs include paced rhythms, artifacts, and cardiac resuscitation tracings. Analyze each tracing according to the systematic approach outlined in Chapter One and formulate an interpretation. Check your answer with the suggested interpretations beginning on page 182.

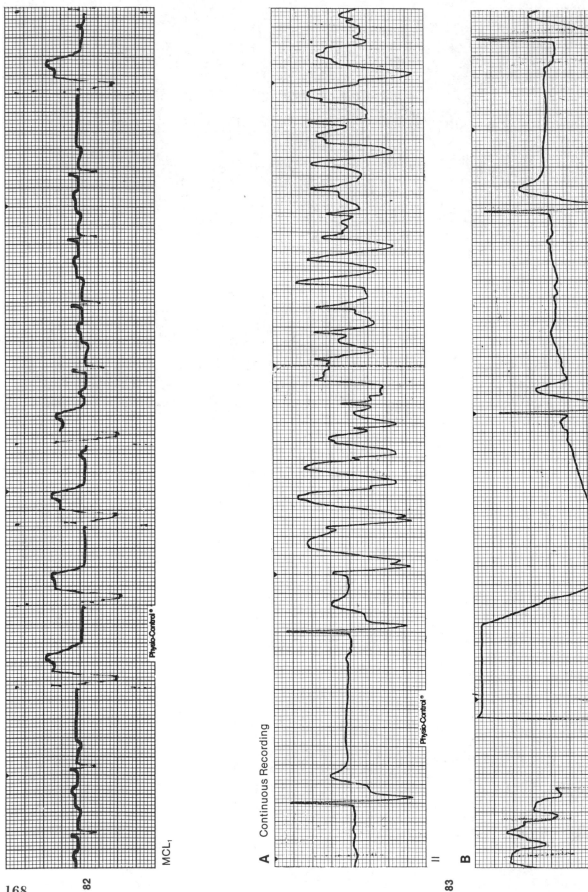

MCL₁

82

A Continuous Recording

II

83

B

II

P

X

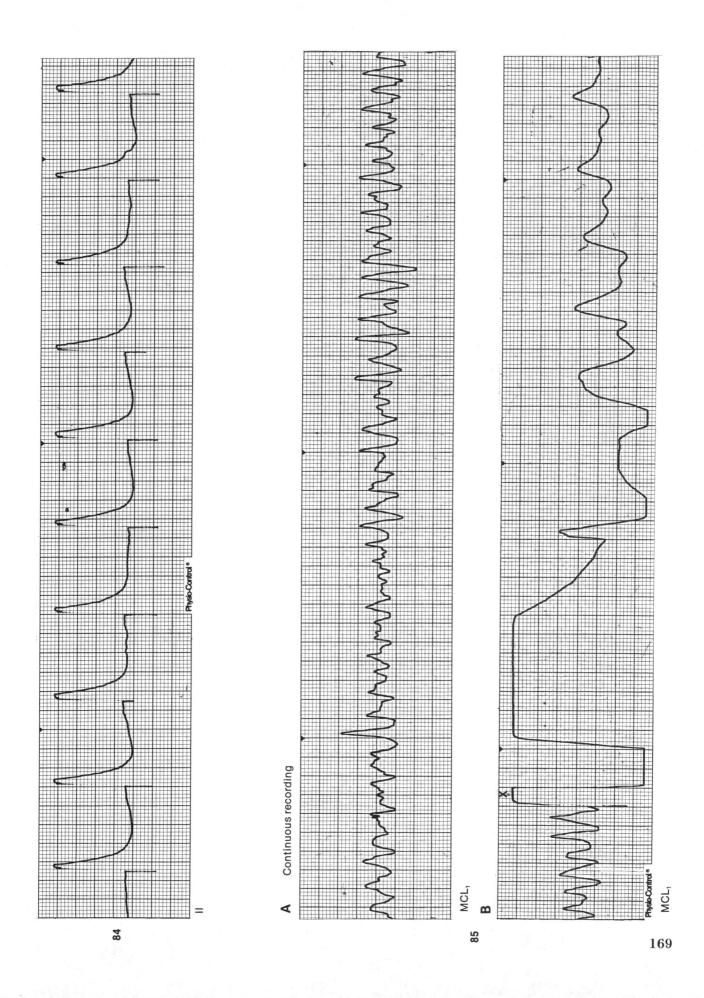

II

84

Physio-Control®

A   Continuous recording

MCL₁

B

85

Physio-Control®

MCL₁

169

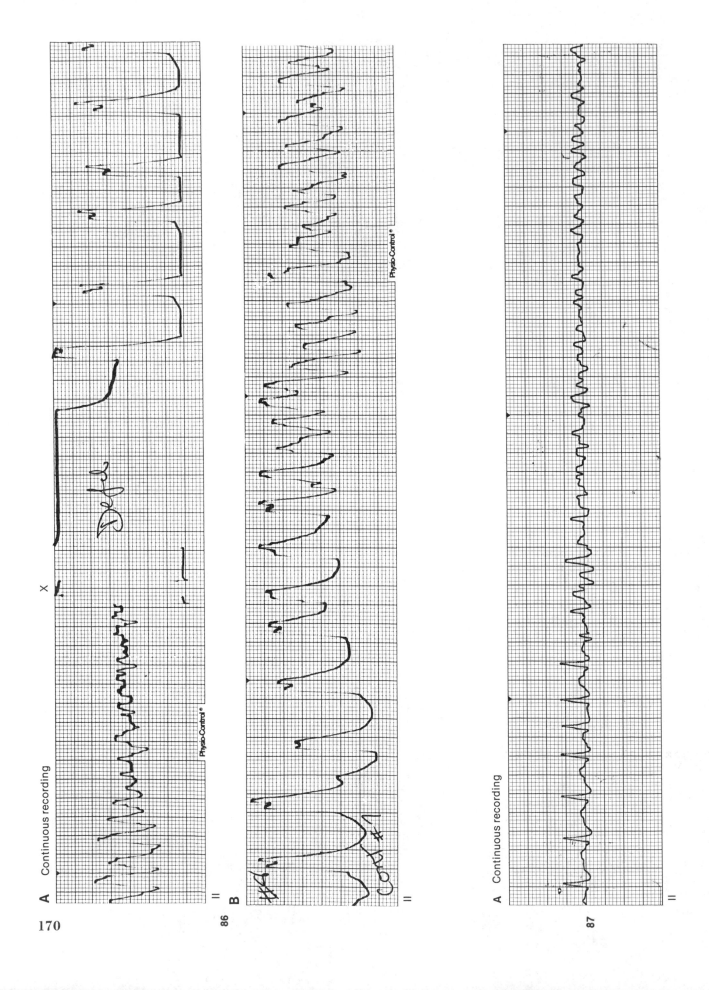

A   Continuous recording

X

Defib

=

B

=

A   Continuous recording

=

170

86

87

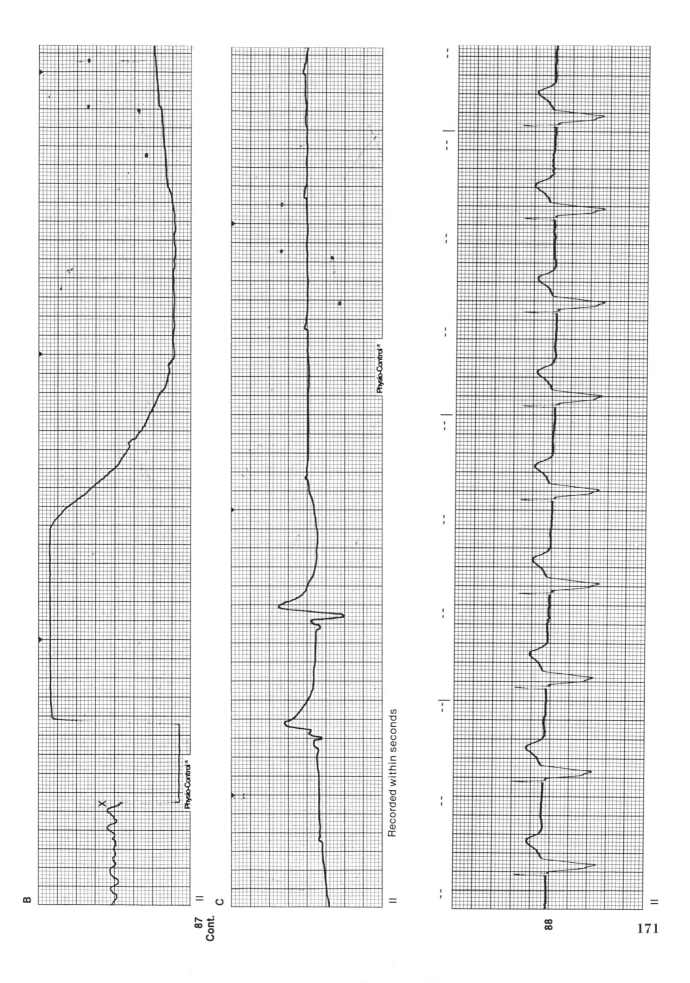

Recorded within seconds

B

87
Cont.

C

Physio-Control®

Physio-Control®

88

171

Continuous recording

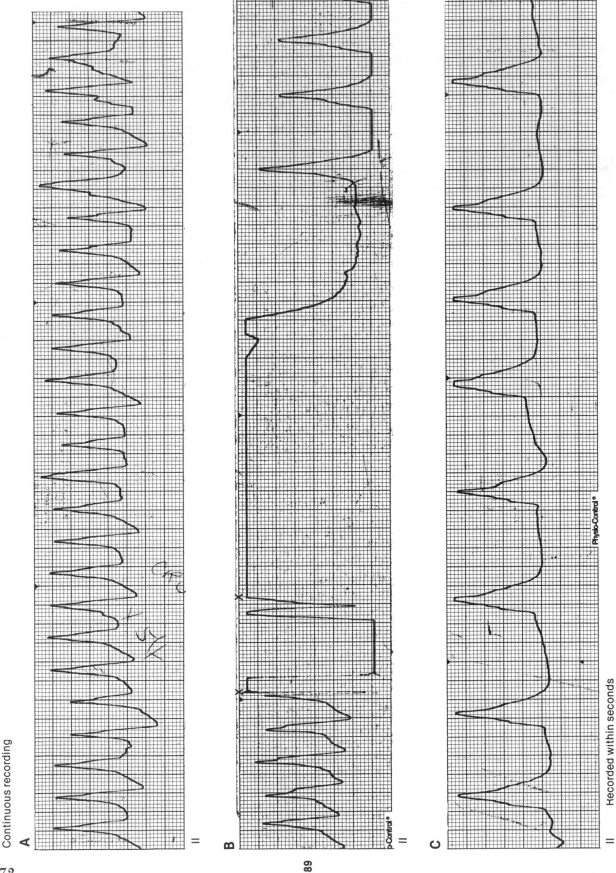

A

II

B

II

C

II

Recorded within seconds

Physio-Control®

Physio-Control®

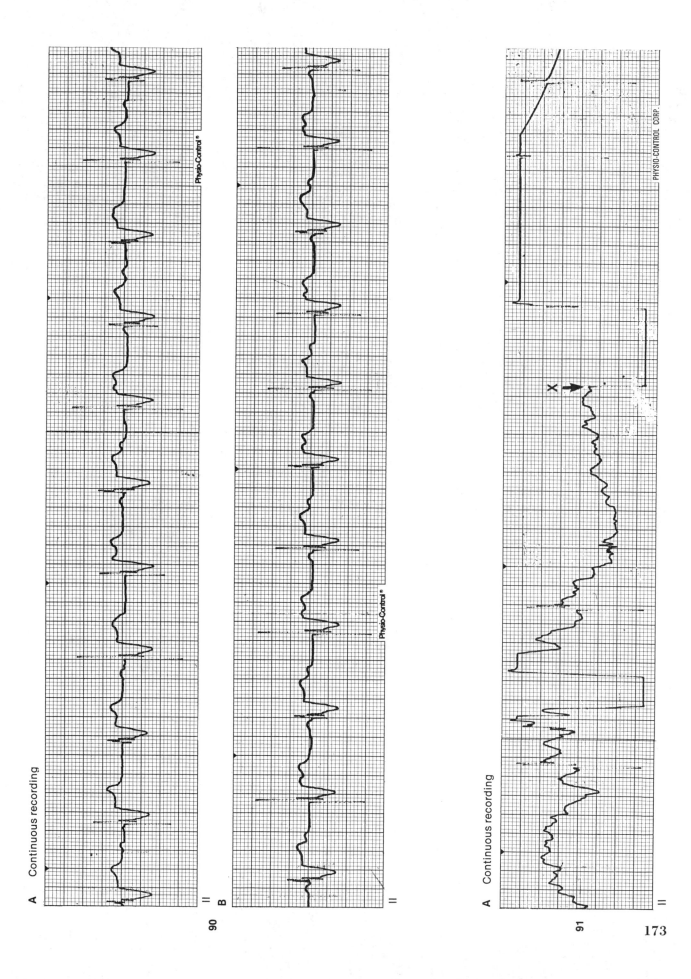

A Continuous recording

B

A Continuous recording

90

91

173

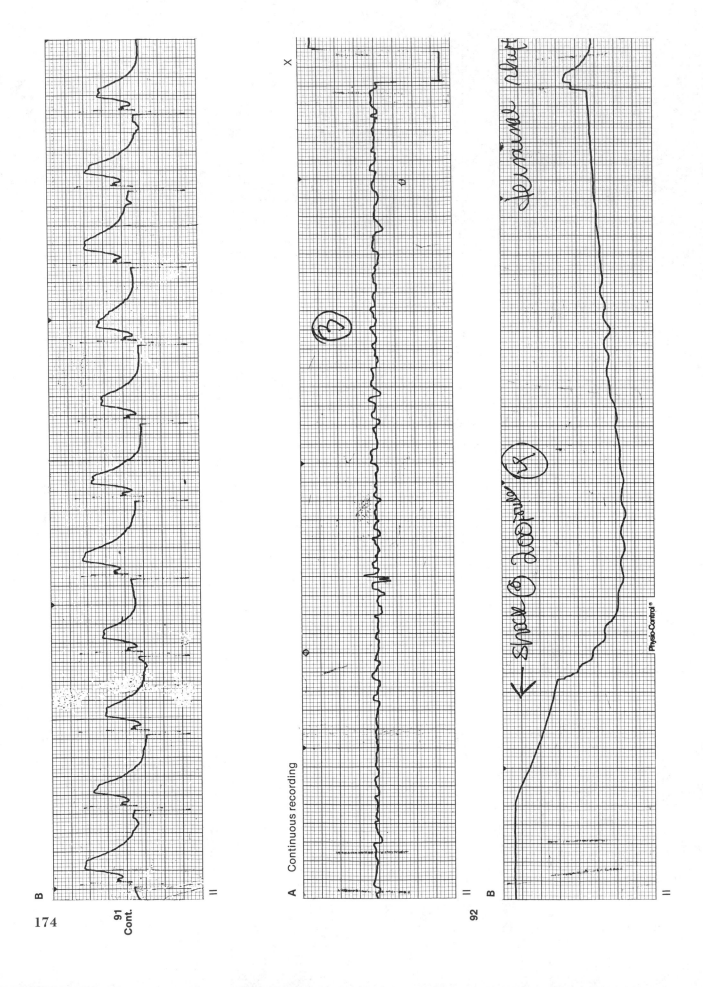

B

II

174

91
Cont.

A   Continuous recording

X

II

92

B

II

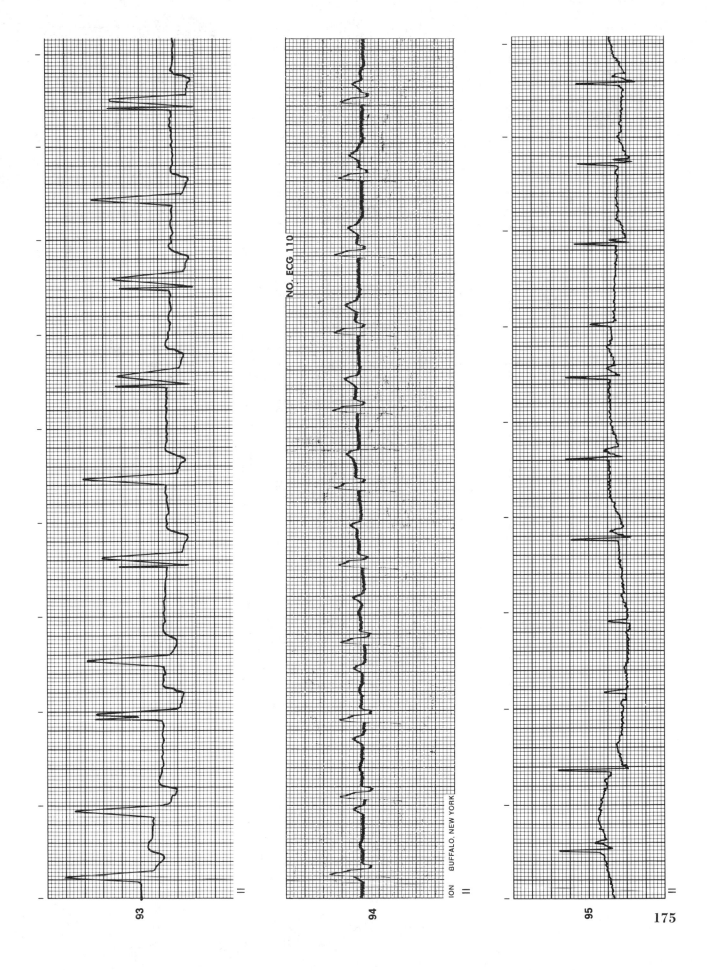

NO. ECG 110

ION   BUFFALO, NEW YORK

93

94

95

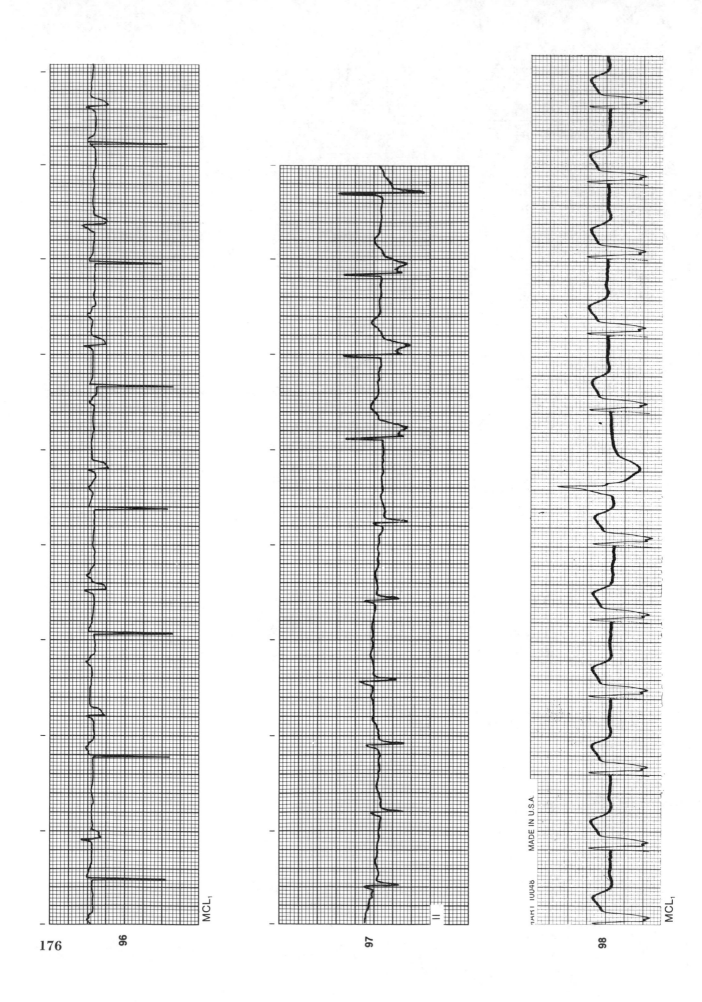

96

MCL₁

97

II

98

MADE IN U.S.A.

MCL₁

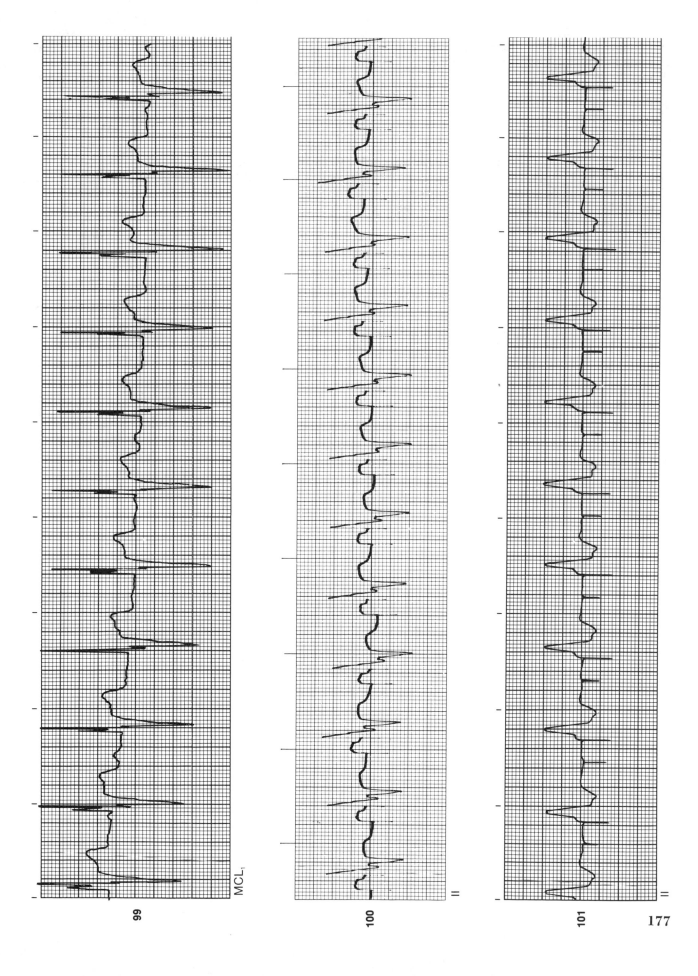

99

100

II

101

II

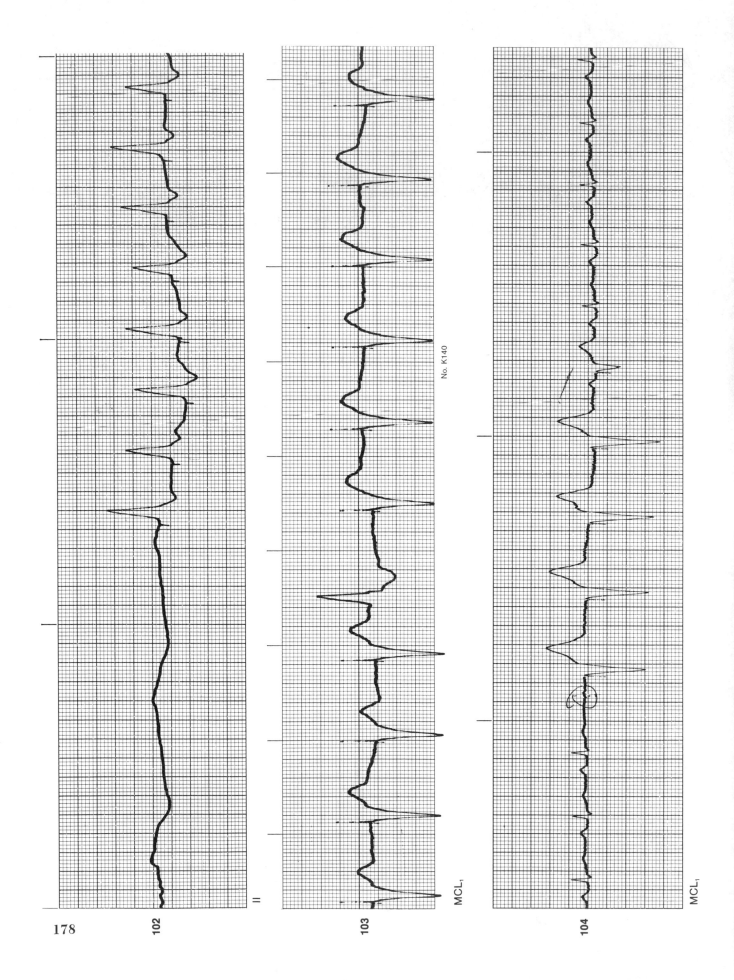

178

102

II

103

MCL₁

No. K140

104

MCL₁

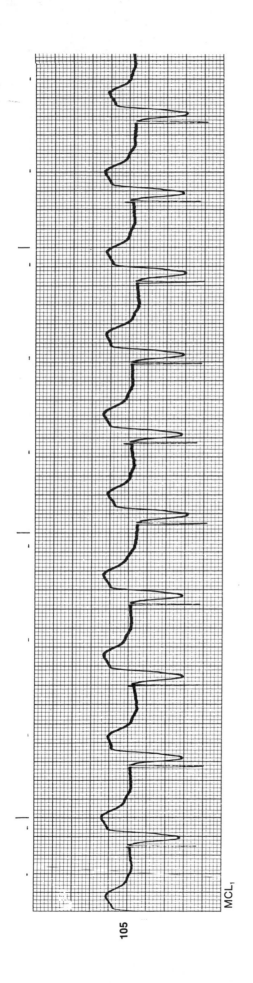

MCL₁

105

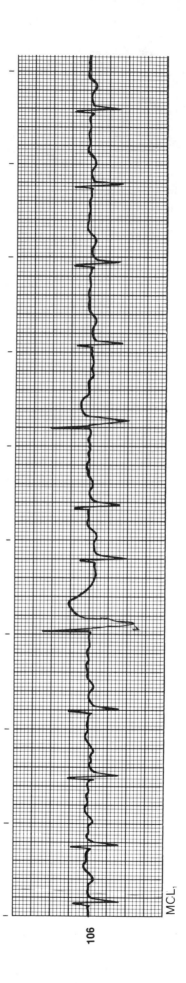

MCL₁

106

179

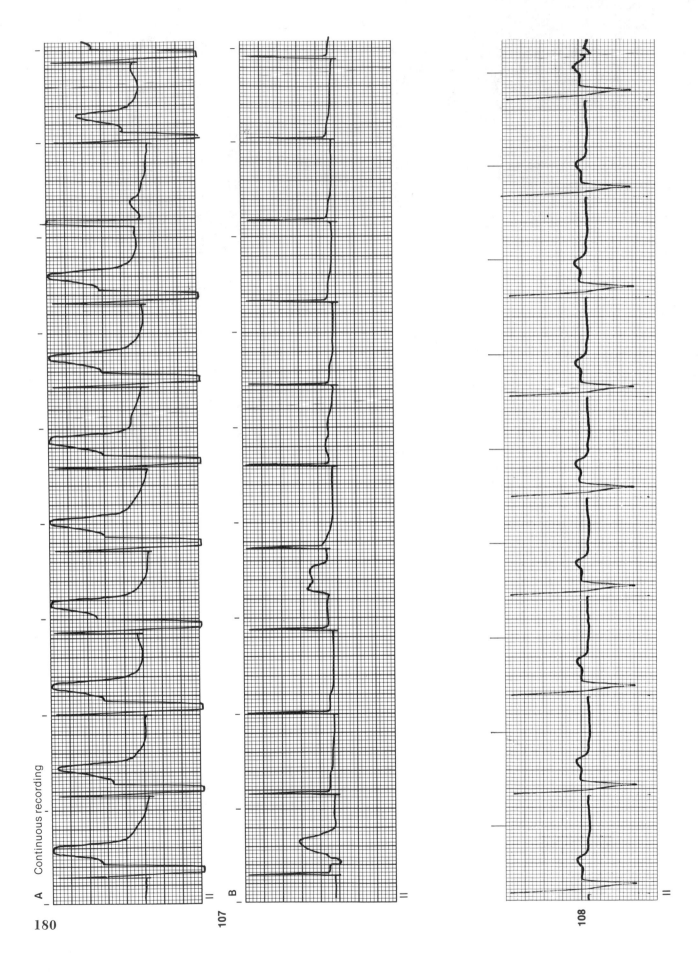

A Continuous recording

II

B

II

II

180

107

108

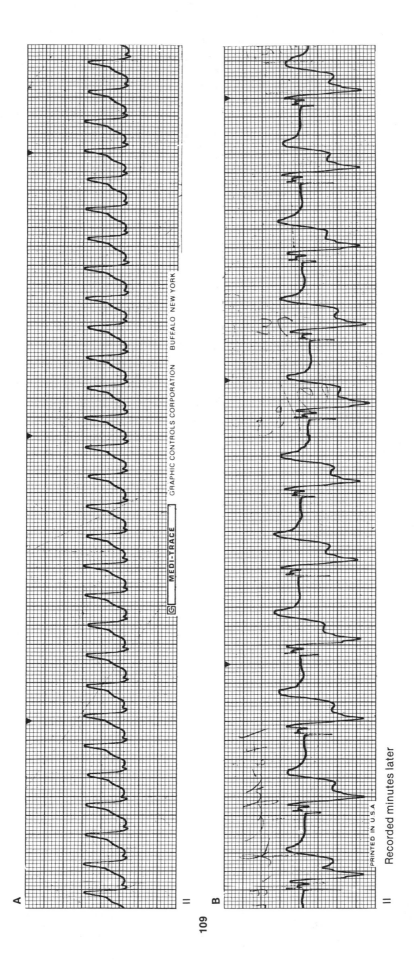

A

II

109

B

II

Recorded minutes later

MEDI-TRACE   GRAPHIC CONTROLS CORPORATION   BUFFALO NEW YORK

PRINTED IN U.S.A

181

ANSWERS TO PRACTICE ECG TRACINGS 82 TO 109

82

other artificial pacer beats occur after the first (see Tracing 82 Answer). Sinus activity returns after the fourth pacer beat. The second set of artificial pacemaker beats occurs after another pause in sinus activity following beat 10.

Rate <u>sinus 85</u> /min.
<u>pacer 72</u> /min. Rhythm <u>irregular</u>
<u>sinus 0.08</u> s.
QRS Duration <u>pacer 0.16</u> s. P-R Interval <u>0.24</u> s.
AV Conduction Ratio <u>sinus 1:1</u>

Interpretation: **The underlying rhythm is sinus with a first degree AV block. An artificial pacemaker rhythm (1:1 capture) occurs at two points when the long R-R intervals reflect a slowing of SA node activity.** (The device has a sensor which turns the pacer on whenever it detects a sinus rate below 73/minute. At other times when the sinus node is above this rate, the artificial pacemaker remains in a standby mode and doesn't discharge.)

Rationale: On initial viewing, we see ventricular activity of two types: some tall and others short. The shorter complexes are sinus beats. The ventricular rhythm is irregular. Just ahead of the QRS complexes are P waves in a 1:1 AV conduction ratio. The first artificial pacemaker spike (beat 3) occurs after an R-R interval of 0.84 second (which corresponds to a rate of 72/min). Three

83

Rate <u>sinus 30</u> /min. Rhythm <u>irregular</u>
<u>sinus 0.12</u> s.
QRS Duration <u>PVC 0.28</u> s. P-R Interval <u>sinus 0.32</u> s.
AV Conduction Ratio <u>sinus 1:1</u>

Interpretation: **Sinus bradycardia with first degree AV block that develops into ventricular fibrillation-tachycardia following two consecutive PVCs.**

Rationale: The first five beats in strip A are sinus because the QRS complexes are narrow and preceded by upright P waves at a fixed interval. A rate of 30/minute is extremely slow for the SA node to be discharging. The P-R interval of 0.32 second indicates a slowed conduction velocity resulting in delayed ventricular activation. Two wide and aberrant beats appear right after the second sinus beat. This leads to the development

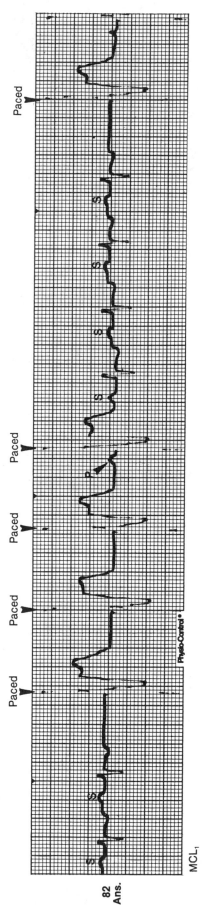

MCL₁
S = sinus beat

82 Ans.

Paced   Paced   Paced   Paced   Paced

184

of a ventricular fibrillation-tachycardia that shows distorted QRS complexes. In strip B, the dysrhythmia is terminated quickly by the application of countershock. The defibrillation converts the rhythm to supraventricular activity.

84

Rate __spikes 72__ /min. Rhythm __absent__ P-R Interval __absent__ s.
QRS Duration __absent__ s.
AV Conduction Ratio __absent__

Interpretation: Noncapturing artificial pacemaker rhythm. No atrial or ventricular activity associated with the pacemaker spikes exists. The patient's inherent rhythm is asystole.

Rationale: No ventricular or atrial complexes are present. Each pacemaker complex begins with a sharp initial negative deflection. The impulse generator is discharging at a fixed rate of 72 impulses per minute, but the heart tissue is not responding (noncapture). Since the myocardium must contract in order to eject blood, cardiac arrest exists.

85

Rate __absent__ /min. Rhythm __absent__ P-R Interval __absent__ s.
QRS Duration __absent__ s.
AV Conduction Ratio __absent__

Interpretation: Ventricular fibrillation refractory to countershock.

Rationale: Strip A shows absence of regular cardiac activity. Instead, chaotic baseline represents ventricular fibrillation. An attempt to terminate the cardiac arrest is made at point X. The sudden deflection of the stylus off the ECG paper and

its slow return to midline is recognizable as defibrillation artifact. The dysrhythmia resumes in strip B.

Discussion: Immediately following defibrillation a check for a palpable pulse should be made. This may be apparent to most but often the resuscitation team becomes preoccupied with the ECG, and they ignore assessing the patient. Even if an adequate rhythm appears following defibrillation, checking for a pulse is essential to determine if electromechanical coupling exists. A pulseless victim with NSR still requires CPR.

86

Rate __absent__ /min. Rhythm __absent__ P-R Interval __absent__ s.
QRS Duration __absent__ s.
AV Conduction Ratio __absent__

Interpretation: ECG recorded during a cardiac resuscitation. **The initial portion shows ventricular fibrillation, which is countershocked at point X. Following defibrillation, there is a brief episode of an accelerated idioventricular rhythm.**

Rationale: This organized rhythm lasts for only a short period, after which ventricular fibrillation reappears.

87

Rate __absent__ /min. Rhythm __absent__ P-R Interval __absent__ s.
QRS Duration __absent__ s.
Conduction Ratio __absent__

Interpretation: **These strips chronicle the rapid decline of sinus rhythm to ventricular fibrillation, then to ventricular standstill.**

Rationale: In strip A sinus rhythm is disrupted by a ventricular ectopic beat at (1). Ventricular fibrillation follows and is countershocked at 400 watt-seconds at X. For the most part, the remainder of strip B and strip C show regular P waves without corresponding QRS complexes. Two isolated idioventricular beats are seen in the bottom tracing. The activity is labeled in Tracing 87 Answer.

88

Rate ___60___ /min. Rhythm ___regular___
QRS Duration ___0.20___ s. P-R Interval ___absent___ s.
AV Conduction Ratio ___absent___

Interpretation: An artificial pacemaker rhythm with 1:1 capture (60/minute).

Rationale: The ventricular rhythm is regular. Each QRS complex, which is wide, is preceded by a tall, upright pacer spike. Atrial activity is missing.

89

Rate ___A) 170___ /min.
___C) 60–70___ /min. Rhythm ___irregular___
___A) 0.20___ s.
QRS Duration ___C) 0.40___ s. P-R Interval ___C)___
AV Conduction Ratio ___absent___

Interpretation: The top tracing shows ventricular tachycardia. Midway through strip B, cardioversion converts the rhythm to a ventricular rhythm at a much slower rate.

Rationale: The ventricular rhythm is slightly irregular with wide and distorted QRS complexes. The ventricular rate is about 170/minute in strip A. The absence of P waves means that atrial activity is missing. The sinus node is no longer the pacemaker; the heart is being stimulated by a rapid ventricular focus. Following cardioversion the rate of the idioventricular rhythm is about 60 to 70/minute. The rhythm becomes irregular, with wider QRS complexes than seen previously in strip A.

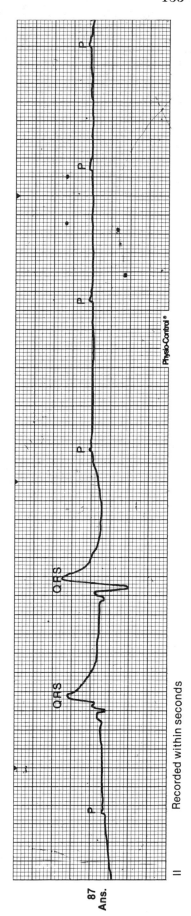

87 Ans.

QRS   QRS   P   P   P   P   P

II   Physio-Control®   Recorded within seconds

186

90

Rate 74 /min. Rhythm regular P-R Interval absent s.
QRS Duration 0.20 s.
AV Conduction Ratio absent

Interpretation: Artificially paced rhythm with 1:1 capture. The patient's own rhythm shows numerous P waves that are not associated with QRS complexes.

Rationale: The ventricular rhythm is regular. The QRS complexes are preceded by biphasic pacemaker spikes. P waves can be observed, but they are not conducted. Each pacemaker spike is associated with a QRS complex, so 1:1 capturing exists.

91

Rate pacer 74 /min. Rhythm pacer–regular P-R Interval absent s.
QRS Duration absent s.
AV Conduction Ratio absent

Interpretation: Strip A: Coarse ventricular fibrillation with superimposed noncapturing artificial pacemaker spikes. The rhythm is converted in B into an artificial pacemaker rhythm after two defibrillations are delivered in quick succession (marked X). A pulse accompanied the rhythm seen in B.

Rationale: Tracing A shows the chaotic configuration of ventricular fibrillation. Also seen are tall artificial pacemaker spikes unaccompanied by QRS complexes. The myocardial fibers are refractory to the paced impulses. Following the return of the stylus to baseline after defibrillation, a steady paced rhythm occurs in B. The rhythm is regular with bizarrely shaped QRS complexes.

Discussion: The treatment of a patient in cardiac arrest is not altered because of the pacemaker. In this case, the underlying rhythm is ventricular fibrillation, so the patient is quickly defibrillated.

92

Rate absent /min. Rhythm absent P-R Interval absent s.
QRS Duration absent s.
AV Conduction Ratio absent

Interpretation: Fine amplitude ventricular fibrillation is countershocked at point X, but the dysrhythmia is refractory. A single agonal idioventricular beat appears in B.

Rationale: Strip A shows fine ventricular fibrillations characterized by a low voltage wavy baseline that lacks constant atrial or ventricular beats. At point X defibrillation is administered which causes the stylus to be pushed briefly to the top of the tracing. When it returns to the middle of the paper, the ECG shows a resumption of fibrillation with one agonal idioventricular beat toward the end of strip B. Asystole quickly follows.

93

Rate 60 /min. Rhythm irregular P-R Interval absent s.
pacer 0.16 s.
QRS Duration instrinsic 0.12 s.
AV Conduction Ratio variable

Interpretation: Atrial fibrillation with a demand ventricular pacemaker at a rate of 60/min with 1:1 capture. Beats 3, 5, 7, 8, and 10, are paced complexes, each occurring following pauses of 1.0 second in the intrinsically conducted atrial impulses.

Rationale:

The ventricular rhythm is irregular. QRS complexes have two configurations, depending on whether they are paced beats or if they are atrial beats conducted through the AV node. The QRS duration is prolonged to different degrees in both instances: paced (0.16 second) and intrinsic (0.12 second). Paced complexes can be recognized by their large positive spikes in front of and merging with the QRS complexes. Atrial activity consists of a fine wavy irregular baseline. Since P waves are absent, AV conduction ratios are not measurable.

94

Rate   atrial 80 /min.
       pacer 73 /min.   Rhythm   pacer–regular
QRS Duration   0.14   s.   P-R Interval   absent   s.
AV Conduction Ratio   absent

Interpretation: Artificial ventricular pacemaker rhythm showing 1:1 capture at a rate of 73/minute.

Rationale: The ventricular rhythm is regular, consisting of pacer spikes followed by QRS-T complexes. The atrial rhythm shows regular P waves occurring at 80/minute. The P waves show no relationship to the QRS complexes because the atria and ventricles are completely dissociated.

95

Rate   pacer 72 /min.   Rhythm   irregular
       sinus 0.06 s.
QRS Duration pacer 0.16 s.   P-R Interval   0.16   s.
AV Conduction Ratio   sinus 1:1

Interpretation: Sinus rhythm with a sinus dysrhythmia and a demand pacemaker at 72/minute with 1:1 capture. Beats 4 and 8 represent normally conducted sinus impulses. When the sinus rate slows below 72/minute, the pacemaker is triggered. At intrinsic rates above 72/minute the pacer is inhibited.

Rationale: The ventricular rhythm is irregular. The R-R interval between consecutive pacer spikes is regular. Sinus beats have a QRS duration of 0.06 sec while that of the paced beats (2, 3, 5, 6, 7, 9, 10, and 11) is 0.12 to 0.16 sec. Each pacer spike is followed by a wide QRS-T complex. P waves are seen before beats 3, 4, and 8. Beat 3 has a much taller QRS complex than the rest of the sinus beats. The reason is that this complex is a fusion beat, meaning that it is formed from the simultaneous activation of the ventricle by an intrinsic as well as a paced beat. The P-R interval for beats 3 and 4 is 0.12 sec and for beat 8 is 0.20 sec.

187

96

Rate   atrial 70 /min. / ventricular 47/min. / pacer 46 /min.   Rhythm regular

QRS Duration ventricular 0.20 s.

P-R Interval absent s.

AV Conduction Ratio absent

Interpretation: Complete AV heart block, idioventricular escape rhythm, and fixed rate pacemaker failing to stimulate the ventricle. Regular pacemaker spikes are evident at 46/min but not associated with QRS-T complexes (see Tracing 96 Answer).

Rationale: The intrinsic ventricular rhythm is slow (47/minute), with small, wide QRS complexes (0.16 sec). Atrial activity consists of notched P waves occurring at 66/minute. No AV conduction exists, as all the atrial impulses are blocked. Failure of the pacer to stimulate the heart is evidenced by the absence of QRS-T complexes following the large negative spikes.

97

Rate   intrinsic 72 /min. / pacer 70 /min.   Rhythm intrinsic-irregular / pacer-regular

QRS Duration intrinsic 0.08s. / pacer 0.12 s.   P-R Interval absent s.

AV Conduction Ratio intrinsic-variable

Interpretation: Atrial fibrillation with a demand pacemaker (beats 7, 8, 9, and 10) with 1:1 capture. The first six beats, representing intrinsic activity, are irregular and narrow. The demand pacemaker discharges when the intrinsic ventricular rate falls below 70/minute.

Rationale: The ventricular rhythm of the paced complexes is regular. The QRS complexes of the paced beats are wider than those of intrinsic beats. No P waves exist and atrial activity consists of fine fibrillatory waves.

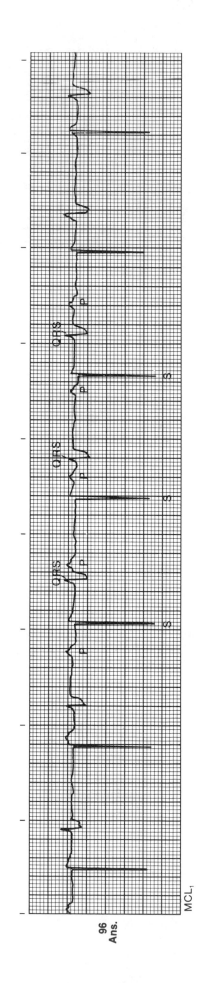

96
Ans.

MCL$_1$

QRS complexes are wide (0.20 second) and distorted. Atrial activity shows P waves at a rate of 90/minute. No AV conduction exists.

98

Rate __pacer 75__ /min. Rhythm __irregular__
__intrinsic 0.20s.__
QRS Duration pacer 0.20 s. P-R Interval __absent__ s.
AV Conduction Ratio __absent__

Interpretation: **Demand pacemaker rhythm with 1:1 capture that is inhibited and reset by a PVC (beat 7).**

Rationale: A regular pacemaker-induced rhythm exists at a rate of 75/minute, that is, at intervals of 0.80 sec. The QRS complexes are wide (0.16 second) and distorted. The PVC is followed by a pause of 0.80 second representing inhibition and resetting of the demand pacemaker. No atrial activity is present.

99

Rate __pacer 72__ /min. Rhythm __regular__
QRS Duration __0.16__ s. P-R Interval __absent__ s.
AV Conduction Ratio __absent__

Interpretation: **Sinus rhythm with complete AV heart block and a regular pacemaker rhythm (1:1 capture).**

Rationale: The ventricular rhythm is regular with pacemaker spikes occurring at a rate of 72/min. The

100

Rate __paced 79__ /min. Rhythm __regular__
QRS Duration __0.20__ s. P-R Interval __0.16__ s.
AV Conduction Ratio __1:1__

Interpretation: **Artificial AV sequential pacemaker rhythm with 1:1 capture.** The first pacemaker spike stimulates the atria, producing a P wave, and the second spike produces a QRS-T complex (ventricular activation).

Rationale: Gross inspection reveals a rhythm whose appearance differs markedly from NSR. The ventricular activity is recognized as the first tall, positive spike (see Tracing 100 Answer) that is part of the wide QRS complex. The QRS duration is about 0.16 second. Atrial activity regularly occurs prior to each QRS complex and consists of a typical, rounded upright P wave. But it differs from NSR in that it is also preceded by a large, negative pacer spike. The AV conduction pattern is normal (1:1), as is the

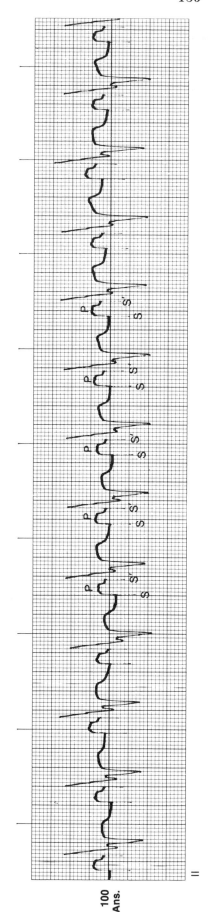

100
Ans.

190

P-R interval. The ventricles and atria are stimulated by separate synchronized artificial pacing electrodes.

101 Rate __paced 74__ /min. Rhythm __regular__ P-R Interval __absent__ s.
QRS Duration __0.20__ s.
AV Conduction Ratio __absent__

Interpretation: **Artificial AV sequential pacemaker rhythm with failure to capture the atria. Ventricular pacing shows 1:1 capture.**

Rationale: Each cardiac complex shows a pair of pacer spikes. The ventricular rhythm is regular with wide bizarre QRS complexes which include pacer spikes (see Tracing 101 Answer). A second pacer spike occurs ahead of the QRS complex at a distance of 5 mm (0.20 second). It is generated via an atrial lead, but it fails to stimulate atrial depolarization. The P waves are missing because the atrial electrode has lost contact with the right atrial endocardium.

102 Rate __pacer 93__ /min. Rhythm __regular__ P-R Interval __absent__ s.
QRS Duration __0.20__ s.
AV Conduction Ratio __absent__

Interpretation: **The initial half of the tracing shows asystole, which is followed by an artificially generated ventricular pacemaker rhythm with 1:1 capture.** (This ECG tracing was recorded during a resuscitation attempt in which asystole occurred. During closed chest cardiac massage, an electrode was passed via the internal jugular vein and superior vena cava into the right ventricle. When connected to an external pacemaker generator, it paced the ventricles at 94/minute).

Rationale: The initial half of the tracing shows an essentially flat line and no electrical activity. Ventricular activity is evident during the latter half of the tracing as wide, distorted QRS-T complexes. Each complex is preceded by a small negatively deflected pacer spike. Atrial activity is missing.

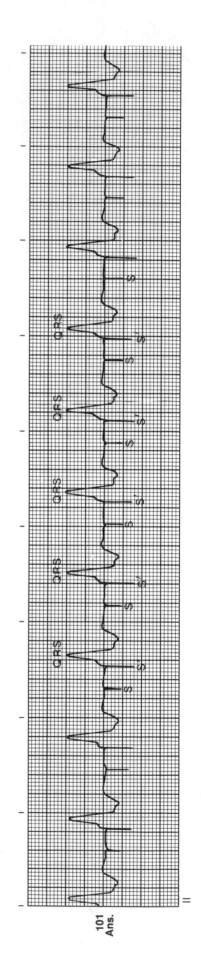

101 Ans.

103

Rate __paced 72__ /min. Rhythm __irregular__
QRS Duration __PVC 0.28__ s. __pacer 0.20__ s. P-R Interval __absent__ s.
AV Conduction Ratio __absent__

Interpretation: **An artificially paced ventricular rhythm with a 1:1 capture inhibited and reset by a PVC (beat 5).** The pacemaker is discharging at a rate of 72/minute (R-R intervals of 0.84 second), representing sensing, inhibition, and resetting of the demand pacemaker.

Rationale: All ventricular complexes except beat 5 consist of a positively deflected pacer spike followed by a wide QRS-T complex. Atrial activity is absent. The PVC is wide and distorted.

104

Rate __sinus 90–100/min.__ __pacer 74__ /min. Rhythm __irregular__
QRS Duration __paced 0.20__ s. __sinus 0.08__ s. P-R Interval __0.20__ s.
AV Conduction Ratio __sinus 1:1__

Interpretation: **Sinus rhythm and an artificially generated pacemaker rhythm with 1:1 capture (beats 4, 5, 6, 7, and 14).** When a pause in ventricular activity equals 0.80 second (rate of 75/minute) as seen following beats 3 and 13, the pacer fires.

Rationale: The ventricular complexes show two distinct shapes: sinus beats 1, 2, 3, 9, 10, 11, 12, and 13 have narrow QRS complexes while the pacer beats are wide and distorted. Beat 8 shows a slightly distorted QRS complex because it was initiated by an intrinsic sinus impulse but was partially activated by a pacer spike, too. Atrial activity, consisting of P waves, occurs prior to all sinus complexes and is missing before the pacer beats.

105

Rate __72__ /min. Rhythm __regular__
QRS Duration __0.24__ s. P-R Interval __absent__ s.
AV Conduction Ratio __absent__

Interpretation: **Artificial ventricular pacemaker rhythm with 1:1 capture at a rate of 72/minute.**

Rationale: Ventricular activity shows wide, distorted QRS complexes consisting of large, negatively deflected pacer spikes and QRS-T complexes. No intrinsic atrial or ventricular impulses are seen.

106

Rate __intrinsic 70–90__ /min. Rhythm __grossly irregular__
QRS Duration __pacer 0.20 s.__ __intrinsic 0.08__ s. P-R Interval __absent__ s.
AV Conduction Ratio __variable__

Interpretation: **Atrial fibrillation with two artificially stimulated pacer complexes (5 and 8) which occur after pauses in ventricular activity of 0.84 second.**

Rationale: The ventricular rhythm is irregularly irregular and, except for beats 5 and 8, has narrow QRS complexes. Beats 5 and 8 consist of tall, positively deflected pacer spikes followed by wide QRS-T complexes. No organized atrial activity is seen, just a fine fibrillatory baseline.

107

Rate ___72___ /min. Rhythm ___irregular___

___intrinsic 0.08___ s.

QRS Duration ___paced 0.24___ s. P-R Interval ___sinus___ s.

AV Conduction Ratio ___1:1___

Interpretation: **A: Artificially paced ventricular rhythm with a 1:1 capture except for beat 9, which is a sinus initiated complex. Several minutes later strip B was recorded. B shows artificially stimulated pacer spikes with no ventricular stimulation or capture. The myocardium fails to respond to the pacer spikes. Two intrinsic ventricular complexes are seen following—but not related**

to—spikes 1 and 4. They do not represent effective depolarizations.

Rationale:

In strip A all the pacer spikes are followed by QRS-T complexes. In strip B none of the spikes depolarize the ventricles. The myocardium is gravely damaged and cannot respond (see Tracing 107 Answer). Two agonal intrinsic beats arising from a ventricular focus are noted (↑).

Discussion:

Noncapture can occur if the pacer electrode does not make adequate contact with the cardiac tissue or in the event of a grossly diseased and unresponsive myocardium.

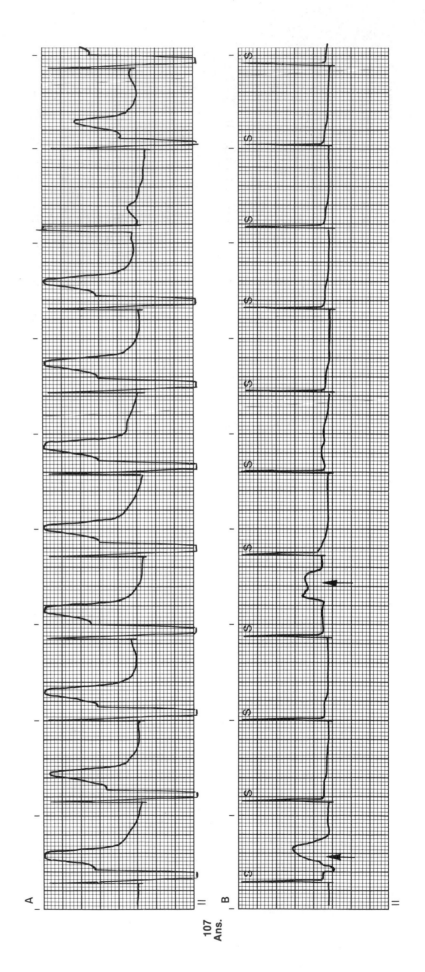

107
Ans.

191

108

Rate __57__ /min. Rhythm __regular__ P-R Interval __absent__ s.
QRS Duration __0.16__ s.
AV Conduction Ratio __absent__

Interpretation: **Artificial ventricular pacemaker rhythm with 1:1 capture, discharging at 57/minute.** (If the pacemaker had been programmed to discharge at a faster rate, this slow rhythm would indicate pacemaker failure, which is usually caused by battery depletion.)

Rationale: The ventricular activity consists of regular pacer spikes followed by wide QRS-T complexes. No atrial activity is seen.

109

Rate __A) 185__ /min.
__B) 72__ /min. Rhythm __A & B) regular__
__A) 0.26__ s.
QRS Duration __B) 0.40__ s. P-R Interval __absent__ s.
AV Conduction Ratio __A & B) absent__

Interpretation: **A: The pacemaker rhythm is inhibited by a rapid tachydysrhythmia. B: Following treatment, return of a normally functioning pacemaker rhythm is evident by pacemaker spiked QRS-T complexes.**

Rationale: No pacemaker spikes are seen in A. The rapid rhythm consists of wide QRS-T complexes. It is either ventricular tachycardia or a PSVT with aberrant conduction. Both dysrhythmias are capable of inhibiting the demand pacemaker due to their rapid rates. In B, the wide bizarre QRS-T complexes are preceded by pacer spikes.

Section 2

MASTERING DYSRHYTHMIAS: ADDITIONAL SELF-ASSESSMENT TRACINGS

Chapter Six

EXERCISE E: SELF-ASSESSMENT ECG TRACINGS 110 to 129

This chapter has a variety of ECG dysrhythmias including atrial dysrhythmias, atrioventricular blocks, and ventricular disturbances for you to practice analyzing. The answers begin on page 207.

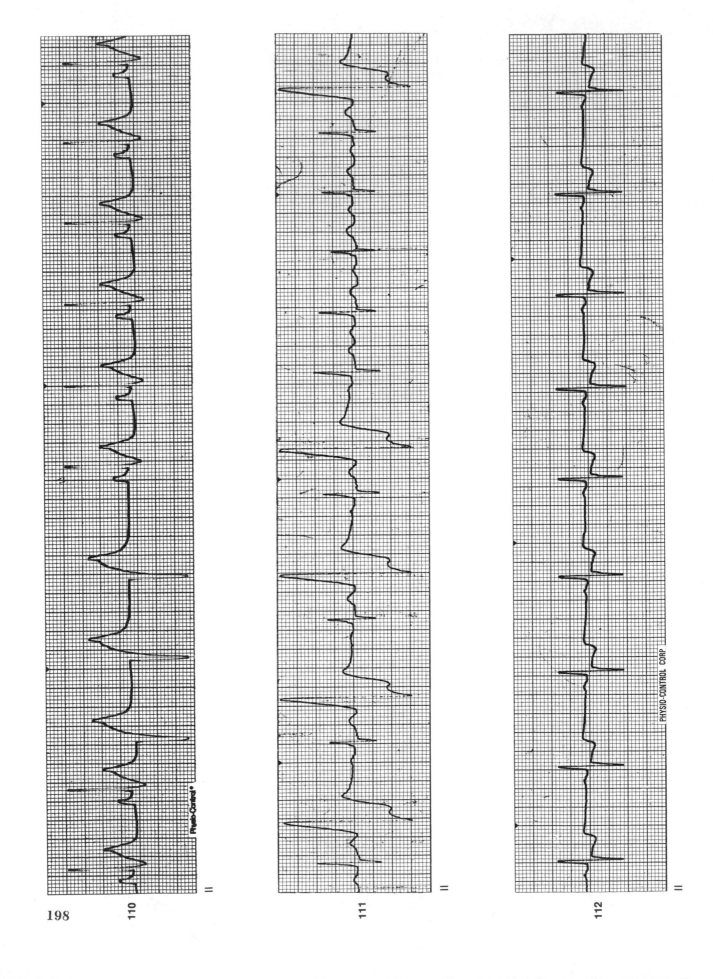

198

110

111

112

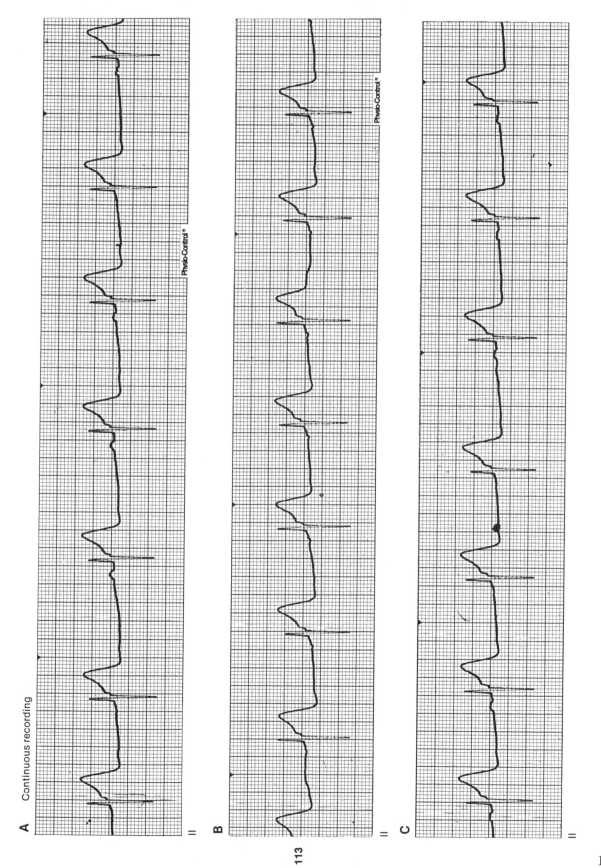

A Continuous recording

B

C

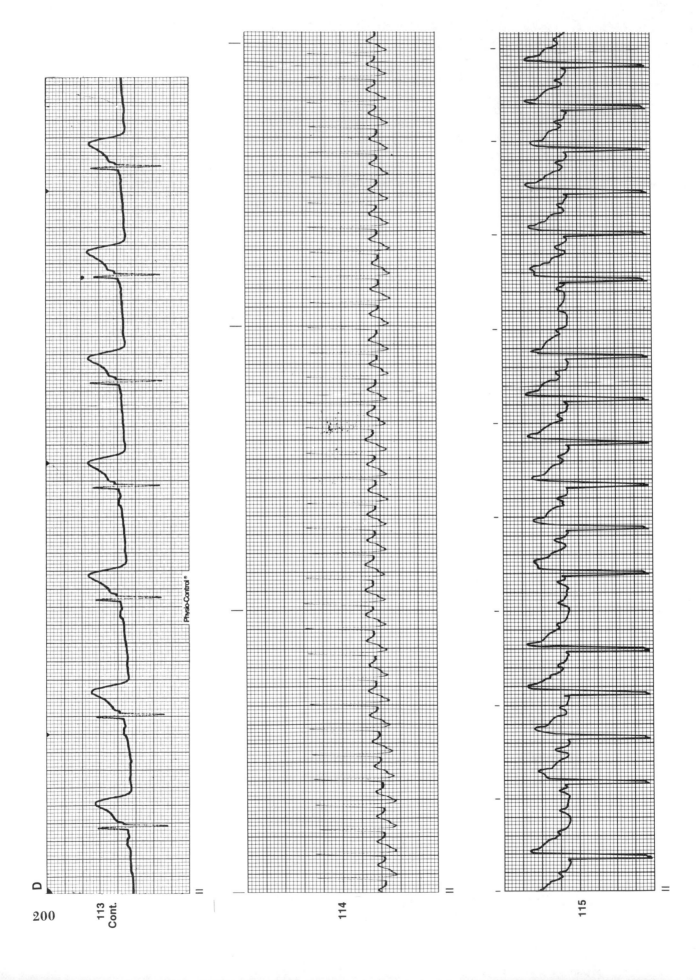

D

113
Cont.

II

Physio-Control®

114

II

115

II

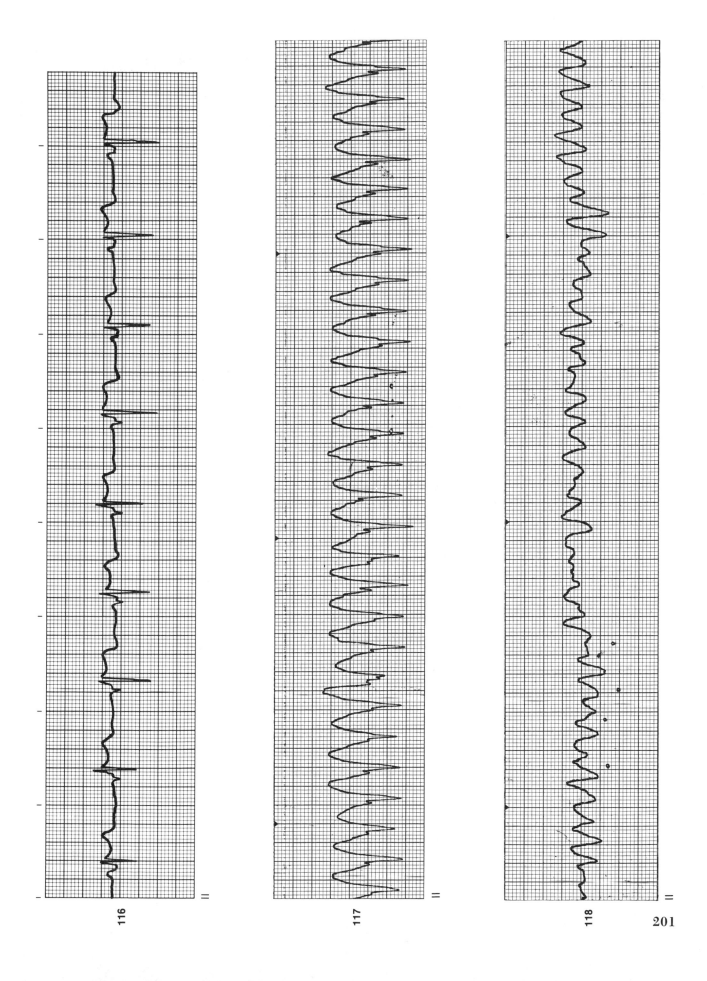

116

117

118

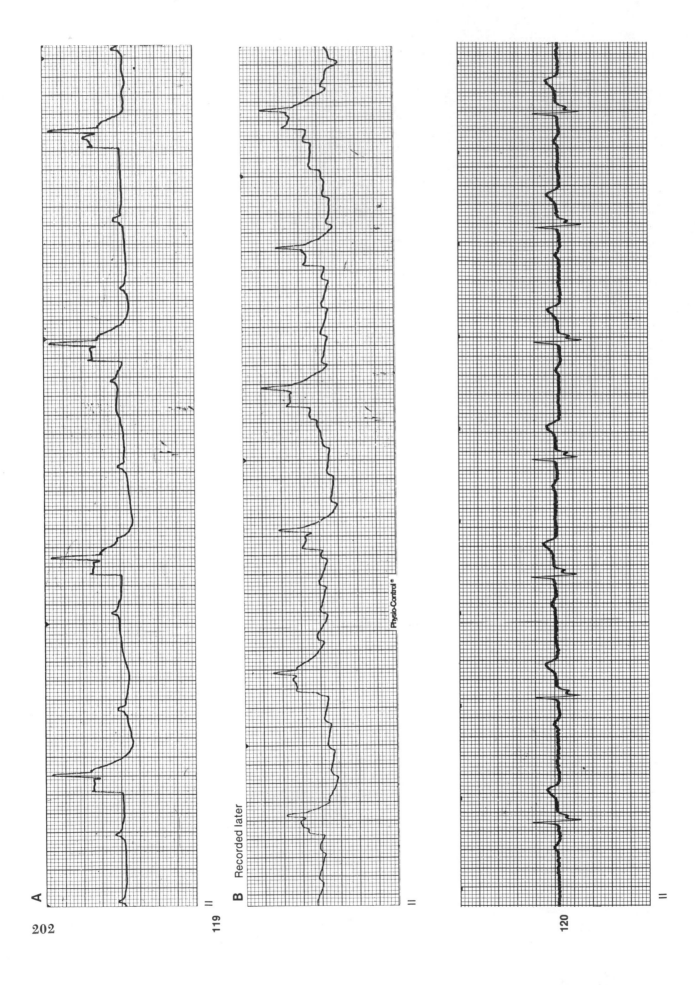

A

II

B Recorded later

Physio-Control®

II

II

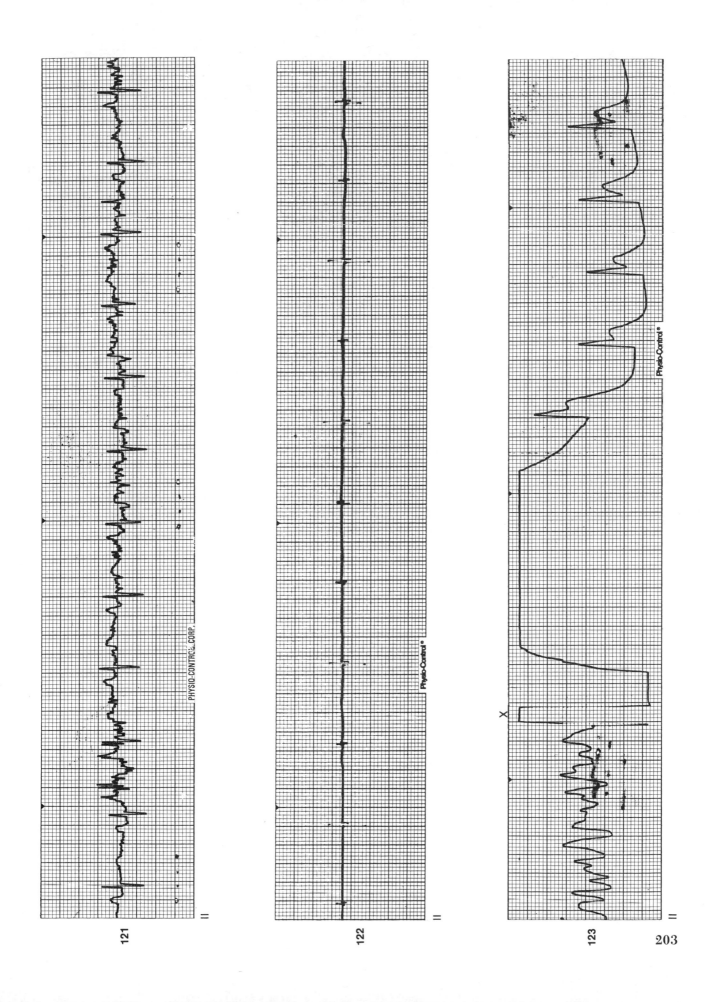

121

PHYSIO-CONTROL CORP.

II

122

Physio-Control®

II

123

Physio-Control®

X

II

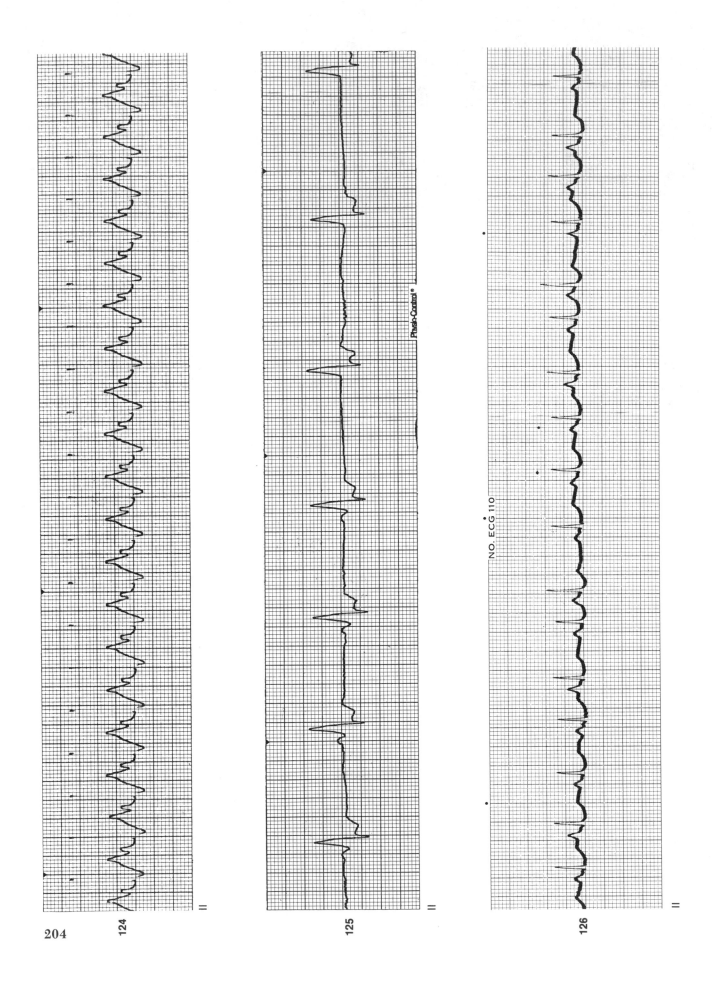

204

124

125

126

NO. ECG 110

II

II

II

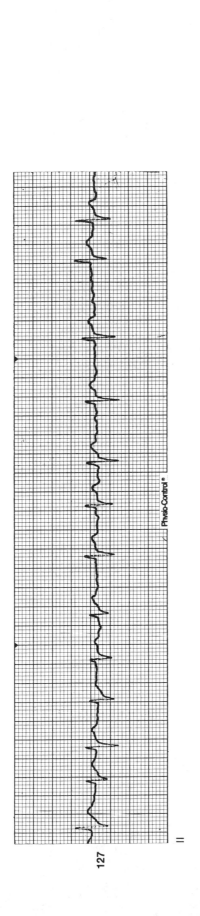

127

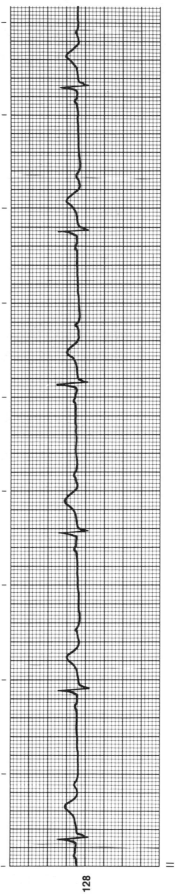

128

205

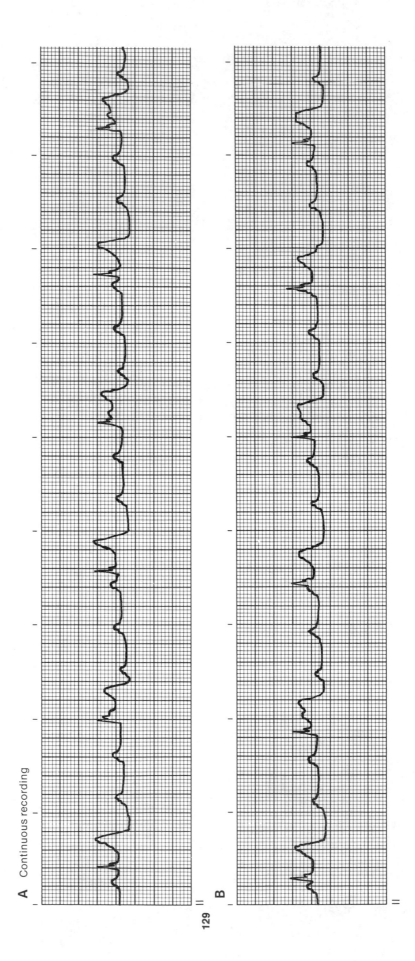

A Continuous recording

B

II

II

ANSWERS TO PRACTICE ECG TRACINGS 110 TO 129

110

Rate _____70_____ /min. Rhythm ___irregular___
_____ sinus 0.08 _____ s.
QRS Duration ventricular 0.14 s. P-R Interval _____0.16_____ s.
AV Conduction Ratio _____1:1_____

Interpretation: Sinus rhythm with a brief run of accelerated idioventricular rhythm.

Rationale: Aside from the aberrant beats (4, 5, and 6), the rhythm shows sinus rhythm. The three successive aberrant beats show typical ventricular characteristics:

- Wide QRS complex
- Lack of P waves
- Discordant T waves

The ectopic beats occur at a rate of 70/min, which is less than the 100/minute needed to classify this dysrhythmia as ventricular tachycardia.

Terminology: The American Heart Association defines ventricular tachycardia as three or more consecutive ventricular beats at a rate of 100/minute or greater. This dysrhythmia is too slow to meet these criteria. Because the rate is faster than the ordinary intrinsic rate of ventricular pacemakers, it is termed accelerated.

Significance: Accelerated idioventricular rhythms commonly develop during the days following a myocardial infarction. They have generally been thought of as benign. Recently, however, this dysrhythmia has been considered as a potential forerunner of more malignant ventricular disorders, but the evidence is not conclusive.

111

Rate _____90_____ /min. Rhythm ___irregular___
_____ sinus 0.08 _____ s.
QRS Duration PVC 0.20 s. P-R Interval _____0.20_____ s.
AV Conduction Ratio _____1:1_____

Interpretation: Sinus rhythm with frequent uniformed PVCs. There is a short sequence of ventricular bigeminy.

Rationale: Concentrating on the sinus beats, we see the normal sequence of P-QRS-T waves. The regularity of the R-R intervals is disturbed by the premature beats. The PVCs lack P waves, have wide distorted QRS complexes, and are followed by compensatory pauses. Each of the first four PVCs occur alternately with a sinus complex (ventricular bigeminy). The PVCs have fixed coupling intervals to the previous T wave of the sinus beat.

112

Rate _____57_____ /min. Rhythm ___regular___
QRS Duration _____0.10_____ s. P-R Interval _____0.16_____ s.
AV Conduction Ratio _____1:1_____

Interpretation: Sinus bradycardia.

Rationale: Ventricular and atrial activity are normal. Atrioventricular conduction ratio is 1:1. Slow discharge of the SA node is the only deviation from NSR.

113

Rate see discussion   Rhythm   irregular
QRS Duration   0.08   s.   P-R Interval   0.20   s.
AV Conduction Ratio   1:1

Interpretation: **The continuous tracing initially shows a sinus bradycardia at a slow rate of about 42 beats/minute and the later development of an AV junctional escape pacemaker at a slightly faster rate of 50/minute.**

Rationale: The QRS complexes for both pacemakers are identical, confirming that the ventricles are being stimulated in an identical manner from the AV bundle onward. It is not uncommon to see a latent pacemaker discharge as the sinus depolarizes at a slower rate. The range of automaticity for the AV junction is between 40 to 60/minute while the normal range for sinus activity is between 60 to 100/minute. Enhanced vagal tone is often the cause of sinus depression. This dysrhythmia is usually transient and subsides as soon as the sinus node accelerates. The R-R intervals are 1.40 sec between sinus beats, and the interval for junctional complexes is 1.20 sec. Atrial activity is absent in many complexes, and only the QRS complexes can be seen. When P waves are seen, they appear just before the QRS complexes, as expected for sinus beats. The waves are labeled in Tracing 113 Answer to indicate the sinus and junctional beats.

114

Rate   230   /min.   Rhythm   regular
QRS Duration   0.06–0.08   s.   P-R Interval   absent
AV Conduction Ratio   1:1

Interpretation: **Supraventricular tachycardia.**

Rationale: Regular ventricular activity is present. The QRS complexes are narrow with sharp waves. Clearly identifiable P waves are not seen, so an AV relationship cannot be detected. (The upright deflections seen just before the R waves are the T waves from the complexes just preceding the QRS complexes.) As the rate increases, the T-P interval correspondingly shortens, and the complexes appear closer together. The rate is too rapid for sinus activity. Also, because the QRS complexes are too narrow to be idioventricular, an SVT is the most logical dysrhythmia.

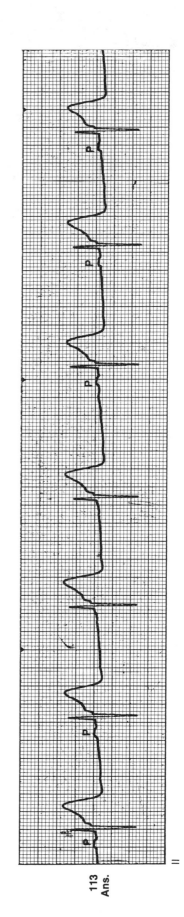

113
Ans.

II

Definition: Wandering atrial pacemaker is characterized by frequently changing P wave shapes and P-R intervals in the setting of a normal heart rate range between 60 and 100/minute. The changing ECG pattern reflects shifts of pacemaker activity from the SA node to the AV junction and other atrial sites. This is believed to be caused by increased automaticity of the ectopic pacemakers. WAP is encountered in healthy individuals as well as in patients with digitalis excess and organic heart disease. It does not significantly alter cardiac function and is not a serious dysrhythmia. (If the same findings occur when the heart rate is over 100/minute, the term "multifocal atrial tachycardia" is applied.)

Rationale: The ventricular complexes are normal and identical regardless of pacemaker origin. Each QRS complex is preceded by a P wave, but the shapes of the atrial depolarization waves differ. Along with varying sizes of P waves, the ectopic beats have differing P-R intervals. Still, the AV conduction ratio is 1:1. The conclusion is that intraventricular conduction is identical for the complexes even though the site of initiation varies.

115

Rate averages 120 /min.   Rhythm irregular

QRS Duration 0.08 s.   P-R Interval 0.12 s.

AV Conduction Ratio 1:1

Interpretation: Atrial flutter with variable AV conduction and an average ventricular response of 120/min. See Tracing 115 Answer for labeled waves.

Rationale: The ventricular rhythm is irregular, with identical QRS complexes. Characteristic atrial flutter waves are unmasked when CSM exposes the F waves hidden in the QRS complexes. AV conduction ratio varies among 2:1, 3:1, and 4:1 at various points.

116

Rate averages 64 /min.   Rhythm regular

QRS Duration 0.08 s.   P-R Interval sinus 0.16 s. atrial 0.12 s.

AV Conduction Ratio 1:1

Interpretation: Wandering atrial pacemaker (WAP). Beats 1, 7, 8, and 9 are sinus complexes, and beats 2 through 6 arise from an ectopic atrial focus and display biphasic P waves. For about 3 seconds, pacing activity shifts from the sinus node to an atrial site.

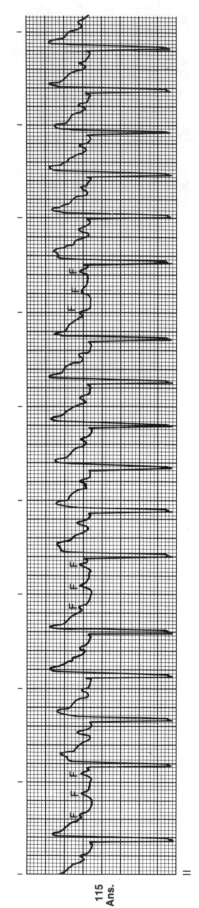

115
Ans.

II

Don't confuse WAP with the emergence of an escape rhythm caused by sinus dysfunction. In escape rhythms, the ectopic pacemaker emerges after a pause that is **longer** than the normal R-R interval and represents a backup system to stimulate the heart. In WAP, the sinus rate is adequate and this dysrhythmia is benign, just as in the development of PACs.

117

Rate ___180___ /min. Rhythm ___regular___
QRS Duration ___0.20–0.28___ s. P-R Interval ___absent___
AV Conduction Ratio ___absent___

Interpretation: Ventricular tachycardia.

Rationale: This dysrhythmia resembles a string of PVCs linked together. In essence, we have continuous ventricular complexes at a rapid rate. The ventricular activity is slightly irregular and the QRS complexes are distorted and wide. Atrial activity is not viewed.

Discussion: Wide, aberrant QRS complexes are also seen in SVTs with abnormal intraventricular conduction defect caused by bundle branch fatigue. We **cannot** be absolutely certain that SVT with aberrant ventricular conduction is not the dysrhythmia present.

118

Rate ___absent___ Rhythm ___absent___
QRS Duration ___absent___ P-R Interval ___absent___
AV Conduction Ratio ___absent___

Interpretation: Coarse ventricular fibrillation.

Rationale: No QRS complexes or P waves exist. The erratic tracing reflects fibrillation.

119

Rate A) ___atrial 70/min.   ventricular 24/min.___
      B) ___atrial 260/min.   ventricular 40/min.___
Rhythm A and B) ___regular___
QRS Duration A) ___over 0.20___ s.   B) ___over 0.20___ s.
P-R Interval A) ___absent___   B) ___absent___
AV Conduction Ratio A) ___absent___   B) ___absent___

Interpretation: **Both tracings show complete AV block, but the atrial rates differ considerably.** The ventricular rate in *A* is about 30/minute, while in *B* it is about 40/minute. Atrial activity occurs at 75/minute in *A* and 260/minute in *B*. Atrial flutter has developed in the AV dissociated state shown in *B*.

Note: Neither of these dysrhythmias generated a pulse, and the patient died soon afterward. Electrical activity without contraction is known as electromechanical dissociation. In such grave situations our attention must be directed toward establishing pulses and accelerating the ventricular activity.

120

Rate ___47___ /min. Rhythm ___regular___
QRS Duration ___0.12___ s. P-R Interval ___0.32___ s.
AV Conduction Ratio ___1:1___

Interpretation: **Sinus bradycardia with first degree AV block.**

Rationale: The ventricular and atrial activity is normal. The deviations from normal sinus rhythm are a P-R interval beyond 0.20 second and the slow sinus rate. The prolonged conduction time indicates that activation of the ventricles begins later than normal. No P waves are actually blocked; they are only delayed briefly. Eventually all P waves pass through the AV node. Increased vagal tone causes sinus node depression and decreased conduction velocity.

212

121

Rate __75__ /min. Rhythm __regular__ P-R Interval __0.16__ s.
QRS Duration __0.08__ s.
AV Conduction Ratio __1:1__

Interpretation: **Regular sinus rhythm is disguised by artifact caused by patient movement.** The artifact distorts the baseline and makes it difficult to see the P and T waves for most of the strip. The QRS complexes, however, can still be identified. Superficially, the artifact mimics the wavy baseline of atrial fibrillation. Unlike atrial fibrillation however, the R-R interval remains constant, and P waves can be seen.

122

Rate __absent__ Rhythm __absent__ P-R Interval __absent__
QRS Duration __absent__
AV Conduction Ratio __absent__

Interpretation: **Pacemaker spikes without capture. The patient's intrinsic rhythm is asystole.**

Rationale: The tracing shows the artifact created by a pacemaker pulse generator. It is not accompanied by capture of the myocardium. The heart is electrically silent.

123

Rate __75__ /min. Rhythm __regular__ P-R Interval __absent__
QRS Duration __0.20–0.28__ s.
AV Conduction Ratio __absent__

Interpretation: **Ventricular fibrillation is countershocked at point X into an accelerated idioventricular or AV junctional rhythm.**

Rationale: Ventricular fibrillation is easy to detect in the early part of the strip because of the chaotic wave form. The defibrillation charge displaces the recording stylus to the top of the tracing, after which it returns to show a regular rhythm. The rhythm is characterized by wide QRS complexes that lack P waves. The rate of 75 is faster than the expected automatic focus in **either the** AV junction or the bundle branches-Purkinje network. The elevated ST segment distorts the QRS complexes, making it impossible to distinguish between a junctional or idioventricular focus.

124

Rate __132__ /min. Rhythm __regular__ P-R Interval __0.16__ s.
QRS Duration __0.08__ s.
AV Conduction Ratio __1:1__

Interpretation: **Sinus tachycardia.**

Rationale: This tracing fulfills the requirements for sinus tachycardia as follows:

• Ventricular activity: normal QRS shape, regular R-R intervals, and a rate of over 100/min.
• Atrial activity: normal P wave shape, regular P-P intervals, and a rate of over 100/min.
• AV relationship is normal; there is one P wave for each QRS complex.

125

Rate __46__ /min. Rhythm __irregular__ P-R Interval __0.16__ s.
QRS Duration __0.16__ s.
AV Conduction Ratio __1:1 (for sinus)__

Interpretation: **The initial portion of the tracing shows a sinus rhythm that abruptly changes to an AV junctional escape rhythm following failure of the sinus node to pace the heart.**

Rationale: The ventricular activity consists of wide QRS complexes—even those associated with P

213

ing and have been replaced by a fine wavy baseline. The relationship of the fibrillatory waves to the QRS complexes (AV conduction) is variable. No fixed conduction ratio exists because the atrial waves arrive at the AV node in a random fashion. As a result, the AV node has different degrees of refractoriness and can transmit only a fraction of the impulse into the ventricle.

128

Rate atrial 75 /min. ventricular 37 /min. Rhythm regular P-R Interval 0.16 s.
QRS Duration 0.08 s.
AV Conduction Ratio 2:1

Interpretation: Sinus rhythm with second degree AV block (2:1 conduction ratio). The ventricular rate is about 37/minute.

Rationale: The ventricular rhythm is regular. The QRS complexes are normal in appearance. The atrial rhythm is regular. There are two P waves to each QRS complex. The conduction ratio is 2:1, with a slow ventricular response (37 beats/minute).

Note: With a 2:1 AV block it is not possible to know whether Mobitz type 1 (Wenckebach) or Mobitz type 2 is present. In 2:1 block, we cannot determine if the P-R intervals are fixed or progressively increase. For this reason, some authors prefer to term it Mobitz type: Nonspecific. To interpret a Mobitz type 1, at least **two consecutive** conducted P-R intervals must be observed before the blocked QRS complex occurs.

---

waves (beats 1 through 6). The R-R intervals differ, depending on whether they are sinus or junctional. Atrial activity can be observed only for the first six beats. The last three beats show no P waves and therefore must have arisen in the AV junction. We know this because the QRS complexes are identical to the sinus beats. The latent pacemaker activity of the AV junction discharges only when the ventricles fail to be stimulated from above.

126

Rate 114 /min. Rhythm irregular P-R Interval 0.16 s.
QRS Duration 0.08 s.
AV Conduction Ratio 1:1

Interpretation: Sinus tachycardia with multiformed PACs (also known as multifocal atrial tachycardia).

Rationale: The QRS complexes generally look the same, except for the two that are slightly taller than the rest. The striking features are the irregular R-R intervals and the fluctuating shapes of P and P' waves. In multifocal atrial tachycardia there are three or more P wave shapes and no dominant R-R intervals.

127

Rate 110 /min. Rhythm grossly irregular P-R Interval absent
QRS Duration 0.10 s.
AV Conduction Ratio absent

Interpretation: Atrial fibrillation with a ventricular response slightly over 100 beats/minute.

Rationale: The QRS complexes are generally similar in shape, but the ventricular rhythm is grossly irregular. Clearly discernible P waves are lack-

214

Discussion: Ventricular pacemakers are considerably slower and more unreliable than sinus sites. The width of the QRS complex varies with the location of the focus in the ventricles and the conduction velocity. Generally it will be narrow if it originates close to the AV node; that is, high in the ventricular system before the His bundle bifurcates. As the pacemaker focus moves more distal from the AV node, the wider the QRS complex is. This reflects the longer time needed to activate both ventricles because the impulse must depolarize the ventricles separately rather than simultaneously.

129

Rate atrial 150 /min. ventricular 39/min.   Rhythm regular

QRS Duration 0.12 s.   P-R Interval absent

AV Conduction Ratio absent

Interpretation: **Third degree AV block with a ventricular rate of 39/min.**

Rationale: The ventricular rhythm is slow and regular. The distorted QRS complexes are wide and notched. Atrial rhythmicity is regular and rapid. The P waves appear to "march through" the QRS complexes because atrioventricular dissociation exists. Many P waves are in the ST segment and T waves, making them hard to see. The P waves activate the atria but are blocked before the ventricles can be reached. An independent pacemaker originates in the ventricles. No fixed AV relationship exists.

Chapter Seven

EXERCISE F: SELF-ASSESSMENT ECG TRACINGS 130 TO 150

This chapter has a variety of ECG dysrhythmias including atrial dysrhythmias, atrioventricular blocks, and ventricular disturbances for you to practice analyzing. The answers begin on page 226.

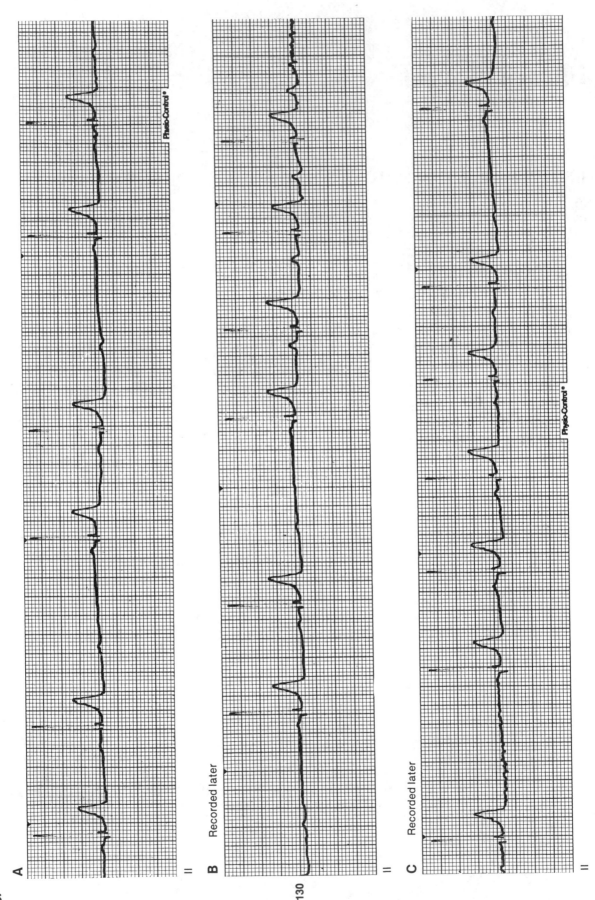

A

=

B   Recorded later

130

=

C   Recorded later

=

216

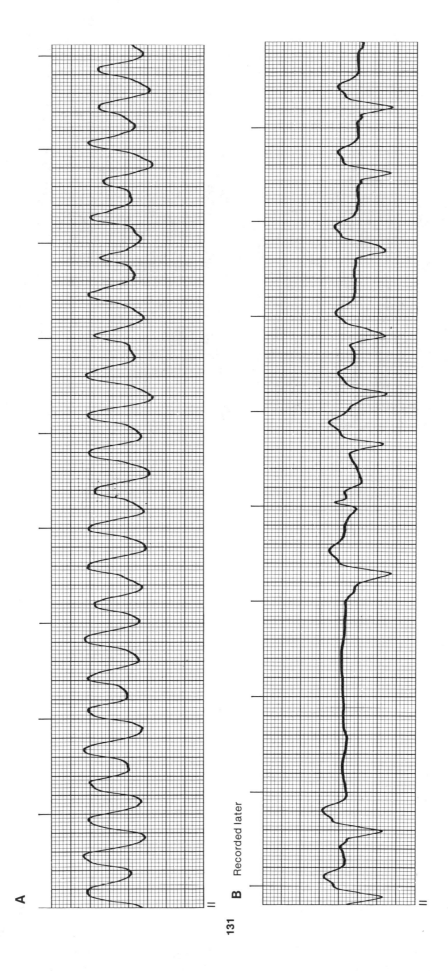

A

B Recorded later

131

217

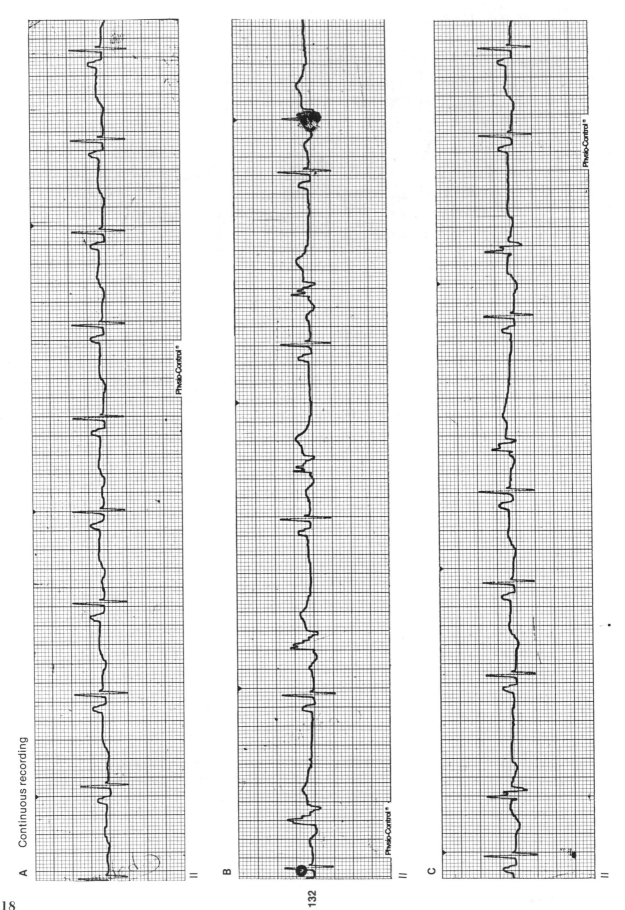

A   Continuous recording

II

B

132

II

C

II

218

Physio-Control®

Physio-Control®

Physio-Control®

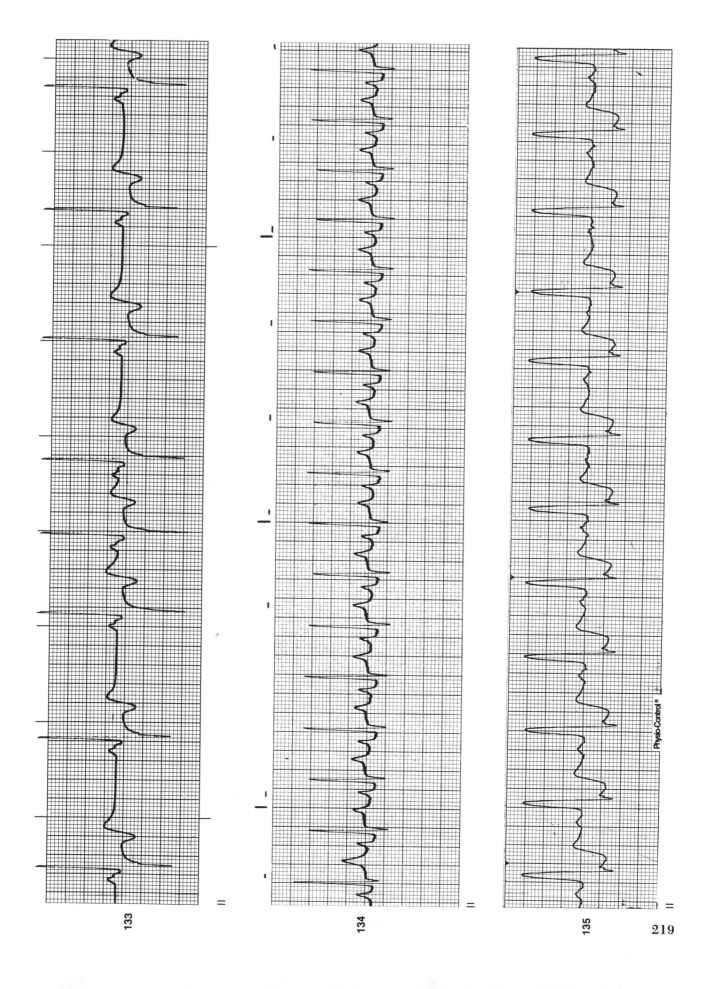

133

II

134

II

135

II

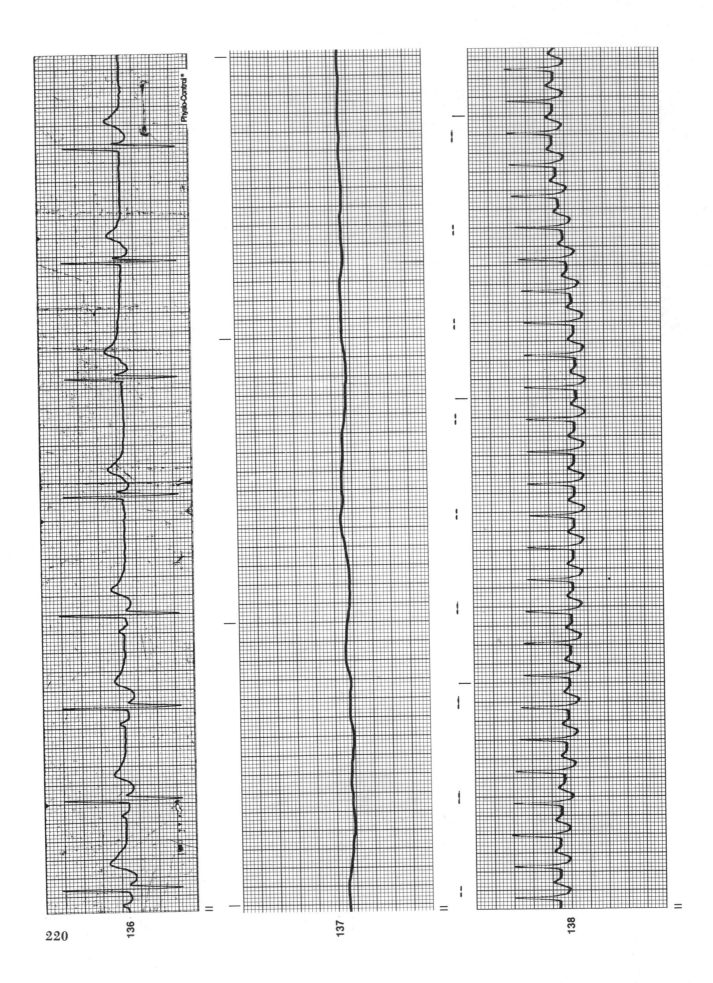

136

137

138

Physio-Control®

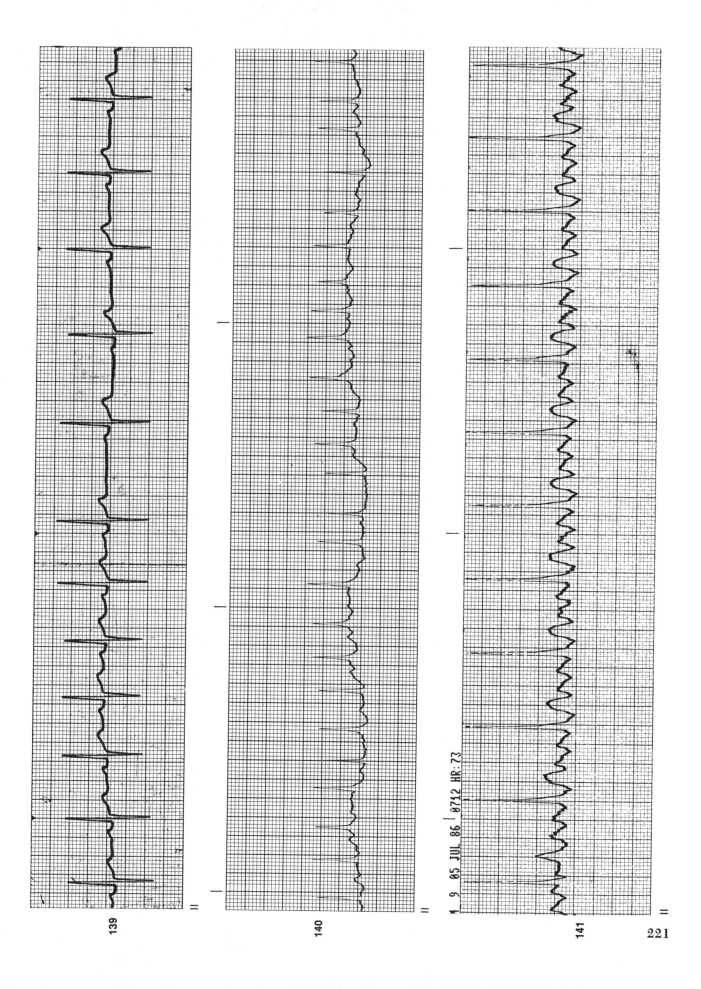

9 05 JUL 86 0712 HR:73

139

140

141

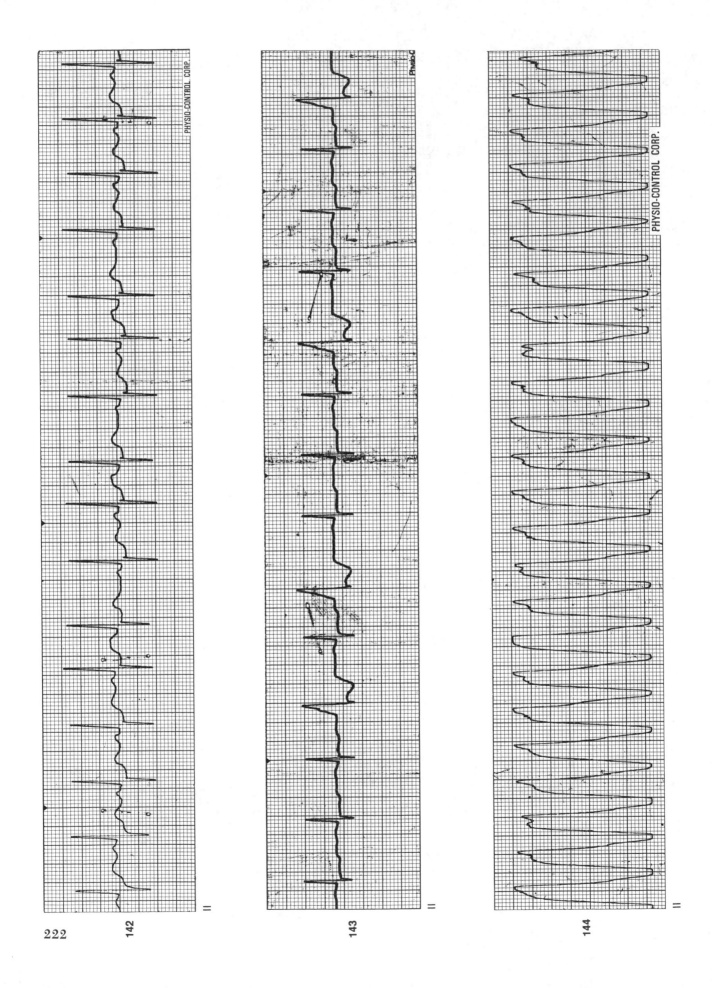

142

143

144

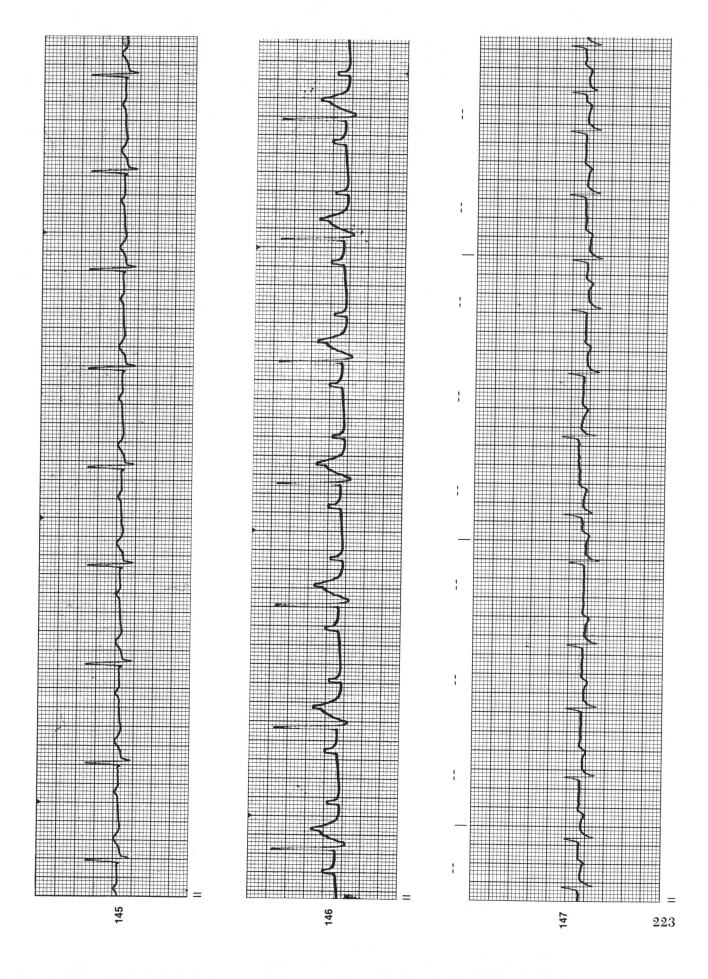

145

146

147

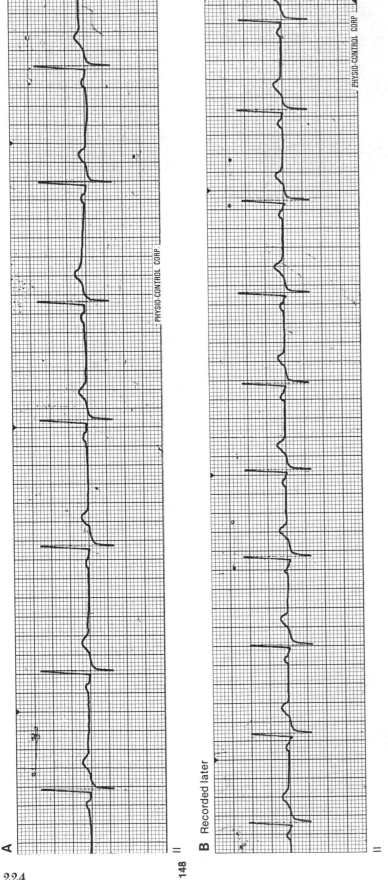

A

B Recorded later

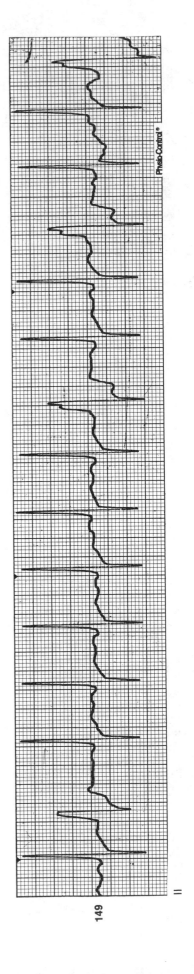

II

II

II

II

224

148

149

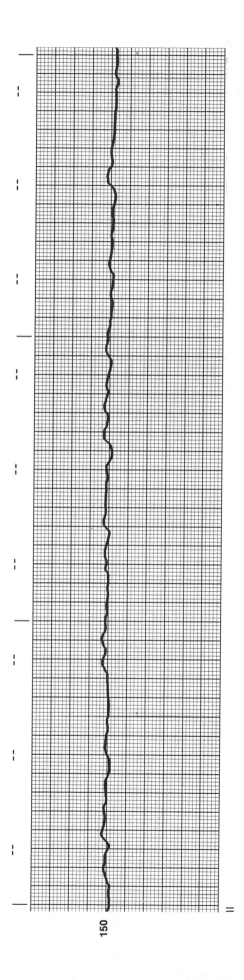

150

ANSWERS TO PRACTICE ECG TRACINGS 130 TO 150

130

Rate average 36 /min. Rhythm irregular

QRS Duration 0.10 s. P-R Interval 0.20, 0.28 s. dropped beat

AV Conduction Ratio 3:2, 5:4, 6:5

Interpretation: Sinus rhythm with second degree AV heart block; Mobitz type 1 (Wenckebach). The AV conduction ratio varies among 3:2, 5:4, and 6:5.

Rationale: In strip A, there is irregular ventricular activity with narrow QRS complexes occurring as grouped beats. The first P wave is not conducted and a QRS complex is missing. The second and third P waves are conducted, with progressive delay of the P-R interval, until the fourth P wave is not conducted. The cycle then repeats itself (see Tracing 130 Answer). In B, we see two more 3:2 cycles followed by a 5:4 AV conduction ratio, that is, five P waves but only four QRS complexes. C shows both a 6:5 and a 3:2 AV conduction ratio.

131

Rate A) 150 /min. Rhythm A) regular
B) 60 /min. B) irregular

QRS Duration A) 0.36 B) 0.24–0.36 s.

P-R Interval A and B) absent

AV Conduction Ratio absent

Interpretation: Ventricular tachycardia/flutter is present in strip A. Several minutes later strip B was obtained. They show deterioration of the ventricular focus into a slow, irregular rhythm. An asystolic period exists for about 2 seconds, followed by distorted ventricular complexes with varying shapes.

Rationale: The wide and distorted QRS complexes, lacking P waves, indicate a ventricular dysrhythmia. In strip A, the rhythm looks like a regular sine wave and is sometimes termed ventricular flutter. Strip B shows a less organized rhythm. Shortly afterward, cardiac standstill occurred.

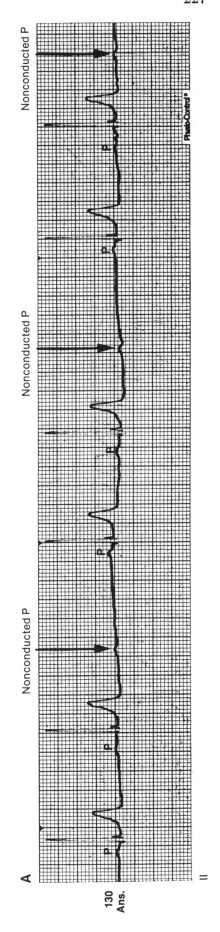

A

Nonconducted P   Nonconducted P   Nonconducted P

II

130 Ans.

132

Rate A) 60 /min. Rhythm A) regular
B) 60 /min. B) irregular
QRS Duration A) 0.10 s. sinus 0.10 s.
PVC 0.20 s. P-R Interval PVC 0.20 s.
AV Conduction Ratio 1:1

Interpretation: Strip *A* shows regular sinus rhythm, and in strip *B* each sinus beat is followed by a premature ventricular complex. The PVCs show different forms. In *C*, the PVCs do not occur after every other beat, but they happen after every third or fourth sinus beat.

Rationale: The sinus beats are recognized by the normal P-QRS-T complexes. The aberrant beats are early, wide, and distorted. They are followed by compensatory pauses and lack P waves, indicating a ectopic ventricular focus. In *B*, ventricular bigeminy is present. This type of grouped beating is due to a reentry of the sinus beat back into the ventricular tissue to reexcite the heart.

Discussion: The clinical information reveals that not all QRS complexes correspond to a forceful ventricular contraction. Since the pulse is only 30/minute, the premature depoloraizations must be occurring before ventricular filling is completed. As a result, the stroke volume is diminished.

133

Rate 45 /min. Rhythm irregular
QRS Duration 0.10 s. P-R Interval PAC 0.16 s. sinus 0.20 s.
AV Conduction Ratio 1:1

Interpretation: Sinus bradycardia with two successive premature atrial complexes (beats 5 and 6).

Rationale: The ventricular rhythm is irregular in the middle of the ECG strip owing to two early beats.

All QRS complexes show the same normal shape. Atrial activity shows P waves that are irregular at the same point as noted for ventricular complexes. P or P' waves are observed before every R wave, indicating that they are supraventricular impulses. Every R wave has a single P wave before it, revealing a 1:1 AV conduction. The P-R intervals are constant. The T waves are biphasic, and the P waves are notched. Therefore, sinus bradycardia exists with two premature atrial complexes.

134

Rate 110 /min. Rhythm regular
QRS Duration 0.08 s. P-R Interval 0.16 s.
AV Conduction Ratio 1:1

Interpretation: Sinus tachycardia.

Rationale: Each cardiac complex consists of a normal appearing sequence of P-QRS-T waves. The SA node is discharging at a rate greater than 100/minute. Sinus tachycardia usually exists in the range of 100 to 150/minute. In certain cases the rate may even rise to 180.

135

Rate 75 /min. Rhythm regular
QRS Duration 0.16 s. P-R Interval 0.20 s.
AV Conduction Ratio 1:1

Interpretation: Normal sinus rhythm.

Rationale: The ventricular rhythm is regular (constant R-R intervals). The QRS complexes are wide, but the depressed ST segment makes an exact measurement difficult. P waves occur before each QRS complex. A fixed 1:1 conduction ratio of atrioventricular impulses exists. Normal sinus rhythm is present.

138

Rate __170__ /min. Rhythm __regular__
QRS Duration __0.10__ s. P-R Interval __absent__
AV Conduction Ratio __absent__

Interpretation: Supraventricular tachycardia.

Rationale: The ventricular rhythm is precisely regular and the QRS complexes are narrow. The QRS duration of 0.06 to 0.08 second signifies that (1) the lower cardiac chambers must be activated along the normal intraventricular pathway normally and (2) that the impulse must have originated from above the bifurcation of the His bundle. Supraventricular sites (sinus, atrial, or junctional) are located proximal to the His bifurcation. Distinct atrial waves are not visible. Upright deflections seen between the R waves are probably T waves (and not P waves). Since we cannot determine an exact focus, we term it supraventricular tachycardia.

Remember: Be suspicious of the possibility that atrial flutter at a rate of 340/minute with 2:1 AV conduction may also yield a ventricular rate of 170/minute. Be sure to scrutinize tracings in this range for flutter waves between the QRS complexes.

Discussion: This dysrhythmia is considered too fast for a sinus focus in addition to the lack of P waves. On rare occasions, the sinus could discharge at 170/minute, but it is not usual. The range between 150 and 250 is common for an atrial focus outside the sinus node. The most common rate for SVT is 170 to 220/minute, which this example shows.

136

Rate A) sinus __60__ /min. B) AV __48__ /min. Rhythm __regular__
QRS Duration AV __0.08__ s. sinus __0.08__ s. P-R Interval AV __absent__ sinus __0.16__ s.
AV Conduction Ratio __sinus 1:1__

Interpretation: Cessation of sinus activity causes the regular sinus rhythm to change to an AV junctional rhythm.

Rationale: The initial portion shows narrow and normal appearing QRS complexes. The P-R interval is within normal limits. The R-R intervals for the first four beats are constant and measure five large boxes. Then the pacemaker site shifts: the fifth QRS, lacking a P wave, arises after an R-R interval (1.24 seconds) that is longer than the dominant rhythm (1.0 second). The sinus arrest permits the AV junction to fire spontaneously. The last five beats show normal QRS complexes that appear identical to the sinus beats. The only difference is the longer R-R intervals and missing P waves. The pacemaker shifts when the ventricles fail to be stimulated from above. The junctional escape rhythm occurs at a rate of about 48/minute which agrees with the degree of automaticity for that region (40 to 60/minute).

137

Rate __absent__ Rhythm __absent__
QRS Duration __absent__ P-R Interval __absent__
AV Conduction Ratio __absent__

Interpretation: Asystole.

Rationale: The absence of all electrical activity in this heart is revealed by a flat ECG. No current is flowing, and as a result, the cardiac cycles are missing.

139

Rate ___78___ /min. Rhythm ___irregular___
QRS Duration ___0.08___ s. P-R Interval ___0.16___ s.
AV Conduction Ratio ___1:1___

Interpretation: **Sinus dysrhythmia.**

Rationale: This dysrhythmia differs from NSR only in the regularly irregular impulse formation of the sinus node. As a result, we see a regular variation in the P-P and R-R intervals. The P waves and QRS complexes are normal. AV conduction ratio is 1:1 with a normal P-R interval. Although this is technically a dysrhythmia, it actually is a physiologic variation of NSR.

140

Rate ___150___ /min. Rhythm grossly irregular
QRS Duration ___0.06–0.10___ s. P-R Interval ___absent___
AV Conduction Ratio ___absent___

Interpretation: **Atrial fibrillation with an uncontrolled ventricular response of 150/min.**

Rationale: The R-R rhythm is grossly irregular. The QRS complexes are within normal ranges in terms of width and shape. Atrial activity is evidenced by small fibrillatory f waves. These f waves convert the normally flat baseline to a collection of small, uneven waves. The AV conduction ratio is too irregular to calculate a relationship.
Hallmark findings of atrial fibrillation:
• Normal QRS complexes
• Irregularly irregular ventricular rhythm
• Small irregular fibrillatory baseline
• f waves replacing P waves

141

Rate atrial 300/min.
Rate ventricular 75/min. Rhythm ___regular___
QRS Duration ___0.08–0.12___ s. P-R Interval ___absent___
AV Conduction Ratio ___4:1___

Interpretation: **Atrial flutter with 4:1 AV conduction.**

Rationale: The ventricular rhythm is regular and the QRS complexes show a consistently narrow shape. Atrial activity is characterized by tall and peaked "flutter" waves. There are four F waves for every QRS complex. The atrial rate is 300/minute, while that of the ventricles is only 75, or a quarter of the atrial focus.

142

Rate ___96___ /min. Rhythm ___irregular___
QRS Duration ___0.08___ s.
P-R Interval ___sinus 0.16___ s.
PAC not measurable
AV Conduction Ratio ___1:1___

Interpretation: **Sinus rhythm with three PACs (beats 6, 9, and 12).**

Rationale: The otherwise regular rhythm is interrupted by three early complexes. The ventricular and atrial activity for the sinus beats are normal. The PACs show P′ waves that distort the preceding T waves. The QRS complexes of the PACs are identical to the sinus beats because, once formed, the impulses activate the ventricles normally.

Discussion: The PACs are easy to distinguish from PVCs because atrial ectopic beats have the following characteristics:

- P' waves before the QRS complexes
- QRS complexes identical to sinus beats
- Noncompensatory pauses
- T wave direction the same as QRS complexes

143

Rate __90__ /min. Rhythm __irregular__
QRS Duration __sinus 0.08__ s. __PVC 0.20__ s. P-R Interval __sinus 0.16__ s.
AV Conduction Ratio __1:1__

Interpretation: Sinus rhythm with frequent unifocal PVCs.

Rationale: If we cover the aberrant ventricular beats, the rest of the rhythm looks regular and normal. The sinus beats show a P-QRS-T complex with flattened P and T waves. The ectopic impulses occur frequently, have wide QRS complexes, and lack P waves. The pauses after the PVCs are fully compensatory, and the T waves slope away from the abnormal QRS direction. Thus, the abnormal complexes are PVCs, which are uniform and occur frequently (greater than 5/minute), disrupting the sinus rhythm.

144

Rate __150__ /min. Rhythm __regular__
QRS Duration __0.24__ s. P-R Interval __absent__
AV Conduction Ratio __absent__

Interpretation: Ventricular tachycardia.

Rationale: The ventricular activity shows wide and bizarre QRS complexes occurring at fixed R-R intervals. Atrial activity is not evident. Therefore, this tachydysrhythmia is originating within the ventricles.

145

Rate __57__ /min. Rhythm __regular__
QRS Duration __0.08__ s. P-R Interval __0.36__ s.
AV Conduction Ratio __1:1__

Interpretation: Sinus bradycardia with a first degree heart block.

Rationale: The QRS complexes are narrow and occur regularly. Each is preceded by a P wave with a fixed P-R interval. The P-R interval is prolonged beyond 0.20 second indicating a delay in the start of ventricular activation. In a first degree heart block no QRS complexes are actually dropped, they only take longer to appear. Normally, the AV node has the greatest degree of refractoriness of the conduction system and delays the sinus impulse before permitting it to activate the ventricles. Intranodal delays are the most common cause of first degree AV blocks, although a delay anywhere in the atria could prolong the P-R interval.

146

Rate __sinus 100/min.__ __ventricle 50__ /min. Rhythm __regular__
QRS Duration __0.10__ s. P-R Interval __0.28__ s.
AV Conduction Ratio __1:1__

Interpretation: Sinus rhythm with second degree AV block with 2:1 AV conduction. The type is nonspecific, meaning we cannot decide which Mobitz type exists (see below).

Rationale: The ventricular activity is slow but regular. The QRS complexes appear narrow and normal. The P-P interval is regular, with P-R intervals of 0.28 second for the P waves that are conducted. The AV conduction ratio is 2:1; only one QRS complex occurs for every two P waves. The second P wave of each cycle is pre-

232

vented from stimulating the ventricles. As a result, the atrial rate is 100/minute but the ventricles beat at half that rate (50/minute).

Terminology: In a 2:1 block it is **not** possible to tell with certainty if Mobitz 1 or Mobitz 2 is present because there is only one visible P-R interval before the dropped QRS. The second P-R interval could be prolonged, but we cannot determine this from a surface ECG. Many erroneously call this type 2 because they assume that the P-R intervals are fixed; this is only true if two consecutively conducted P waves are seen. It is possible to make an educated guess as to the type based on other findings in the tracing besides conduction ratio.

We can make an educated guess about which form of second degree block is present by examining the:

1. **P-R interval.** A P-R interval greater than 0.20 second is found in classical Wenckebach Mobitz type 1. It signifies the block is likely to be intranodal, or within the AV node proper. Type 1 does not usually progress to more advanced form of AV block.

2. **QRS duration.** A QRS duration greater than 0.12 sec is characteristic of Mobitz type 2. It suggests that the delay is distal to the AV node and may involve the His bundle, the bundle branches, the branch fasicles, or a combination of these. Type 2 is more likely to progress to higher grades of block. Tracing 146 does **not** show widened QRS complexes, and this is further evidence that type 1 exists.

147

Rate 90–100 /min. Rhythm grossly irregular
QRS Duration 0.08 s. P-R Interval absent
AV Conduction Ratio 1:1

Interpretation: **Atrial fibrillation with a ventricular response of 90 to 100/minute.**

Rationale: The R-R intervals are grossly irregular and consist of normal QRS complexes. P waves are not seen; instead, a flat baseline is present. This is because the fibrillatory waves are not detected in all leads. In this strip the waves are so small as to appear almost flat. The clue to atrial fibrillation is the irregularity of ventricular activity caused by concealed AV conduction of the f waves.

148

Rate A) 46 /min. Rhythm A and B) regular
B) 67 /min.
QRS Duration A) 0.08 s. P-R Interval A) 0.16 s.
B) 0.08 s. B) 0.16 s.
AV Conduction Ratio A) 1:1
B) 1:1

Interpretation: **Strip A: Sinus bradycardia. Strip B: Regular sinus rhythm.**

Rationale: A normal sequence of P-QRS-T complexes is seen at a rate below 60/minute. Ventricular rhythmicity is regular with normal QRS shapes. P waves precede each QRS and are constant in contour. The P-P and P-R intervals are constant; therefore, AV conduction is normal.

In strip B the same basic pattern is noted but the rate now falls within the normal range (60 to 100/minute).

149

Rate ___95___ /min. Rhythm ___irregular___

sinus 0.10 s.

QRS Duration PVC ___0.16___ s. P-R Interval ___0.16___ s.

AV Conduction Ratio ___1:1___

The aberrant beats are:

- Premature (early in the R-R cycle)
- Wide and distorted
- With compensatory pauses
- Without P waves
- With QRS complexes that differ in shape from each other (multiformed).

Interpretation: Sinus rhythm with multiformed PVCs.

Rationale: The underlying rhythm is sinus because:

- Each QRS has the same shape and is within normal duration.
- Each QRS is preceded by a P wave.
- The P waves are upright and of the same shape.
- Each P wave is followed by a QRS complex.
- The P-R interval is normal.
- The rate of cardiac cycles is just slightly under 100/minute.

150

Rate ___absent___ Rhythm ___absent___

QRS Duration ___absent___ P-R Interval ___absent___

AV Conduction Ratio ___absent___

Interpretation: Low-voltage (fine amplitude) ventricular fibrillation. The tracing is almost flat enough to be considered asystolic.

Rationale: No ventricular or atrial complexes are noted. The wavy baseline has very small waves not exceeding 3 mm.

Chapter Eight

EXERCISE G: SELF-ASSESSMENT ECG TRACINGS 151 TO 170

This chapter has a variety of ECG dysrhythmias including atrial dysrhythmias, atrioventricular blocks, and ventricular disturbances for you to practice analyzing. The answers begin on page 245.

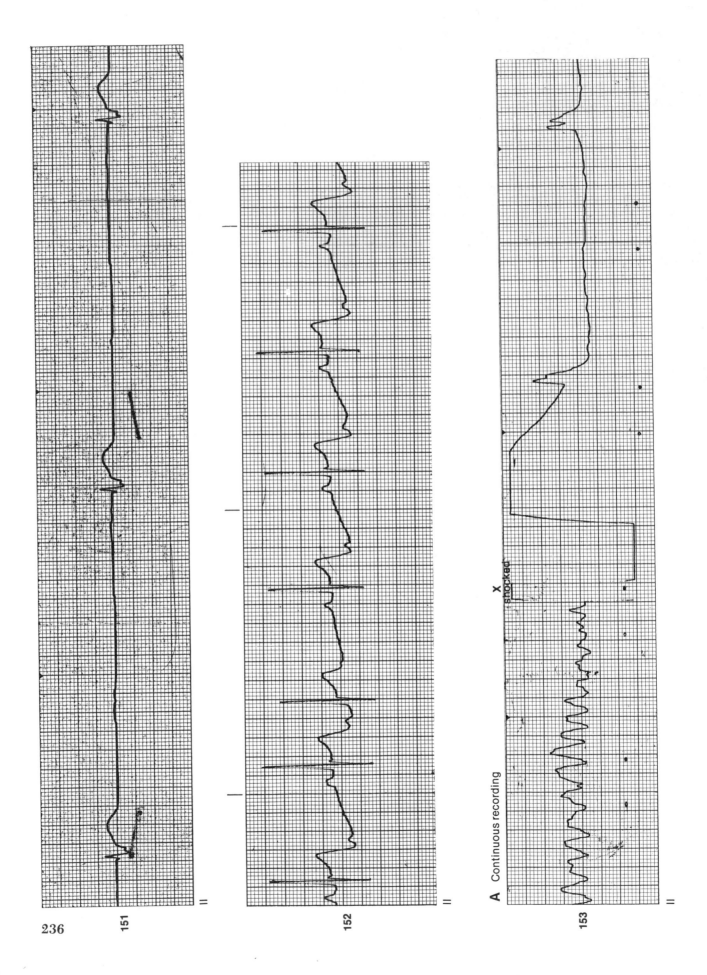

A Continuous recording

151

152

153

236

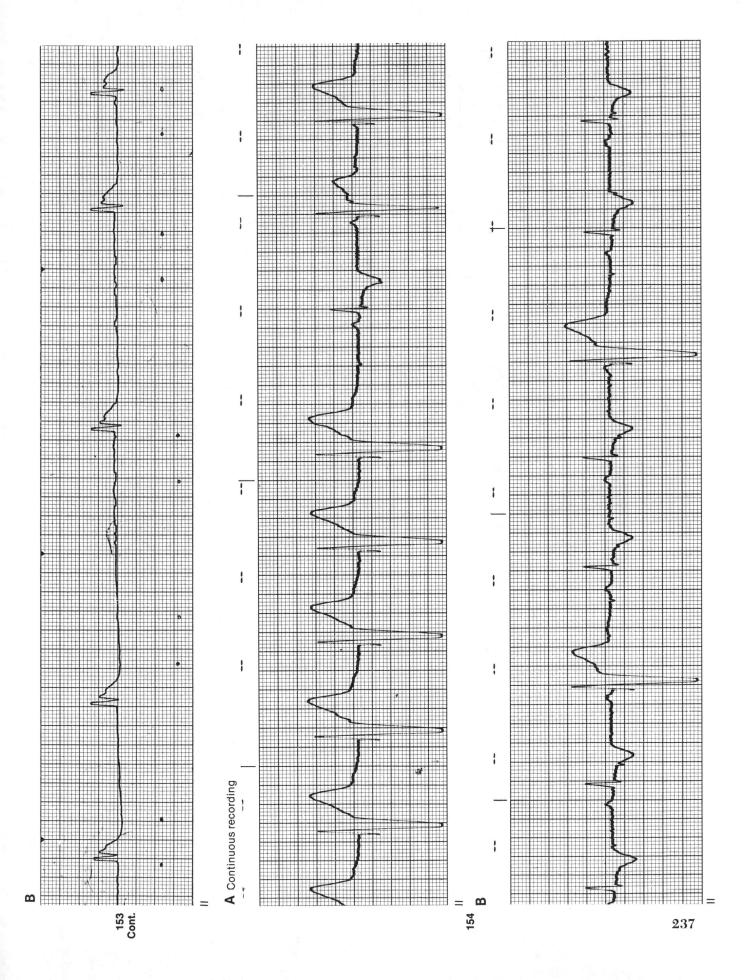

B

153
Cont.

A Continuous recording

154

B

237

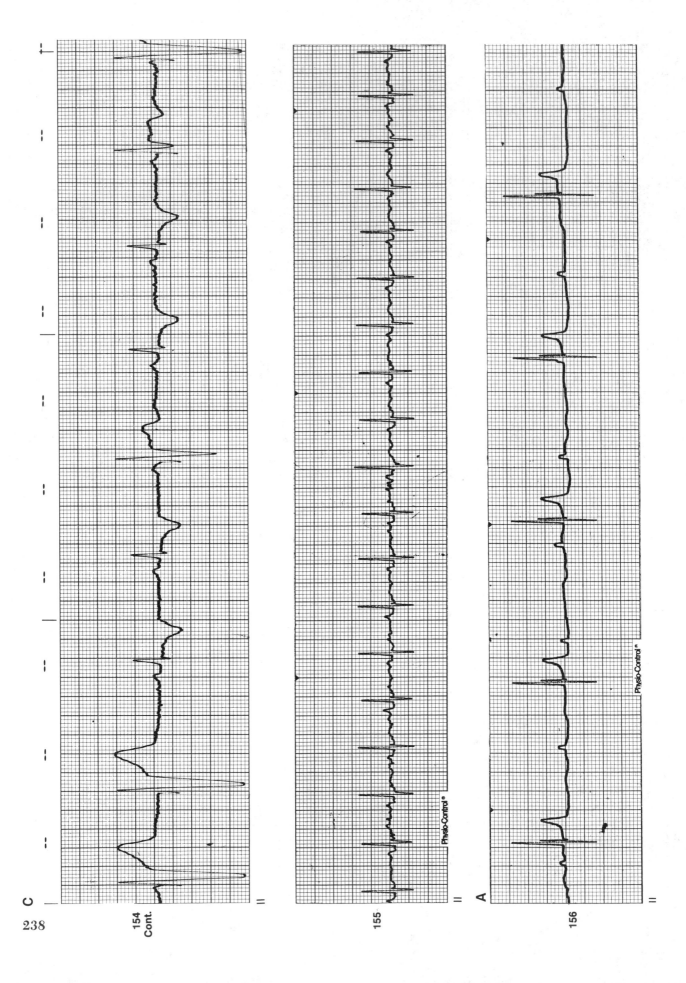

C

154
Cont.

II

155

II

A

156

II

Physio-Control®

Physio-Control®

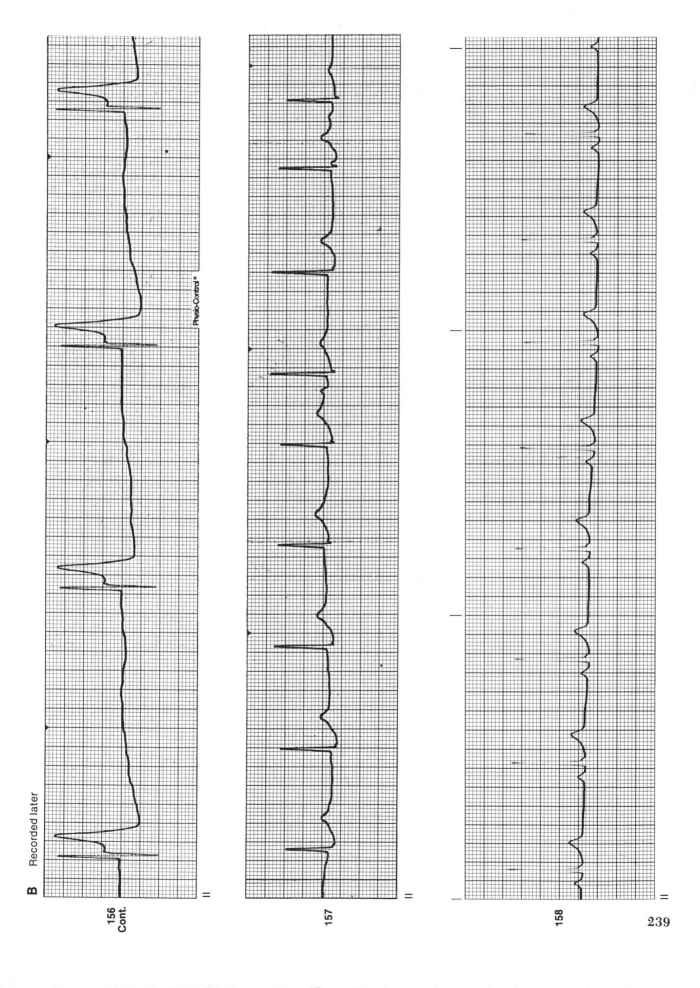

B Recorded later

156
Cont.

157

158

Physio-Control®

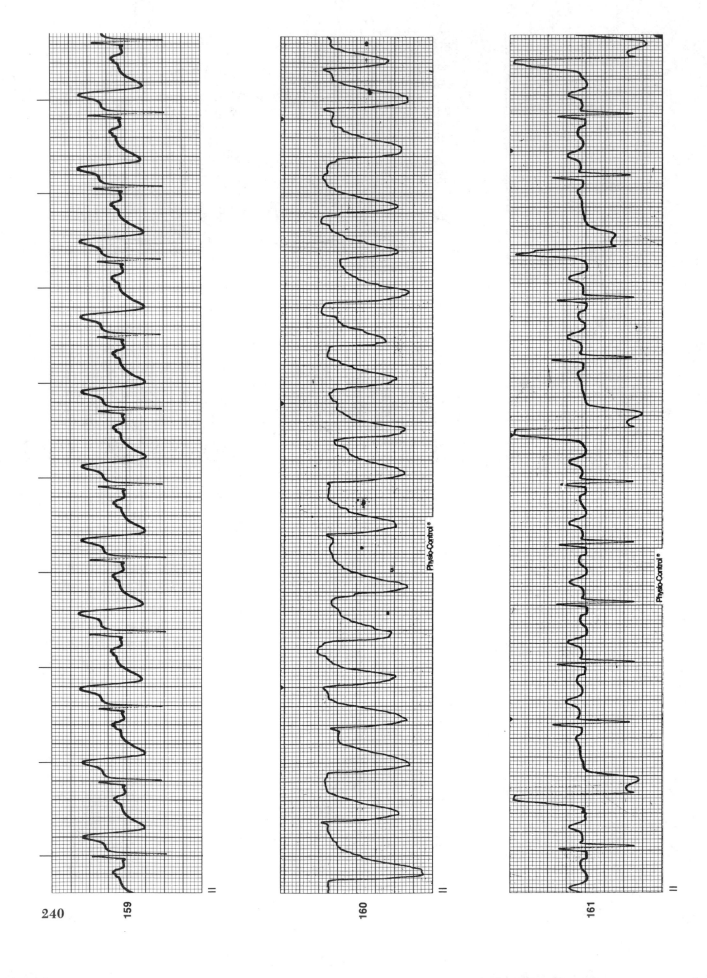

240

159

160

Physio-Control®

161

Physio-Control®

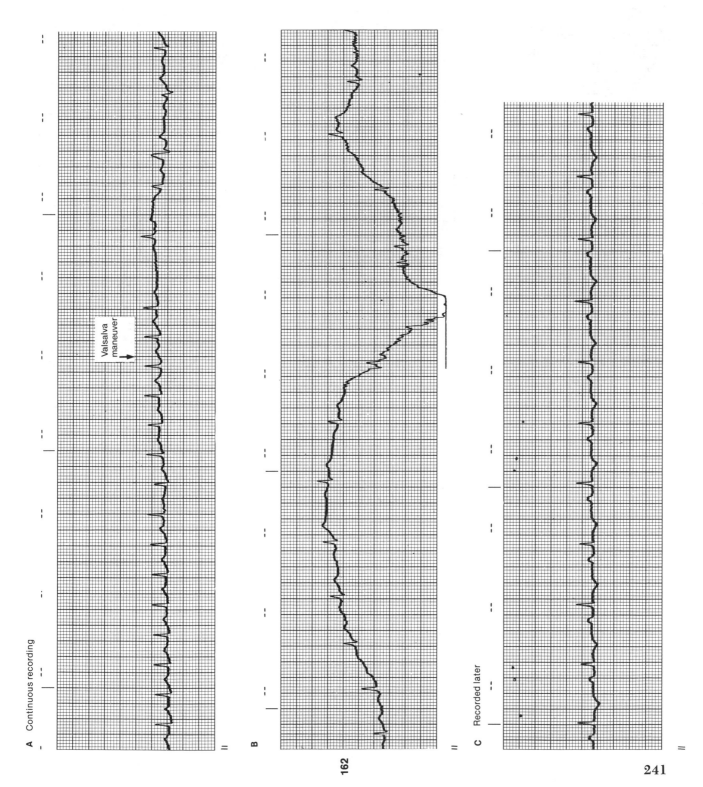

A Continuous recording

Valsalva
maneuver →

B

162

C Recorded later

241

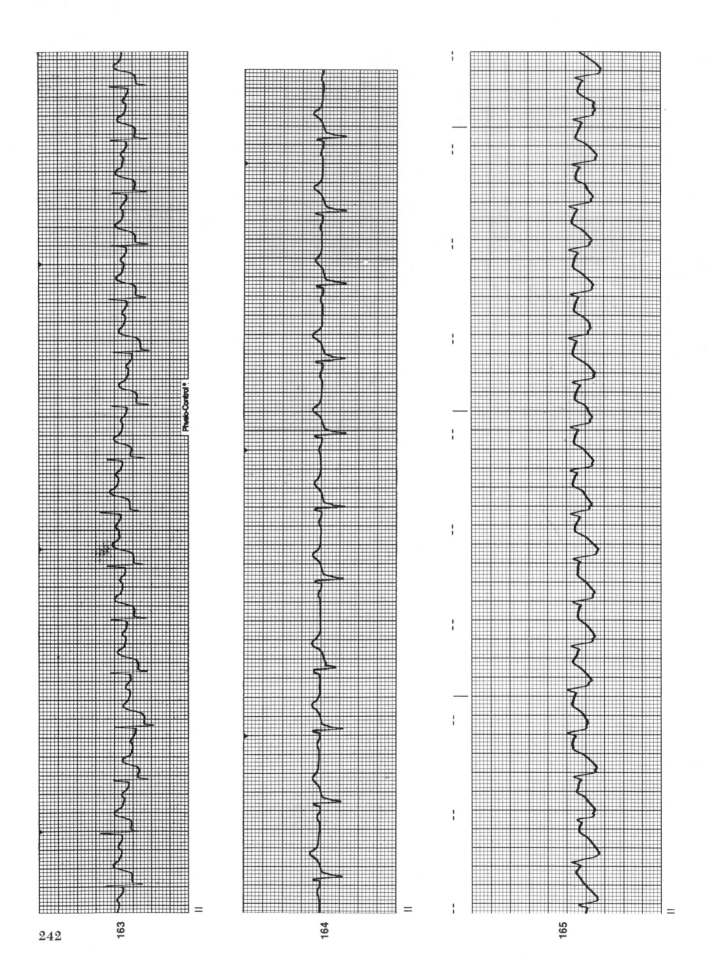

242

163

164

165

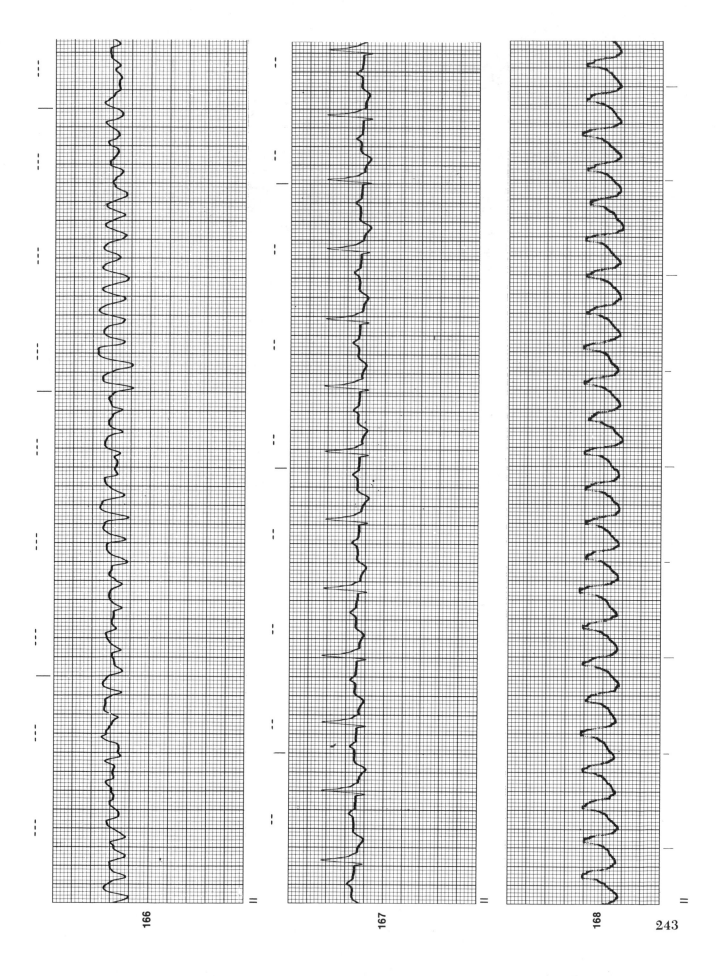

166

167

168

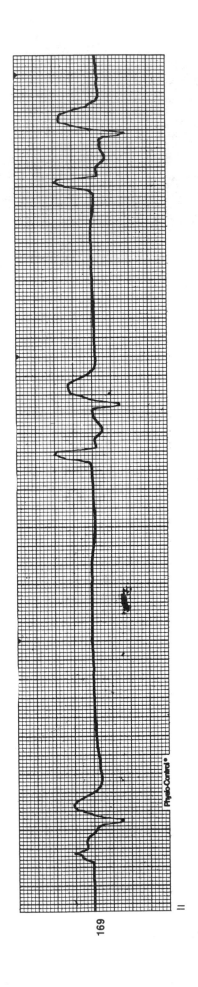

169

Physio-Control®

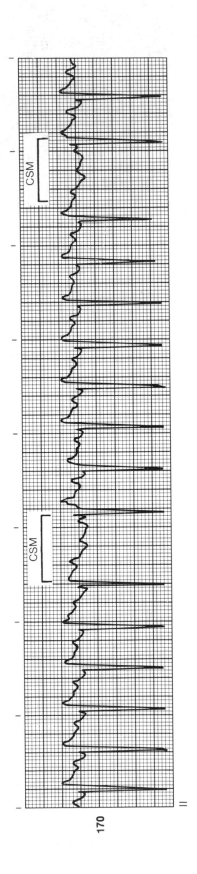

CSM

CSM

170

244

ANSWERS TO PRACTICE ECG TRACINGS 151 TO 170

151
Rate __15–20__ /min. Rhythm __regular__ P-R Interval __absent__
QRS Duration __0.12__ s.
AV Conduction Ratio __absent__

Interpretation: Slow idioventricular (agonal) rhythm.

Rationale: The extremely slow rate of cardiac cycles strikes the interpreter's eye immediately. The QRS complexes are wide and occur at regular R-R intervals. Atrial activity is not present. Since death follows unless therapy is effective, this has come to be known as a premorbid or an agonal dysrhythmia. This dysrhythmia does not usually generate a pulse because of damage in the excitation contraction coupling mechanism.

152
Rate __50__ /min. Rhythm __irregular__
P-R Interval __0.16__ s. for rest, 0.24 s. for beat 3,
QRS Duration __0.10__ s.
AV Conduction Ratio __2:1, 3:2__

Interpretation: Sinus rhythm with second degree AV block Mobitz type 1 (Wenckebach).

Rationale: If the AV conduction was only 2:1, we could not determine if Mobitz type 1 or 2 were present because we could not examine the P-R intervals to see if they lengthen before the dropped beat. In this case, however, the fourth P wave is conducted and we see the classical prolongation of the P-R interval. The ventricular rhythm is irregular because of beat 3. If the block was 2:1, the rhythm would be constant. Aside from beat 3, there are two P waves for each QRS complex.

153
Rate __absent__ /min. Rhythm __absent__ P-R Interval __absent__
QRS Duration __absent__
AV Conduction Ratio __absent__

Interpretation: Ventricular fibrillation being countershocked into a slow idioventricular rhythm.

Rationale: Strip A shows ventricular fibrillation. At point X defibrillation takes place with a direct current countershock. When the stylus returns to the middle of the paper, wide and bizarre QRS complexes occurring at a slow rate can be observed. In strip B the disordered rhythm is irregular and attests to the unreliability of idioventricular pacemakers. The last complex in B has a P wave and may be a supraventricular beat.

154
Rate __63__ /min. Rhythm __irregular__ P-R Interval __0.16__ s.
QRS Duration sinus __0.08__ s. paced 0.20 s.
AV Conduction Ratio __1:1 for sinus beats__

Interpretation: Shows a sinus bradycardia with an artificial pacemaker rhythm occurring when the sinus node slows, that is, when the R-R interval is greater than 1.08 seconds.

Rationale: In A all but the eighth beat are pacemaker complexes with 1:1 capture, meaning that each pacer spike is associated with a ventricular complex.

In B, beats 1, 2, 4, 5, 7, 8, and 9 are sinus beats with a first degree AV block. Beats 3 and 6 are pacemaker initiated complexes; however, P waves are noted before the QRS complexes. This is because they are fusion beats, consisting of a sinus P wave and a ventricular complex stimulated by a pulse generator. These combined beats show characteristics of both pacemaker sites.

155

Rate ___120___ /min. Rhythm ___regular___ P-R Interval ___0.16___ s.
QRS Duration ___0.08___ s.
AV Conduction Ratio ___1:1___

Interpretation: **Artifact due to patient tremor, which causes the sinus tachycardia to mimic atrial fibrillation.**

Rationale: The clue that this is not atrial fibrillation rests with the regular rhythmicity of ventricular activity. In fibrillation, the random AV node conduction causes irregular ventricular rhythm, exhibited by totally irregular R-R intervals. This tracing, on the other hand, shows a precisely ordered R-R interval. Patient movement distorts the baseline.

156

Rate ___atrial 50–60___ /min.
A) ventricular ___35___ /min.
B) ventricular ___23___/min. Rhythm ___A and B) regular___
QRS Duration A) ___0.10___ s.
B) ___0.12–0.16___ s.
P-R Interval ___A) and B) absent___
AV Conduction Ratio ___A) and B) absent___

Interpretation: **Strip A: Sinus rhythm with third degree AV block. Strip B: Idioventricular rhythm at a rate of 23/minute.**

Rationale: In A, the ventricular rhythm is regular with normal QRS complexes. They are not associated with P waves. The atrial rhythm is irregular with 50 to 60 P waves/minute. The P waves are not related to the QRS complexes. Therefore, third degree AV block is present.

In B, only a slow, regular QRS rhythm (23/minute) is present. No P waves are seen. The slow degree of automaticity reflects a ventricular pacemaker.

157

Rate ___54___ /min. Rhythm ___irregular___
QRS Duration ___0.10___ s.
P-R Interval ___0.20 s (beats 7 and 10)___
AV Conduction Ratio ___1:1 (beats 7 and 10)___

Interpretation: **An AV junctional rhythm with two sinus capture beats (7 and 10). Sinus arrest allows the AV junction to pace the heart.**

Rationale: The ventricular rhythm is irregular at the points where the sinus node discharges. Aside from beats 7 and 10, the R-R intervals are regular. The shapes of the sinus and junctional QRS complexes are identical. The atrial activity of the junctional complexes is absent; P waves can only be seen before the two sinus beats. The two sinus beats are said to capture the heart because they occur at points when the ventricles are polarized and able to conduct an impulse. The sinus node is discharging at a slow rate and allows the AV junction (intrinsic rate 40 to 60/minute) to emerge as pacemaker. The QRS complexes are identical for both the sinus and junctional complexes because conduction through the intraventricular pathways is the same.

158

Rate **55** /min. Rhythm **regular** P-R Interval **0.16** s.
QRS Duration **0.08** s.
AV Conduction Ratio **1:1**

Interpretation: **Sinus bradycardia.**

Rationale: Ventricular complexes have a normal appearance and regular R-R intervals. Atrial activity consists of typical P waves and regular P-P intervals. Each P wave is followed by a QRS complex. The AV conduction ratio is 1:1, and the P-R interval is normal. The rate of sinus activity is slightly slower than occurs in NSR (60 to 100/minute).

159

Rate **75** /min. Rhythm **regular** P-R Interval **0.20** s.
QRS Duration **0.10** s.
AV Conduction Ratio **1:1**

Interpretation: **Normal or regular sinus rhythm (NSR or RSR).**

Rationale: The ventricular and atrial activity is normal with a 1:1 AV conduction ratio. No deviations from NSR are found. The ST segment is elevated and the T wave is inverted.

160

Rate **120** /min. Rhythm **irregular** P-R Interval **absent**
QRS Duration **0.24–0.28** s. AV Conduction Ratio **absent**

Interpretation: **Ventricular tachycardia.**

Rationale: Ventricular activity consists of wide and bizarre QRS complexes. The R-R intervals are irregular. Atrial activity is missing. This dysrhythmia is beginning to degenerate into an even more chaotic rhythm. It lacks the general regularity of ventricular tachycardia (compare with other examples). In less than 1 minute, ventricular fibrillation occurred.

161

Rate **92** /min. Rhythm **irregular**
sinus **0.10** s.
QRS Duration PVC **0.24** s. P-R Interval **0.20** s.
AV Conduction Ratio **1:1**

Interpretation: **Sinus rhythm with four unifocal PVCs (complexes 4, 10, 13, and 16).**

Rationale: The ventricular rhythm is irregular. The QRS complexes are narrow in the sinus beats but distorted in the PVCs. P waves precede the sinus QRS complexes but not the PVCs. AV conduction is 1:1 for the sinus beats but absent for the PVCs. The coupling intervals for the ectopic beats to the prior T waves are fixed.

162

Rate **A) 160** /min. Rhythm: **A) to C) regular**
C) 75 /min. **A) 0.06–0.08** s.
QRS Duration **C) 0.08** s.
A) absent
P-R Interval **B) 0.20** s.
A) absent
AV Conduction Ratio **1:1**

Interpretation: **A** and **B** are continuous tracings showing a paroxysmal supraventricular tachycardia (rate 160/minute). The Valsalva maneuver was effective in terminating the dysrhythmia at point X. The latter portion of the tracing shows a baseline artifact caused by patient movement. In **C**, taken 1 minute later, sinus activity can clearly be seen.

junctional complexes has three possibilities: before the QRS but inverted, after the QRS, or as in this example, missing because the QRS vector obscures it.

Rationale: In the early portion of A, regular and narrow QRS complexes can be seen. P waves cannot be found. The effectiveness of the vagal stimulations can be seen because the rate slows considerably to 75/minute, and P waves are normal.

163

Rate __108__ /min. Rhythm __regular__
QRS Duration __0.08__ s. P-R Interval __0.16__ s.
AV Conduction Ratio __1:1__

Interpretation: Sinus tachycardia.

Rationale: The ventricular activity shows normal QRS complexes that have regular R-R intervals. Atrial activity shows P waves with a constant shape and a fixed P-R interval. An AV conduction ratio of 1:1 is present. The only difference from NSR is the rapid sinus rate. The ST segment is depressed.

164

Rate __75__ /min. Rhythm __irregular__
QRS Duration sinus 0.10 s. PJC 0.10 s. P-R Interval __0.16__ s.
AV Conduction Ratio __1:1__

Interpretation: Sinus rhythm with a PJC (beat 5).

Rationale: The ventricular rhythm is regular except for the short R-R interval after beat 4. The QRS complexes are normal in shape. P waves can be seen before all the sinus beats but not before the PJC. Sinus beats have P-R intervals which are fixed and within a normal time sequence. The PJC has a QRS identical in shape to the sinus beats but differs in that it lacks a P or P' wave. In lead 2, the shape of the P' waves in

165

Rate __130__ /min. Rhythm __regular__
QRS Duration __0.10__ s. P-R Interval __absent__
AV Conduction Ratio __absent__

Interpretation: AV junctional tachycardia. (SVT).

Rationale: The ventricular rhythm is regular and shows distorted QRS complexes. Abnormalities of the ST-T wave segments do not allow calculation of precise QRS durations. The atrial activity is regular, but it follows—rather than precedes—the QRS complexes. This retrograde P wave indicates that ventricular activation occurs ahead of the atria. The tachycardiac rate is much faster than the intrinsic degree of automaticity expected for the AV junction (40 to 60/minute). Enhanced automaticity of this focus or the establishment of an AV nodal reentry are the likely causes.

166

Rate __absent__ Rhythm __absent__
QRS Duration __absent__ P-R Interval __absent__
AV Conduction Ratio __absent__

Interpretation: Ventricular fibrillation/flutter.

Rationale: Fibrillation is characterized by chaotic ventricular activity. No definite QRS complexes exist, nor are P waves present. Ventricular flutter is applied to a faster form of ventricular tachycardia where the QRS complexes begin to lose their shape; instead they appear to form a con-

...tinuous sine wave. Flutter exists in the brief period during the transition from tachycardia to fibrillation.

167

Rate __82__ /min. Rhythm __regular__
QRS Duration __0.12__ s. P-R Interval __0.24__ s.
AV Conduction Ratio __1:1__

Interpretation: Sinus rhythm with first degree AV heart block.

Rationale: The QRS complexes have a regular rhythm and a wide shape. Each is preceded by a single P wave with constant P-R intervals. The P-P intervals are fixed. The P-R duration of 0.24 sec indicates a prolongation of conduction time before the ventricles are activated. The delay is usually localized to the AV node.

168

Rate __160__ /min. Rhythm __regular__
QRS Duration __0.24__ s. P-R Interval __absent__
AV Conduction Ratio __absent__

Interpretation: Ventricular tachycardia.

Rationale: The rapid ventricular rhythm resembles a series of PVCs. The QRS complexes are wide and bizarre. No atrial activity is evident. P waves are occurring but the independent atrial complexes are lost in the wide QRS complexes.

169

Rate __45__ /min. Rhythm __irregular__
QRS Duration __0.16–0.20__ s. P-R Interval __absent__
AV Conduction Ratio __absent__

Interpretation: Agonal rhythm of coupled idioventricular complexes.

Rationale: The rhythm is slow and irregular and is composed of bizarre QRS complexes. The grouped beating shows idioventricular complexes. The disorganized rhythm is produced by a dying heart.

170

Rate __atrial 250__ /min. Rhythm __irregular__
__ventricular 120__ /min.
QRS Duration __0.08__ s. P-R Interval __absent__
AV Conduction Ratio __2:1__

Interpretation: Atrial flutter with variable AV conduction. Vagal maneuvers are employed to unmask the hidden F waves.

Rationale: It is difficult to detect the 2:1 AV conduction except during CSM. The ventricular rhythm is irregular during CSM. The QRS complexes have a normal duration. The atrial activity is regular but at a rate twice that of the ventricles.

Avoid misinterpreting this dysrhythmia as sinus tachycardia, which is a common error when the flutter waves are not readily apparent. Because the ventricular rhythm is regular, it occurs between 140 and 160 (due to 2:1 AV conduction), and is preceded by an atrial wave, it mimics sinus tachycardia. It is important to use vagal maneuvers when faced with what appears to be a prolonged case of sinus tachycardia.

Chapter Nine

EXERCISE H: SELF-ASSESSMENT ECG TRACINGS 171 TO 200

This chapter has a variety of ECG dysrhythmias including atrial dysrhythmias, atrioventricular blocks, and ventricular disturbances for you to practice analyzing. The answers begin on page 265.

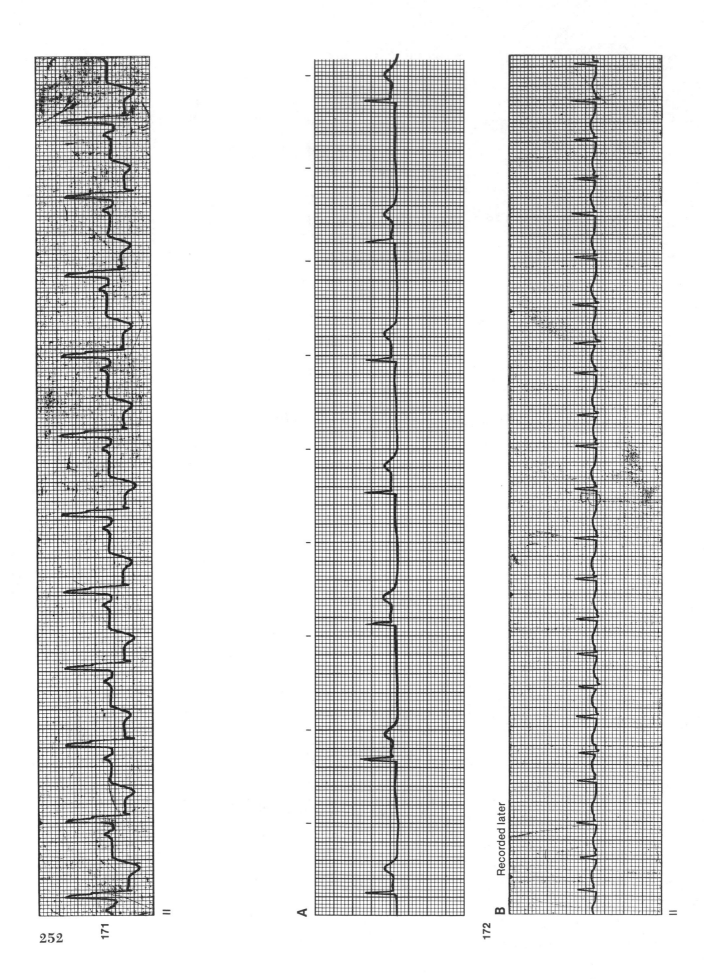

252

171

II

A

B

Recorded later

172

II

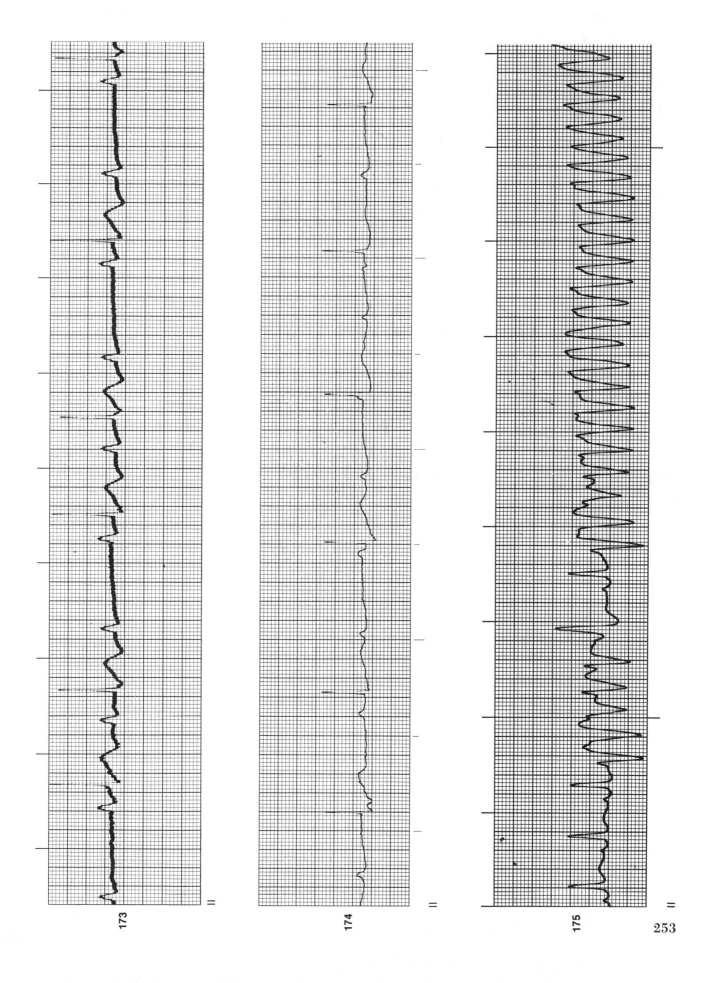

173

174

175

253

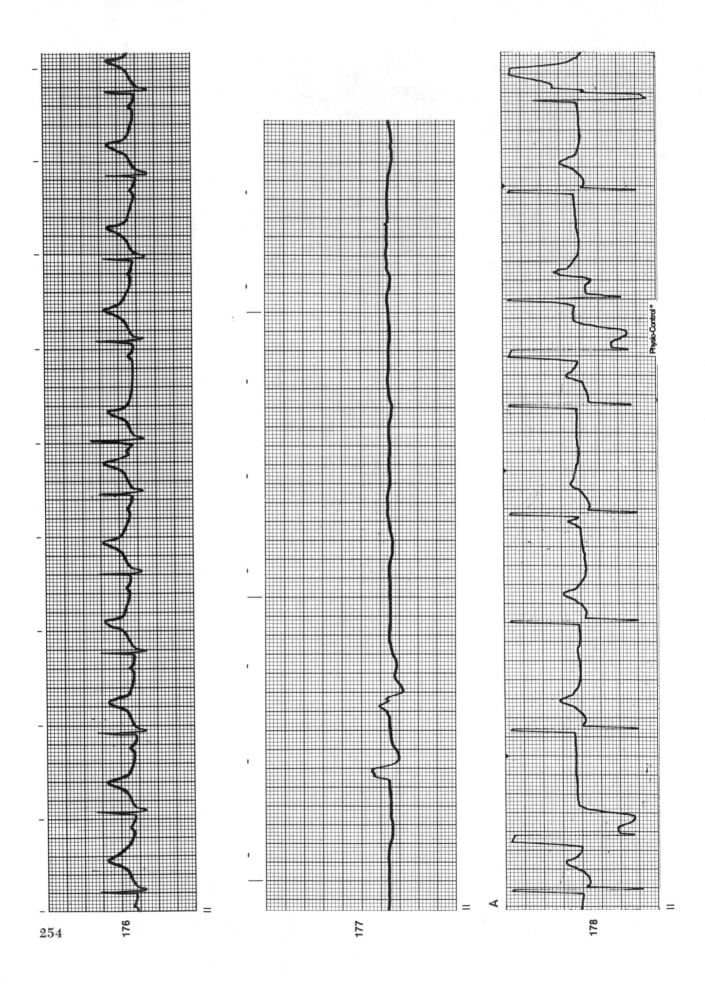

176

II

177

II

A

178

II

PhysioControl®

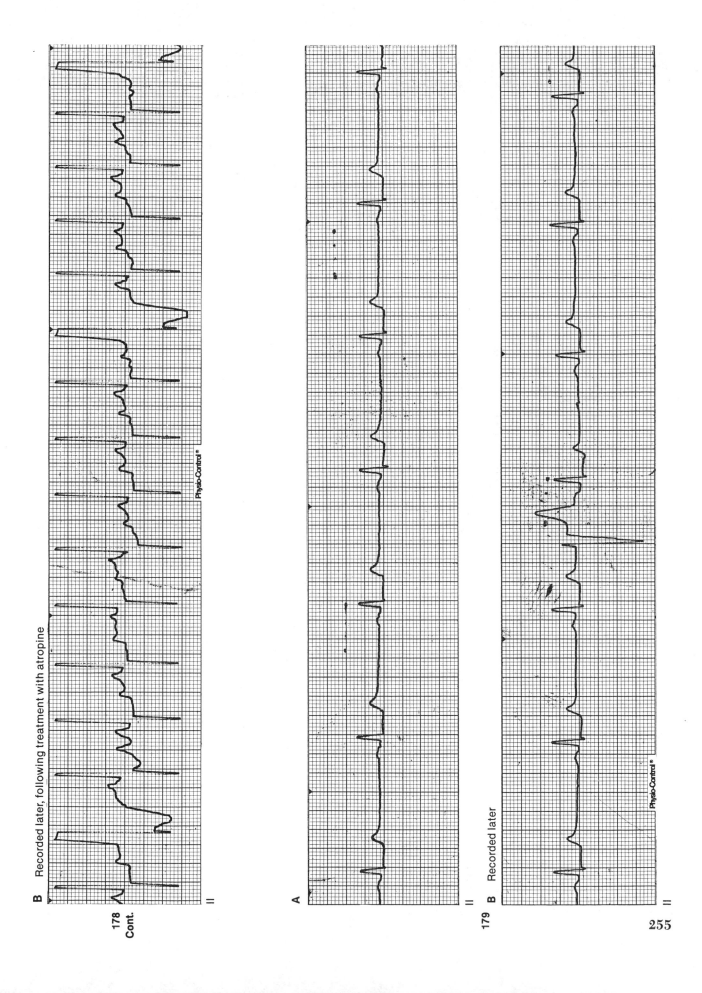

B Recorded later, following treatment with atropine

178
Cont.

II

Physio-Control®

A

II

179 **B** Recorded later

II

Physio-Control®

255

Continuous recording

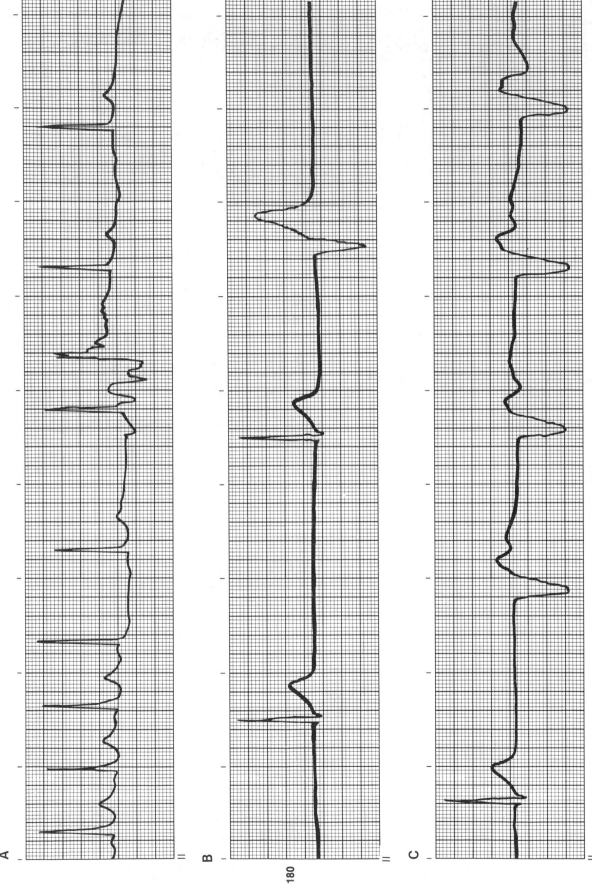

A

B

180

C

II

II

II

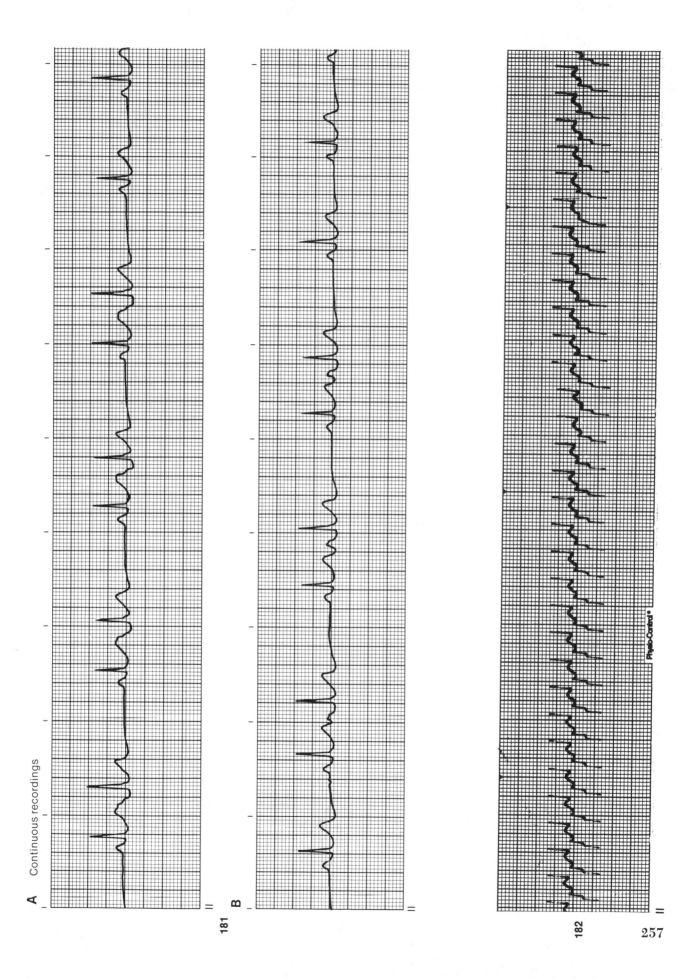

II

B

II

Physio-Control®

II

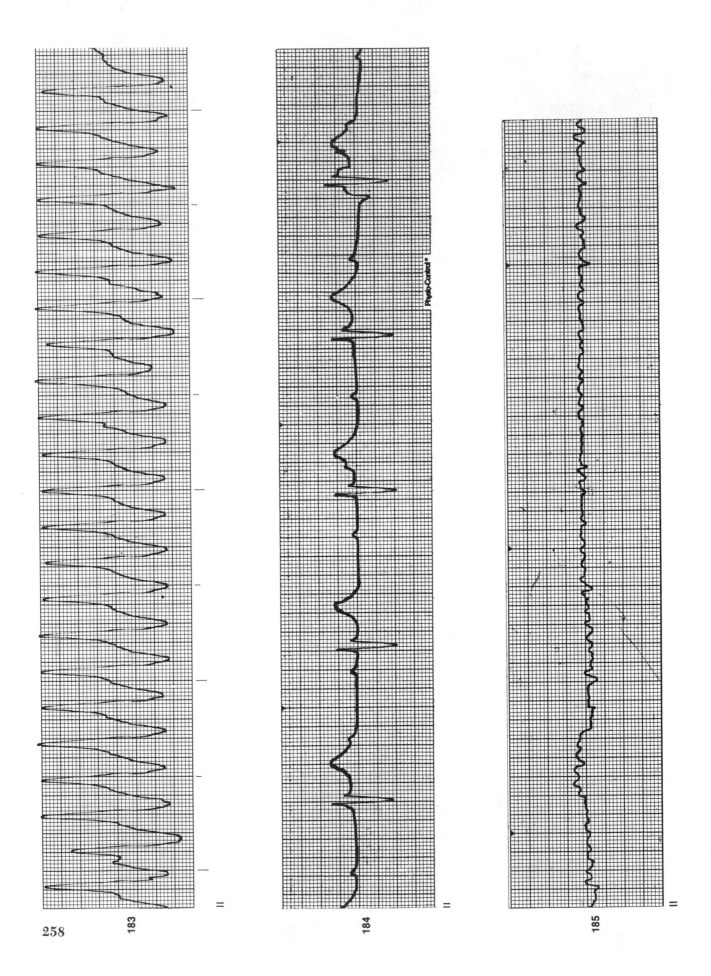

258

183

184

185

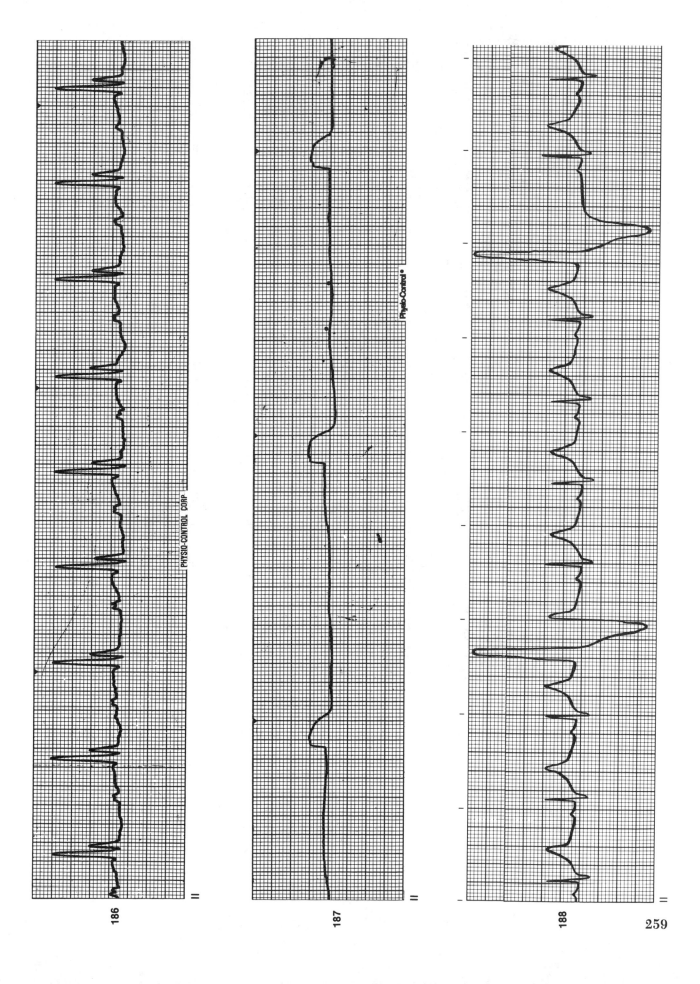

186

187

188

259

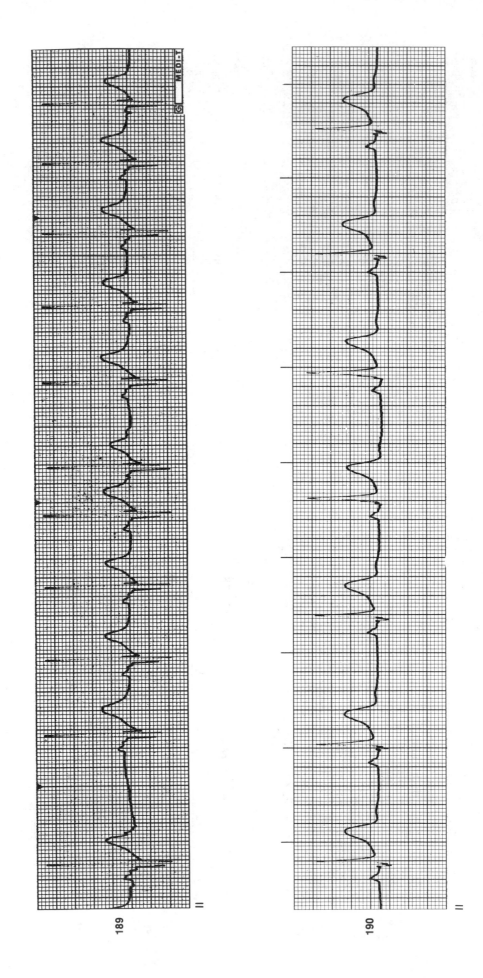

189

190

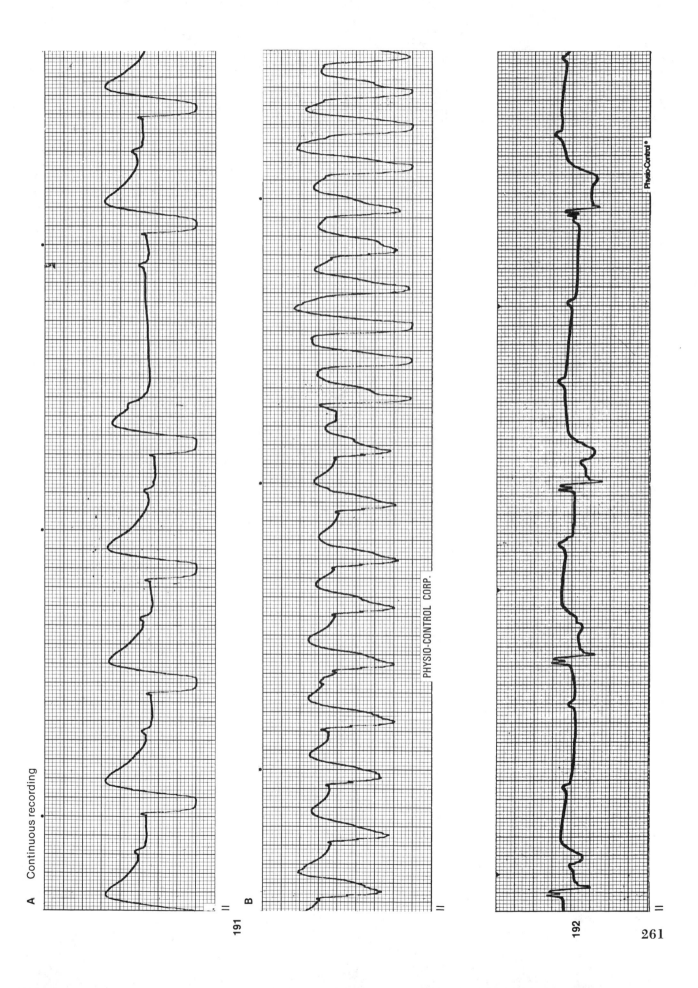

A   Continuous recording

PHYSIO-CONTROL CORP.

Physio-Control®

191

192

261

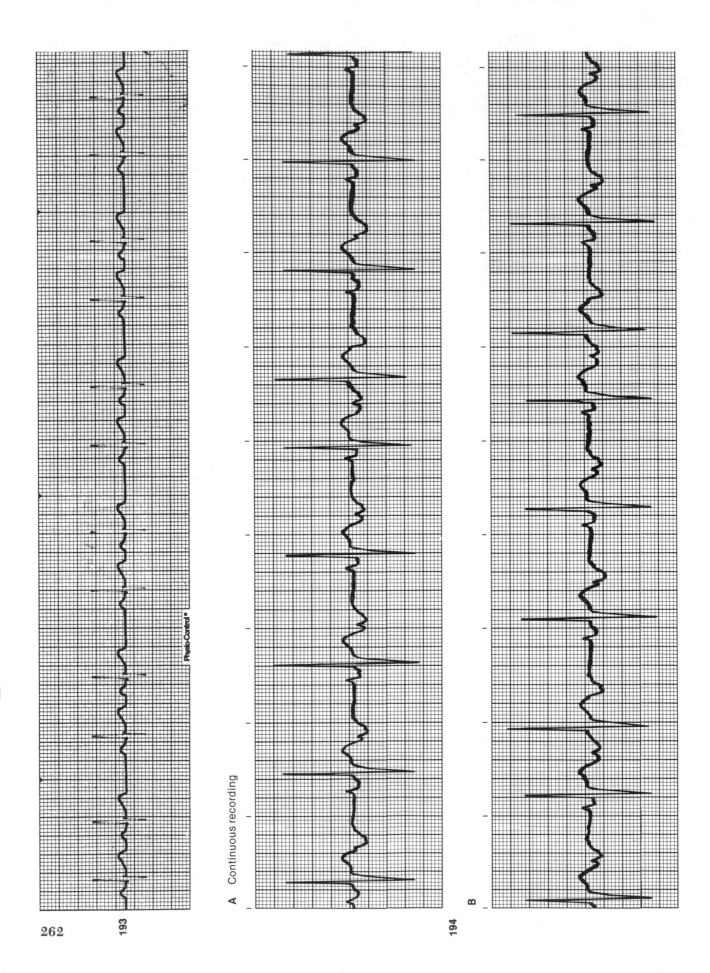

262

193

A Continuous recording

194

B

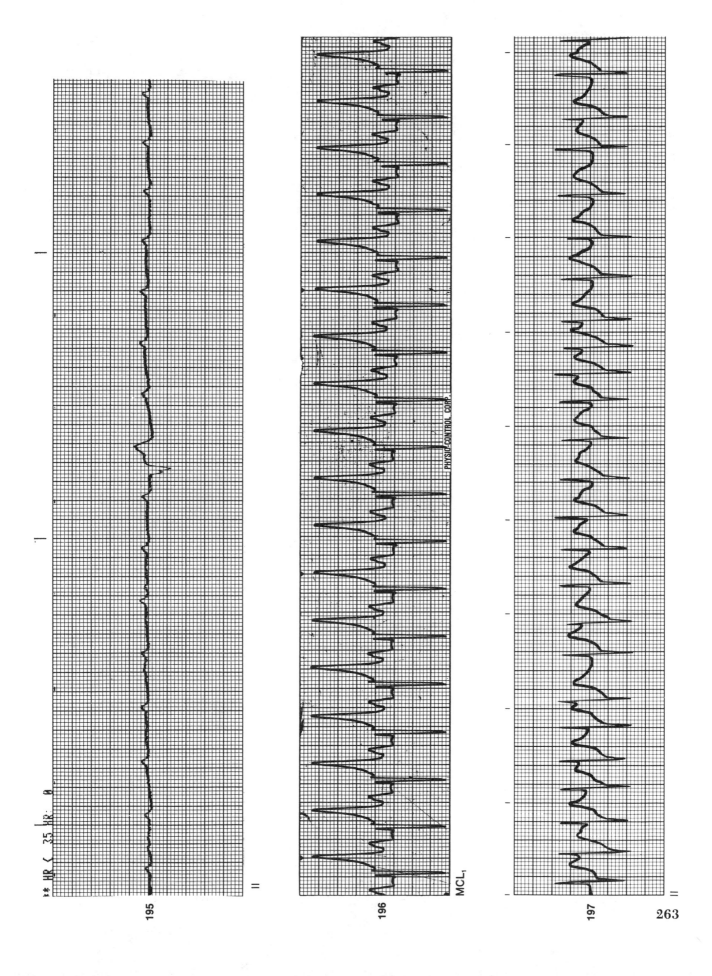

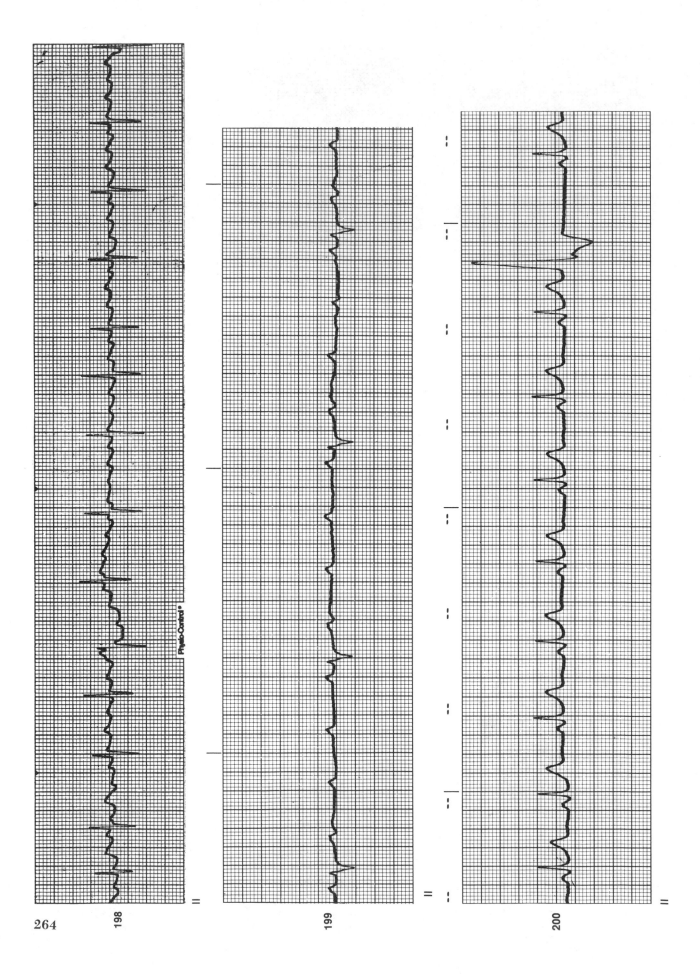

198

199

200

Physio-Control®

ANSWERS TO PRACTICE ECG TRACINGS 171 TO 200

171

Rate ___72___ /min.　Rhythm ___Regular___　PR Interval ___0.16___ s.
QRS Duration ___0.12___ s.
AV Conduction Ratio ___1:1___

Interpretation: Normal or regular sinus rhythm.

Rationale:
- Regular R-R intervals
- Regular P-P intervals
- P waves of the same shape
- Normal P-R interval
- 1:1 AV conduction

This tracing looks different from other examples of NSR because the QRS complex is notched, the ST segment is depressed, and the T wave is biphasic.

172

Rate ___A) 43___ /min.　___B) 150___ /min.　Rhythm ___A) regular___　___B) slightly irregular___
QRS Duration ___A) 0.06___ s.　___B) 0.06___ s.　P-R Interval ___A) absent___　___B) retrograde___
AV Conduction Ratio ___A) absent___　___B) retrograde 1:1___

Interpretation: In A, the AV junctional rhythm is secondary to sinus node failure. In B, AV junctional tachycardia exists.

Rationale: A: The QRS complexes are less than 0.10 second, indicating normal intraventricular conduction of supraventricular impulse. The rhythm is regular and is within the range expected for a pacemaker in the AV junction (40 to 60/minute). There is no evidence of atrial activity because P waves are not seen. Slow sustained AV junctional rhythm occur when sinus node fails to pace the heart.
B: The QRS complexes are narrow, but the rhythm is slightly irregular. The retrogradely conducted P' waves are clearly visible immediately following the QRS complexes. The AV conduction ratio is 1:1, but the order of stimulation is reversed: the atria are activated after the ventricles. The rate is greater than 100/minute and, coupled with the other findings, indicates the dysrhythmia is an AV junctional tachycardia. Junctional tachycardia is one type of a group of tachydysrhythmias known as supraventricular tachycardias (SVT).

173

Rate ___40___ /min.　Rhythm ___irregular___　P-R Interval ___0.28, 0.36___ s.　dropped QRS
QRS Duration ___0.06___ s.
Conduction Ratio ___3:2___

Interpretation: Sinus rhythm with a second degree AV block, Mobitz type 1 (Wenckebach), 3:2 AV conduction, and an average ventricular rate of 40/minute.

Rationale: We observe grouped beating: two QRS complexes followed by a pause. The longest R-R interval is less than twice the shortest one. The P-P intervals are constant indicating regular discharge of the sinus node. Not all the P waves are followed by a QRS; however, all the QRS complexes are preceded by at least one P wave. The P-R intervals show a cyclic variation: 0.28 second, 0.36 second, dropped beat, 0.28 second, 0.36 second, dropped beat, and so forth. The conduction ratio is three P waves to two QRS complexes, indicating that the last P wave of each group is not conducted. The progressive increase in P-R length is the hallmark of a Wenckebach block.

174

Rate atrial 70 /min. ventricular 40/min.   Rhythm regular   P-R Interval absent

QRS Duration 0.06 s.

AV Conduction Ratio absent

Interpretation: Sinus rhythm with third degree AV heart block.

Rationale: The ventricular rhythm is regular but slow (40/min). The QRS complexes look normal. The P-P intervals are regular, but no AV relationship exists between the P waves and QRS complexes. Complete AV dissociation occurs when independent pacemakers control the atria and ventricles.

175

Rate 230 /min.   Rhythm irregular   P-R Interval absent

QRS Duration 0.20 s.

AV Conduction Ratio absent

Interpretation: Sinus tachycardia with an R-on-T phenomenon, causing the development of ventricular tachycardia. The tracing shows a fusion beat (labeled 1) and a capture beat (labeled 2).

Rationale: The initial three beats are sinus, but the fourth beat occurs prematurely and is ventricular in origin. The timing of the ectopic beat occurs during the vulnerable period of the third sinus complex when the fibers have not all repolarized. The premature stimulus strikes during this period of electrical dissimilarity and results in the development of ventricular tachycardia. Ventricular tachycardia can be recognized by distorted QRS complexes that occur at basically regular R-R intervals. The ectopic beats lack associated P waves, so there is no AV relationship.

176

Rate 70 /min.   Rhythm irregular   P-R Interval sinus 0.16 s. PAC 0.12

QRS Duration 0.06 s.

AV Conduction Ratio 1:1

Interpretation: Sinus rhythm with a PAC (beat 7).

Rationale: Aside from the PAC, the rhythm is regular. The QRS complexes are narrow. The P-R intervals are normal for sinus beats. The PAC shows a shortened P-R interval and occurs early in the R-R interval. The AV relationship is 1:1.

177

Rate sporadic /min.   Rhythm irregular   P-R Interval absent

QRS Duration 0.20 s.

AV Conduction Ratio absent

Interpretation: Aside from two agonal idioventricular complexes, asystole is evident.

Rationale: No organized rhythm exists. Two idioventricular beats occur. The rest of the tracing shows a dying flat baseline. This dysrhythmia reflects a dying myocardium, hence the term agonal rhythm is applied.

178

Rate A) 52 /min. B) 98 /min.

Rhythm A) irregular B) irregular

QRS Duration A) 0.08 s. B) 0.20 s.

P-R Interval A) absent B) 0.16 s.

AV Conduction Ratio A) absent B) 1:1

Interpretation: Strip A shows an AV junctional rhythm at a rate of 52/minute that includes several ventricular ectopic complexes. After treatment, sinus impulses return in strip B at a much faster rate. Strip B: Sinus tachycardia with PVCs.

Rationale: Strip A: The third, eighth, and eleventh QRS complexes are PVCs. They are recognized by the wide and distorted QRS complexes. The remainder of the QRS complexes show a narrow shape at a rate of 52/minute. The normal QRS complexes lack P waves and indicate their origination in the AV junction.

Strip B: Atropine is vagolytic and favors an increased firing of the AV junction as well as the SA node. Fortunately, the sinus node resumes the role of pacemaker because of its rapid rate of discharge. The QRS complexes have the same general shape as in A, yet they are now preceded by regular P waves.

179

Rate A) 42 /min. B) 42 /min.

Rhythm A) regular B) irregular

QRS Duration A) 0.08 s. B) 0.08 s.

P-R Interval A) 0.20 s. B) 0.20 s.

PVC 0.16 s.

AV Conduction Ratio A) 1:1 B) 1:1

Interpretation: Marked sinus bradycardia (42/minute) with a single (interpolated) ventricular ectopic beat (beat 5 in B).

Rationale: Strips A and B are identical except for beat 5 in B. The ventricular rhythm is regular except for the PVC. The QRS complexes have a constant appearance except for the bizarre shape of the PVC. All R waves have a P wave ahead of them, except again, the PVC. Unlike most PVCs, this one is not followed by a compensatory pause. It occurs so early in the R-R interval that by the time the next scheduled sinus impulse arrives, the AV node is no longer refractory. As a result, the sinus rhythm is not disturbed. The PVC shows the findings typical for ectopic beats:

- greater voltage QRS complex
- absent P wave
- wide and bizarre QRS
- discordant T waves
- interpolated because the PVC does not disturb the underlying R-R interval.

mal intraventricular conduction. The T waves of the sinus beats that appear just ahead of the PACs are distorted by the P′ waves.

180

Rate A) sinus 86, AV 40/min. B) AV 21/min.
Rhythm A) irregular B) irregular
QRS Duration A) sinus 0.10, AV 0.10 s. B) sinus 0.08, ventricular 0.20 s.
P-R Interval A) sinus 0.16 s. B) absent
AV Conduction Ratio absent

Interpretation: Strip A: Regular sinus rhythm suddenly develops into a sinus arrest. A slower AV junctional pacemaker appears.

Strip B: Shows beats from two pacemaker sites: Beats 1, 2, and 4 are junctional, and 3 is an idioventricular beat.

Strip C: A slow idioventricular rhythm exists.

Rationale: In A we initially see normal appearing P-QRS-T complexes, but after six sinus beats P waves disappear. Instead, the same narrow QRS complexes occur but at a slower rate. In B, the junctional complexes have narrow QRS complexes, missing P waves, and a slow rate. The single idioventricular complex (beat 3) lacks a P wave and has a wide and bizarre QRS complex. In C, the series of beats are all from a ventricular focus.

181

Rate 66/min. Rhythm irregular
QRS Duration 0.08 s. P-R Interval sinus 0.16 s.
AV Conduction Ratio 1:1

Interpretation: Sinus rhythm with frequent PACs. Periods of atrial bigeminy are seen.

Rationale: The early part of this tracing shows a regularly irregular pattern: each sinus beat is followed by a PAC. The QRS complexes of the sinus and ectopic atrial foci are identical, indicating nor-

182

Rate 200/min. Rhythm regular
QRS Duration 0.10 s. P-R Interval absent
AV Conduction Ratio absent

Interpretation: Supraventricular tachycardia.

Rationale: The QRS complexes are normal in shape and duration, indicating normal conduction from a supraventricular focus. The R-R intervals are precisely regular. Atrial activity cannot be identified.

183

Rate 160/min. Rhythm regular
QRS Duration 0.20 s. P-R Interval absent
AV Conduction Ratio absent

Interpretation: Ventricular tachycardia.

Rationale: The ventricular rate (160/min) is slightly irregular. The QRS complexes are wide and bizarre. Atrial activity is not associated with the QSR complexes.

184

Rate atrial 75 ventricular 37/min. Rhythm regular
QRS Duration 0.12 s. P-R Interval absent
AV Conduction Ratio absent

Interpretation: Sinus rhythm with third degree AV block (Complete AV dissociation).

Rationale: The QRS complexes are slow and wide. Regular atrial activity is noted, but complete AV disso-

185

ciation exists. None of the P waves are related to the QRS complexes. The P waves appear to march through the ventricular complexes because of the different rhythms of the independent pacemakers.

Rate absent Rhythm absent P-R Interval absent
QRS Duration absent
AV Conduction Ratio absent

Interpretation: Fine amplitude ventricular fibrillation.

Rationale: This display of ventricular fibrillation shows low-voltage fluctuation of the baseline. No hard rules exist for deciding whether it is fine or coarse. Generally with a properly standardized machine, if the distance from a peak to the next valley of the waves is 3 mm or less, we term it fine. If the size is 4 mm or greater, we label it coarse. To avoid confusion it may be better to mention the actual amplitude of the waves, for instance, "ventricular fibrillation of about 3 mm in height."

186

Rate 57 /min. Rhythm regular P-R Interval 0.40 s.
QRS Duration 0.20 s.
AV Conduction Ratio 1:1

Interpretation: Sinus bradycardia with first degree AV heart block.

Rationale: The ventricular complexes are distorted and wide due to an intraventricular conduction abnormality. All the QRS complexes are pre-ceded by a single P wave. The P-P intervals and P-R intervals are fixed. The P waves show notching. The P-R interval of 0.40 second is very long; a considerable delay exists before ventricular activation occurs. The slow rate and prolonged P-R interval are indicative of enhanced vagal tone.

187

Rate 20 /min. Rhythm regular P-R Interval absent
QRS Duration 0.36 s. absent
AV Conduction Ratio absent

Interpretation: A slow idioventricular rhythm.

Rationale: Ventricular activity: Slow and distorted QRS complexes. Atrial activity: Absent. Escape ventricular pacemakers discharge at rates between 20–40/min.

188

Rate 67 /min. Rhythm irregular
sinus 0.08 s.
QRS Duration PVC 0.20 s. P-R Interval 0.16 s.
AV Conduction Ratio 1:1

Interpretation: Sinus rhythm with two uniformed PVCs (beats 4 and 9).

Rationale: This rhythm is irregular because two beats occur early in the R-R cycles. Since the premature complexes have wide QRS complexes, lack P waves, and are followed by compensatory pauses, they must be ectopic ventricular beats. The sinus complexes have P-QRS-T waves that are normal. The coupling intervals of the PVCs to the previous sinus beats are constant.

189

Rate ___75___ /min. Rhythm ___irregular___

QRS Duration ___0.10___ s.

___sinus 0.16___ s.

P-R Interval ___PAC   0.12___ s.

AV Conduction Ratio ___1:1___

Interpretation: **Sinus rhythm with premature atrial beats. The pause noted early in the tracing is due to a non-conducted PAC. See Tracing 189 Answer for the labeled events. Two other PACs (beats 8 and 13), both of which are conducted, are seen.**

Rationale: The ventricular rhythm is irregular at the points that the PACs occur. The QRS complexes show the same narrow shape, indicating a supraventricular origin. The pause (long R-R interval) shows a P' wave of the nonconducted PAC distorting the downslope of beat 3's T wave from beat 3. Beats 8 and 13 are premature atrial complexes. They show P' waves and P-R intervals that are different than those of sinus beats. The AV conduction ratio is 1:1 except for the nonconducted PAC, where it is 2:1 for one cycle.

190

Rate ___46___ /min. Rhythm ___regular___

QRS Duration ___0.10___ s. P-R Interval ___0.20___ s.

AV Conduction Ratio ___1:1___

Interpretation: **Sinus bradycardia.**

Rationale: The QRS complexes are normal and the rhythm is regular. The shapes of the P waves and the P-P intervals are constant. The P-R interval is normal and a 1:1 AV conduction ratio exists. The only deviation from NSR is decreased discharge of the sinus node.

191

Rate ___A) 48___ /min. Rhythm A) and B) irregular

___B) 120___ /min.

QRS Duration ___A) 0.24___ s. ___A) 0.40___ s.

___B) 0.24___ s. P-R Interval ___B) absent___

AV Conduction Ratio ___A) 1:1   B) absent___

Interpretation: **Strip A shows a sinus bradycardia with a first degree AV block and one early nonconducted P' wave after the sixth QRS complex. Strip B shows the sudden development of ventricular tachycardia.**

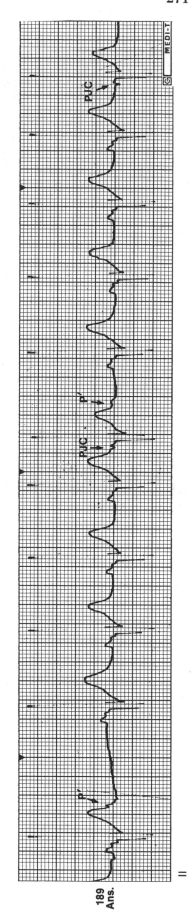

189
Ans.

272

Rationale: The QRS complexes are wide and distorted. Each QRS in *A* is preceded by a P wave. The pause in activity is caused by a premature P' wave that can be seen in the previous ST segment. In *B*, a rapid ventricular rhythm occurs.

192

Rate atrial 75 /min.
ventricular 30/min. Rhythm irregular P-R Interval absent
QRS Duration 0.20 s.
AV Conduction Ratio absent

Interpretation: Sinus rhythm with third degree AV heart block.

Rationale:
• Slightly irregular R-R intervals
• Constant P-P intervals
• No AV Relationship
• Ventricular rate slower than atrial
• Wide, distorted QRS complexes

193

Rate 80 /min. Rhythm irregular
QRS Duration sinus 0.08 PAC 0.08 s. P-R Interval sinus 0.16 s. PAC 0.16 s.
AV Conduction Ratio 1:1

Interpretation: Atrial bigeminy (every other beat is a PAC).

Rationale: The rhythm is regularly irregular. The pattern shows two grouped beats followed by a pause. The QRS complexes are identical. The atrial activity shows two different waves: P and P' configurations. The P' of each group shows a more rounded contour than the P waves. The second P wave of each pair is premature and develops early in the R-R cycle.

Rate 55 /min. Rhythm irregular
QRS Duration 0.12 s. P-R Interval see Rationale
AV Conduction Ratio 2:1, 3:2

194

Interpretation: Sinus bradycardia with second degree AV block, Mobitz type 1 (Wenckebach), 3:2 conduction ratio.

Rationale: The ventricular rhythm is irregular. QRS complexes 6, 11, 15, and 19 have shorter R-R intervals coupled to the prior QRS complexes. Each QRS complex is normal and consistent in shape and duration. Atrial activity occurs regularly with constant P-P intervals. Each P wave has a normal upright and consistent shape (see Tracing 194 Answer). The AV relationship is not normal. Most of the QRS complexes have more than one P wave associated with them (except QRS complexes 6, 11, 15, and 19, which have a 1:1 conduction ratio). Most QRS complexes have a 2:1 conduction ratio; that is, every other P wave is not conducted ("dropped QRS"). This is a second degree AV block. In order to determine whether it is a Mobitz type 1 or 2, we look at the P-R intervals to see if they are constant or changing prior to the dropped QRS complexes. QRS complexes 6, 11, 15, and 19 have longer P-R intervals (0.26 sec) compared to the rest (0.16 second). The P-R cycles show a pattern of 0.16 second, 0.26 second, and then a P wave that is not conducted (see Tracing 194 Answer). Therefore, the conduction ratio for these four cycles is 3:2. In summary, the signs of Wenckebach AV heart block are grouped beating, dropped QRS complexes, and increasing P-R intervals.

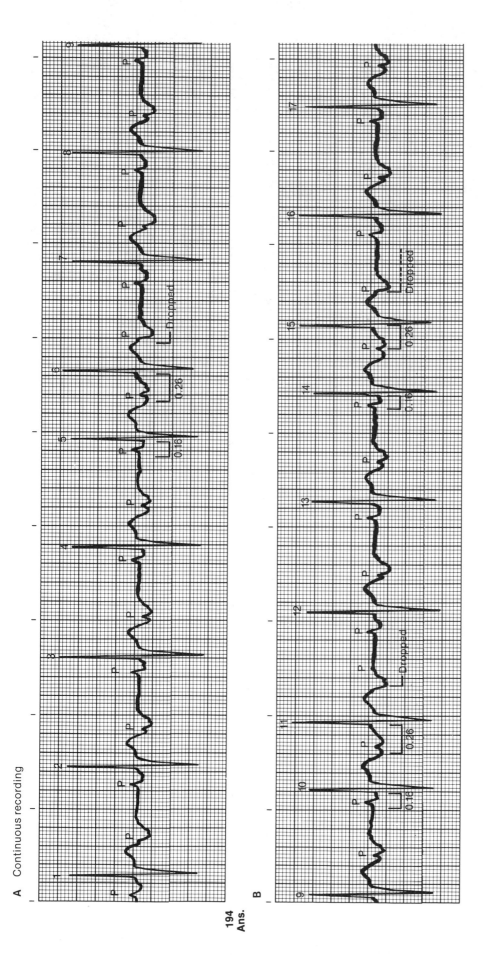

A Continuous recording

B

194
Ans.

195

Rate atrial 105 /min. / ventricular occasional/min. Rhythm atrial regular / ventricular absent
QRS Duration 0.16 s. P-R Interval absent
AV Conduction Ratio absent

Interpretation: Sinus tachycardia and complete AV heart block with ventricular standstill.

Rationale: There is only one wide, bizarrely shaped QRS complex. The lone, agonal complex is not associated with a pulse. In contrast, the atrial rhythm is rapid, regular, and consists of normal appearing P waves. None of the P waves are conducted, so the ventricles remain unstimulated. More than the AV conduction pathway is diseased, or else a stable escape rhythm would have emerged. The only hope of rescuing the agonal rhythm is to insert an artificial pacemaker and hope it is able to capture.

196

Rate 120 /min. Rhythm regular P-R Interval 0.20 s.
QRS Duration 0.08 s.
AV Conduction Ratio 1:1

Interpretation: Sinus tachycardia.

Rationale: Ventricular activity is composed of normally shaped QRS complexes and regular R-R intervals. The P waves are upright, constant in shape, and appear before every QRS complex. P waves at a rate greater than 100/minute indicates sinus tachycardia. The AV relationship is 1:1. The T waves are tall and peaked.

197

Rate 160 /min. Rhythm irregular P-R Interval absent
QRS Duration 0.08 s.
AV Conduction Ratio variable

Interpretation: Atrial fibrillation with a ventricular rate of 160/minute.

Rationale: The ventricular complexes are narrow and normal in appearance. The rhythm of the QRS complexes is grossly irregular. The QRS complexes of normal duration reveals that they are supraventricular in origin. P waves are absent. Based on the narrow QRS complexes and irregular ventricular activity, we can assume that atrial fibrillation is responsible, even though fibrillatory (f) waves are not visible.

198

Rate ventricular average 100/min. / atrial 300 /min. Rhythm irregular P-R Interval absent
QRS Duration 0.08 s.
AV Conduction Ratio 2:1, 3:1, 4:1

Interpretation: Atrial flutter with variable ventricular conduction (2:1, 3:1, 4:1).

Rationale: The QRS complexes look normal in shape and duration. The ventricular rhythm is irregular due to variable AV conduction. The atrial rate is about 300/minute and consists of flutter waves.

199

Rate: atrial 108 /min.
ventricular 27 /min.
Rhythm: atrial regular /min.
ventricular regular
QRS Duration 0.12 s. P-R Interval absent
AV Conduction Ratio absent

Interpretation: Sinus tachycardia and high grade second degree AV block, Mobitz type 2, 4:1 AV conduction, with a ventricular response of 27/min.

Rationale: The ventricular rhythm is regular, and the QRS complexes are slightly widened and distorted. The atrial rhythm is also regular but is about four times faster than the QRSs. This occurs because the AV conduction ratio is 4:1, meaning that three of every four P waves are blocked. One P wave of each cycle is hidden on top of the T wave. While the atria are tachycardic, the ventricles are severely bradycardic. This form of second degree heart block is termed **high grade** because two or more consecutive P waves are blocked. It represents advanced disease of the conduction system and is likely to progress to complete block. This would be a disaster because so far no escape pacemakers have developed in spite of a rate of only 27/min. Insertion of an artificial pacemaker is needed immediately.

200

Rate 76 /min. Rhythm irregular
sinus 0.08 s.
QRS Duration PVC 0.20 s.
P-R Interval 0.16 s.
AV Conduction Ratio 1:1

Interpretation: Sinus rhythm with a single PVC (beat 9).

Rationale: Except for the PVC, the rhythm is regular. The sinus beats have normal sequences of P-QRS-T waves. The PVC, on the other hand, has a wide and distorted QRS with a retrograde P wave (seen in the ST segment). A compensatory pause follows the PVC.

Section 3
APPENDICES

GLOSSARY

Aberrant Conduction:

Abnormal impulse transmission causing the ECG waves to have a distorted shape. Often used when referring to a PAC or SVT with aberration, meaning that the QRS complex, instead of being narrow, is wide and distorted.

Accelerated AV Junctional Rhythm:

Ectopic AV junctional pacemaker discharging at a rate abve 60/minute but below 100/minute.

Accelerated Idioventricular Rhythm:

Ectopic ventricular pacemaker discharging at a rate above 40/minute but under 100/minute. Often incorrectly referred to as "slow ventricular tachycardia."

Accelerated Rhythm:

An ECG rhythm that occurs at a rate faster than the usual intrinsic rate of depolarization for a specific focus. For example, an ectopic pacemaker originating in the ventricles at a rate of 75/minute would be considered accelerated because the usual rate of spontaneous discharge (automaticity) for such a focus is in the range of 20 to 40/minute.

Accessory Bundle

Alternate muscular connection between the atria and ventricles, bypassing the AV node.

Action Potential:

Abrupt phasic changes in the electrical charges of the cell membrane, including polarization, depolarization, and repolarization (see Fig. A–1).

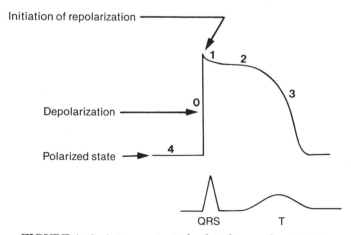

FIGURE A–1. Action potential related to surface ECG.

After-Depolarization: Small electrical impulses, occurring following action potentials, which can cause dysrhythmias if they are large enough to reach threshold.

Agonal Rhythm: ECG rhythm recorded from a dying heart; asystole with several idioventricular complexes.

Anoxia: Absence of oxygen.

Antegrade: Flowing in a forward direction (anterograde).

Antidysrhythmic Drugs: A variety of different types of agents, including oxygen, digitalis, Xylocaine, and propranolol, used to correct disordered cardiac rhythms and rates.

Arrest: Cessation of activity. Sinus arrest: failure of SA node to discharge. Cardiac arrest: stoppage of heart activity.

Arrhythmia: Used synonymously with dysrhythmia but technically less correct. See Dysrhythmia.

Arrhythmogenic: Capable of causing dysrhythmias; examples include ischemia, hypoxia, acidosis, and certain drugs.

Artifact: An artificial disturbance of the ECG signal, commonly caused by electrical (60 cycle) interference or muscular activity.

Artificial Pacemaker: An electrical pulse generator which can substitute on a temporary or permanent basis for a defect in the SA node or conduction paths.

Asystole: Lack of cardiac electrical activity reflected by a flat (isoelectric) line on the ECG and accompanied clinically by absent vital signs (i.e., cardiac arrest). P waves, QRS complexes, and T waves are absent.

Atrial Dysrhythmia: See Supraventricular Dysrhythmia.

Atrial Depolarization: Activation of the resting atrial tissue by an action potential that spreads as an electrical wave. The ECG records this as a P wave.

Atrial Extrasystoles: See Premature Atrial Complex.

Atrial Fibrillation: A tachydysrhythmia characterized by chaotic atrial activity at a rate above 350/min.

Atrial Flutter: Tachydysrhythmia characterized by regular atrial cycles 250 to 350/minute associated with some ratio of conducted and nonconducted atrial beats.

Atrial Repolarization: The process in which the atrial tissues return to their resting state following depolarization. Atrial repolarization is not reflected on the ECG since the larger QRS complex obscures it.

Atrial Tachycardia: See Supraventricular Tachycardia.

Atrioventricular (AV) Block: Disturbance of conduction at or below the AV node. Supraventricular impulses are either temporarily delayed or are unable to activate the ventricles because they are blocked.

Atrioventricular (AV) Dissociation: Independent activation of the atria and ventricles.

Atrioventricular (AV) Junction: The tissue surrounding the AV node, including the atrial tissue, and His bundle, which possesses automaticity.

Atrioventricular (AV) Node: Small mass of conducting tissue lying in the posterior floor of the right atrium connecting the atria and ventricles.

Automaticity: The ability of a cell to spontaneously depolarize without being externally stimulated. Cells with automaticity have the potential to serve as pacemakers.

Bidirectional Ventricular Tachycardia: Known as "torsade de pointes"—the QRS complexes rotate 180 degrees in the same lead.

Bigeminy: ECG rhythm when every other beat is a premature complex (PVC, PJC, or PAC).

Biphasic: Having positive and negative components. For example, a biphasic T wave means that part of the wave is above the baseline while part is below.

Block: A delay or interruption (complete or incomplete) of a cardiac impulse.

Bradydysrhythmias: Group of dysrhythmias sharing a ventricular rate below 60/minute.

Bradycardia: Slow heart rate. In sinus bradycardia the SA node discharges at a rate of less than 60/minute.

Bradycardia-Tachycardia (Brady-Tachy) Syndrome: Subset of patients with sick sinus syndrome who manifest pronounced periods of bradycardia alternating with tachycardia (sinus tachycardia, PSVT, atrial fibrillation, and atrial flutter).

Bundle Branches: A continuation of the AV bundle which divides into right and left conduction branches (paths).

Bundle Branch Block: Disorder in the spread of an impulse through the right and/or left bundle branches.

Bundle of His: Continuation of AV nodal fibers that spreads downward into the ventricles. Also known as the AV bundle.

Bypass Tract: An abnormal bundle of muscle connecting the atria and ventricles but bypassing the AV node. The AV node no longer controls the rate of ventricular stimulation because the atrial impulses follow an alternate pathway.

Capture Complex: Activation of the heart chambers by an impulse. During AV dissociation, a sinus capture complex indicates that a supraventricular beat was able to stimulate the ventricle. Also used when referring to an artificially paced beat, which depolarizes the heart.

Cardiac Cycle: The electrical (P waves, QRS complexes, T waves) and mechanical events (systole and diastole) that compose a single heart beat.

Cardiac Standstill: See Asystole.

Cardioversion: Synchronized electrical discharge used to terminate dysrhythmias that are refractory to drugs, or when an immediate conversion to sinus rhythm is needed.

Cardioverter: Machine used to deliver a synchronized countershock.

Carotid Sinus Massage (CSM): Application of digital pressure to the neck region just lateral to the trachea, thereby stimulating the carotid sinus and causing discharge of parasympathetic impulses to slow tachydysrhythmias and convert them to NSR.

Compensatory Pause: The period following a PVC which compensates for the premature impulse so that the interval between the R wave before the PVC and the one after the PVC is equal to twice the normal R-R interval.

Conductivity: Ability of a cell to transmit an action potential.

Defibrillate: To terminate ventricular fibrillation by electrical countershock.

Deflection: Movement of the ECG stylus from the baseline caused by changes in transmembrane potential.

Delta Wave: Initial slurring of the QRS complex; seen in preexcitation states such as Wolff-Parkinson-White syndrome. As a result, the P-R interval is shortened.

Depolarization: Activation of the heart tissue due to spread of the electrical impulse.

Diastolic Filling Time: Amount of time available for the chambers of the heart to fill with blood between systoles. As the heart rate increases in tachydysrhythmias, the diastolic filling time decreases causing a fall in cardiac output.

Discordant T Waves: T waves that have a deflection opposite to that of the main QRS complex.

Dissociation: Isolation of electrical and/or mechanical activity.

A-V Dissociation: Independent beating of the atria and ventricles.

Electromechanical Dissociation (EMD):   Pathologic state in which an action potential does not result in systole. Organized ECG activity is not accompanied by cardiac contraction.

Dressler Beats: Fusion beats that occur during ventricular tachycardia.

Dropped Beat: A beat that is not conducted.

Dysrhythmia: Any ECG pattern that varies from normal sinus rhythm. A disordered cardiac rhythm due to abnormalities in impulse formation or conduction.

ECG: Abbreviation for electrocardiogram (also known as EKG).

Ectopic Impulse: Originating from a site other than the sinus node (e.g., atrial, junctional, or ventricular); also called extrasystoles.

Ectopic Coupling Interval: The period from the sinus beat until the ectopic complex.

Ectopic Focus: A pacemaker site other than the SA node.

Ectopy: Complexes of ectopic origin.

Electrical Alternans: Variation in the size of every other QRS complex; often seen in chronic lung disease and pericardial effusion.

Electrocardiogram (ECG):   Graphic record of the electrical activity of the heart.

Electromechanical Association: Normal state in which ECG events are coordinated with a pulse and cardiac output.

Enhanced Automaticity:	Increased excitability of pacemaker tissue.
Escape Beat/Rhythm:	The development of latent pacemakers to stimulate the heart when there is sinus node slowing or failure. The atria, AV junction, or ventricles may be the site of a single complex or a sustained rhythm.
Excitability:	The ability of a cell to become depolarized when stimulated.
Exit Block:	Failure of stimulus to activate surrounding structures. For example, in sinoatrial exit block, the sinus impulse is unable to spread to the atrial tissue.
Extrasystoles:	Same as ectopic complexes.
f Waves:	Fibrillatory waves characteristic of atrial fibrillation.
F Waves:	Flutter waves characteristic of atrial flutter.
Fibrillation:	Chaotic electrical cardiac activity that is unable to stimulate coordinated cardiac contractions. As a result, the pumping activity of the atria and/or ventricles is lost. The ECG inscribes an irregular and wavy baseline.
Fibrillation-Flutter:	A hybrid atrial dysrhythmia that contains features of atrial fibrillation and flutter.
Flutter:	Rapid ectopic electrical activity that stimulates cardiac chambers in an organized fashion.
First Degree AV Block:	A delay in AV conduction reflected in a P-R interval greater than 0.20 second.
Focus:	Site of impulse formation. Unifocal refers to one site of origin, as opposed to multifocal, which describes more than a single site.
Fusion Beat:	A complex produced by the simultaneous discharge of two pacemakers as with an atrial and ventricular focus. As a result of the two waves meeting within the ventricles or atria, the two forces somewhat cancel one another, producing a smaller or narrower complex than normal. The hybrid complex shows some characteristics of the PVC and the sinus beat.
His Bundle:	Also called the common or AV bundle, this portion of conducting pathway is a continuation of AV nodal fibers that travel into the ventricles and then divide into bundle branches. It channels sinus impulses to the ventricular muscles.
His-Purkinje Fibers:	Portions of the intraventricular conduction system composed of the tissues of the His bundle, including the fibers of the terminal Purkinje pathways.
Hypoxia:	Low oxygen content.
Idio-:	Prefix meaning from within. An idioventricular rhythm arises in the ventricle and controls only the ventricle. An idiojunctional (nodal) rhythm arises in the AV junction and controls only the ventricles.
Interpolated Beat:	When an ectopic beat occurs so early that it activates the ventricle and it repolarizes by the time the next sinus impulse

arrives. These beats show a noncompensatory pause because sinus activity is not disrupted.

Intraventricular Conduction Defect (IVCD): Abnormal spread of impulse within the ventricles resulting in a bizarre QRS complex or prolonged QRS duration.

Irritability: Increased automaticity, commonly caused by ischemia or hypoxia.

Ischemia: Inadequate blood supply resulting in decreased supply of oxygen relative to demand; leads to anaerobic metabolism.

Isoelectric Line: Flat ECG line found between the waves or cycles.

Isorhythmic AV Dissociation: The atria and ventricles beat independently because the rates of the pacemakers are so close to one another. No actual AV block is present, yet sinus slowing permits the AV junction to discharge and compete for control.

J (Junction) Point: Point at which the QRS complex merges with the ST segment.

Junctional (AV) Tachycardia: An ectopic rhythm originating from the AV junction at a rate above 100/minute.

MCL: Modified (bipolar) chest lead (MCL) system that simulates the pattern found with unipolar leads. For example, $MCL_1 = V_1$ and $MCL_6 = V_6$.

Mobitz Type AV Blocks: See Second Degree AV Block.

Multifocal: Arising from two ectopic sites; more correctly, this should be termed multiformed.

Multifocal Atrial Tachycardia (MAT): A dysrhythmia with a rate over 100/min having three or more differently shaped P waves; associated with pulmonary disease.

Multiformed: Ectopic beats with two different shapes; resulting from different sites of origin or from a single site but following separate paths to activate the heart.

Nodal Rhythm: See Atrioventricular (AV) Junction.

Nodal Tachycardia: See Junctional (AV) Tachycardia.

Noncompensatory Pause: The period following an ectopic beat is less than compensatory; that is, the period from the R wave before an ectopic beat until the R wave that follows is less than twice the normal R-R interval.

NSR: Abbreviation for normal sinus rhythm; used synonymously with regular sinus rhythm.

P Wave: Part of cardiac cycle corresponding to depolarization of the atria.

P' (P Prime) Wave: Label for any ectopic P wave other than a sinus impulse.

PAC: Abbreviation for premature atrial complex.

Pacemaker: The site that controls the heart rate because it has the fastest rate of self-discharge (automaticity).

Pacemaker Undersensing: Malfunction of artificial pacemaker where the normal QRS complexes are not sensed.

Paroxysm: Occurring in bursts or spasms, as in paroxysmal supraventricular tachycardia, in which the onset and termination are abrupt.

Paroxysmal Atrial Tachycardia (PAT): More correctly, this dysrhythmia is now referred to as paroxysmal supraventricular tachycardia.

PJC: Abbreviation for premature junctional complex.

Polarized State: An electrically responsive state in which a cell is able to respond to a stimulus by becoming depolarized.

P-P Interval: Period between consecutive P waves.

P-R Interval: Period of each cardiac cycle corresponding to the time from the start of atrial depolarization until the ventricles are activated.

Premature Atrial Complex (PAC): A premature discharge of an ectopic atrial pacemaker that disrupts regular sinus rhythm.

Premature Junctional (Nodal) Complex (PJC): A premature ectopic beat originating in AV junctional tissue.

Premature Ventricular Complex (PVC): A premature ectopic beat originating in the ventricles.

Purkinje Fibers: The distal portion of the ventricular conduction system.

QRS Complex: Portion of cardiac cycle corresponding to depolarization of the ventricles.

QRS Duration: Measured from the beginning of the Q wave until the end of the S wave, corresponding to the time required for ventricular activation.

Q-T Interval: Period from start of the QRS complex until the end of the T wave; corresponds to ventricular depolarization and repolarization.

Quadrigeminy: Grouping of four beats, usually three sinus beats and a PVC.

Q Wave: Initial negative deflection of the QRS complex. Pathologic Q waves: indicative of a myocardial infarction.

Reentry Mechanism: Cause of dysrhythmias in which the uniform wave of depolarization is split into wavelets owing to varying conduction velocities.

Refractory Period: The time during which a cell is unresponsive to a consecutive stimulus.

Regular Sinus Rhythm (RSR): See Normal Sinus Rhythm.

Repolarization: The process by which a cell, after being discharged, returns to its state of readiness.

R-on-T Phenomenon: When a PVC occurs so prematurely that it lands on the prior T wave (the ventricle's vulnerable period of repolarization) during which ventricular fibrillation or tachycardia may result.

R-R Interval: Period between consecutive QRS complexes.

R Wave:
The first positive deflection of the QRS complex; used also to refer to the entire QRS complex.

SA Node:
Abbreviation for sinoatrial, or sinus, node; the normal pacemaker for the heart.

Second Degree AV Block:
An incomplete form of heart block in which not all the impulses are conducted along the AV pathway. One or more sinus impulses are blocked and are unable to stimulate the ventricles.

Sick Sinus Syndrome:
Syncope and lightheadedness secondary to SA node dysfunction, which causes pronounced sinus bradycardia, brady-tachy syndrome, sinus arrest or block, or sustained AV junctional rhythm.

Sinus Dysrhythmia:
Benign dysrhythmia showing variation in the P-P interval as a result of the effects of breathing on the SA node's regularity.

Sinus Block Arrest:
The sinus impulse fails to originate or fails to be conducted to atrial tissue.

Sinus Bradycardia:
A dysrhythmia consisting of a rate below 60/minute, originating in the SA node.

Sinus Node:
Pacemaker site of the heart; small bundle of tissue in right atrium that paces the heart because it has the fastest rate of automaticity.

Sinus Pause:
Temporary interruption of sinus functioning.

Sinus Rhythm:
See Normal Sinus Rhythm.

Standby Pacing Mode (Demand Mode):
When an artificial pacemaker senses intrinsic cardiac activity and does not discharge. This prevents competition between the artificial pacemaker and sinus activity. The pulse generator discharges only when it senses a long R-R interval.

Stokes-Adams Syndrome:
Syncope caused by third degree AV heart block; it has come to be used in the more general sense to indicate loss of consciousness due to any dysrhythmia.

ST-T Wave Displacements:
Abnormality in repolarization of the ventricles which shifts the ST segment away from the baseline.

Supernormal Period:
See Vulnerable Period.

Supraventricular:
Site above the ventricles, that is, in the SA node, atria, or AV junction.

Supraventricular Dysrhythmia:
A dysrhythmia originating from an ectopic focus above the bifurcation of the AV bundle. Generally, such beats have narrow QRS complexes unless aberrant conduction is present.

Supraventricular Tachycardia:
A general term referring to a group of tachydysrhythmias arising from above the AV bundle bifurcation, including sinus tachycardia, PSVT, atrial flutter and fibrillation, and AV junctional tachycardia.

Tachycardia:
Heart rate greater than 100/minute.

Tachydysrhythmia:
Group of dysrhythmias that share a ventricular rate greater than 100/minute.

Threshold: The minimal amount of stimulus needed to generate an action potential.

Torsade de Pointes: A form of ventricular tachycardia in which the QRS complexes change configuration.

Trigeminy: Grouped beating consisting of three complexes, usually one ectopic beat after two sinus beats.

T Wave: Part of ECG cycle corresponding to ventricular repolarization.

U Wave: An ECG wave sometimes observed following the T wave; thought to be related to late repolarization of the ventricles.

Vagal Maneuvers: A number of actions aimed at increasing parasympathetic tone; for example, carotid sinus massage, orbital massage, and Valsalva maneuver.

Vasovagal Attack (Syncope): Hypotension due to increased parasympathetic (vagal) tone, leading to bradycardia and vasodilation. Referred to as a "simple faint," this condition will correct itself if the patient is allowed to assume a supine position, thereby correcting the transient hypotension.

Ventricular Ectopy: Occurrence of ectopic ventricular complexes; may be either premature or escape ventricular beats.

Ventricular Extrasystole: See Premature Ventricular Complexes.

Ventricular Fibrillation: Life-threatening dysrhythmia characterized by absent cardiac cycles (P-QRS-T waves) and a wildly fluctuating baseline forming a chaotic zigzag ECG pattern, resulting in cardiac arrest.

Ventricular Flutter: An accelerated form of ventricular tachycardia; resembles a continuous sine wave and is observed just before ventricular fibrillation.

Ventricular Standstill: Cessation of QRS activity.

Ventricular Tachycardia: Dysrhythmia caused by the discharge of an ectopic ventricular pacemaker at a rate of over 100/minute; characterized by wide QRS complexes lacking P waves.

VPC: Abbreviation for premature ventricular complex.

Vulnerable Period: Phase of cardiac cycle corresponding to upstroke of T wave; period when the heart is vulnerable to initiating serious ventricular dysrhythmias if a PVC occurs.

Wandering Atrial Pacemaker (WAP): Benign dysrhythmia in which the sinus node temporarily loses pacing function to ectopic atrial foci; the ECG shows P waves of different shapes and varying P-R intervals.

Wenckebach AV Block: See Second Degree AV Block, Mobitz type 1.

Wolff-Parkinson-White (W-P-W) Syndrome: Case of ventricular preexcitation by way of alternate pathway that bypasses the AV node. ECG shows a shortened P-R interval (less than 0.10 second), slurred upstroke of the QRS complex, and a widened QRS complex.

ABBREVIATIONS

AF	Atrial fibrillation
AMI	Acute myocardial infarction
AV	Atrioventricular
BBB	Bundle branch block
bpm	Beats per minute
CPR	Cardiopulmonary resuscitation
CSM	Carotid sinus massage
ECG (EKG)	Electrocardiogram
EMD	Electromechanical dissociation
LBBB	Left bundle branch block
MCL	Modified chest lead
MI	Myocardial infarction
NSR	Normal sinus rhythm
PAC	Premature atrial complex
PJC	Premature junctional complex
PM	Pacemaker
PNC	Premature nodal complex
PSVT	Paroxysmal supraventricular tachycardia
PVC	Premature ventricular complex
RBBB	Right bundle branch block
RSR	Regular sinus rhythm
SA	Sinoatrial
VF	Ventricular fibrillation
VT	Ventricular tachycardia
WAP	Wandering atrial pacemaker
W-P-W	Wolff-Parkinson-White (syndrome)

288

SELF-ASSESSMENT FORMS

Ventricular Activity
QRS Rate_____
QRS Shape_____
QRS Duration_____
R-R Rhythm_____

Atrial Activity
P Wave Rate_____
P Wave Shape_____
P-P Rhythm_____

AV Relationship
P-R Interval _____
Conduction Ratio (P:R)____:____
Pacemaker Site (Dominant)___
Other Sites_____

Other Significant Findings_____
Interpretation_____
_____

Ventricular Activity
QRS Rate_____
QRS Shape_____
QRS Duration_____
R-R Rhythm_____

Atrial Activity
P Wave Rate_____
P Wave Shape_____
P-P Rhythm_____

AV Relationship
P-R Interval _____
Conduction Ratio (P:R)____:____
Pacemaker Site (Dominant)___
Other Sites_____

Other Significant Findings_____
Interpretation_____
_____

Ventricular Activity
QRS Rate_____
QRS Shape_____
QRS Duration_____
R-R Rhythm_____

Atrial Activity
P Wave Rate_____
P Wave Shape_____
P-P Rhythm_____

AV Relationship
P-R Interval _____
Conduction Ratio (P:R)____:____
Pacemaker Site (Dominant)___
Other Sites_____

Other Significant Findings_____
Interpretation_____
_____

INDEX

Italics indicate figures; "t" indicates tables.